Urban Public Health

URBAN PUBLIC HEALTH

A Research Toolkit for Practice and Impact

Edited by Gina S. Lovasi, Ana V. Diez Roux,
and Jennifer Kolker

OXFORD
UNIVERSITY PRESS

OXFORD
UNIVERSITY PRESS

Library of Congress Cataloging-in-Publication Data
Names: Lovasi, Gina S., editor. | Diez Roux,
Ana V. (Ana Victoria), editor. | Kolker, Jennifer, editor.
Title: Urban public health : a research toolkit for practice and impact /
[edited by] Gina S. Lovasi, Ana V. Diez-Roux, Jennifer Kolker.
Description: New York, NY : Oxford University Press, 2021. |
Includes bibliographical references and index.
Identifiers: LCCN 2020017145 | ISBN 9780190885304 (paperback)
Subjects: MESH: Urban Health | Public Health Practice |
Public Health Systems Research—methods
Classification: LCC RA418 | NLM WA 380 | DDC 362.1/042—dc23
LC record available at https://lccn.loc.gov/2020017145

9 8 7 6 5 4 3 2 1

Printed by Marquis, Canada

CONTENTS

CONTRIBUTING AUTHORS

Michael Bader, PhD
Associate Professor, Sociology
and Public Policy & Administration
American University
Washington, DC

Sharrelle Barber, ScD, MPH
Assistant Research Professor
Epidemiology and Biostatistics
Dornsife School of Public Health
Drexel University
Philadelphia, PA

Mary T. Bassett, MD, MPH
François-Xavier Bagnoud Professor
  of the Practice of Health and
  Human Rights
Director, François-Xavier
  Bagnoud Center for Health and
  Human Rights
Department of Social and Behavioral
  Sciences
Harvard T. H. Chan School of
  Public Health
Harvard University
Cambridge, MA

Usama Bilal, MD, PhD, MPH
Assistant Professor
Epidemiology and Biostatistics,
  Urban Health Collaborative
Dornsife School of Public Health
Drexel University
Philadelphia, PA

Jo Ivey Boufford, MD
Clinical Professor of Global Health
College of Global Public Health
New York University
New York, NY

**Bridgette M. Brawner, PhD,
MDiv, APRN**
Senior Fellow at the Center for
  Public Health Initiatives
Assistant Professor of Nursing,
  Family and Community Health
School of Nursing
University of Pennsylvania
Philadelphia, PA

**Waleska Teixeira Caiaffa, MD,
PhD, MPH**
Professor of Epidemiology and
  Public Health
Observatory for Urban Health—Belo
  Horizonte
Universidade Federal de
  Minas Gerais
Belo Horizonte, Brazil

Amy Carroll-Scott, PhD, MPH
Associate Professor, Community
  Health and Prevention
Dornsife School of Public Health
Drexel University
Philadelphia, PA

Jason Corburn, PhD
Director, Institute of Urban and
  Regional Development
Professor, City & Regional Planning
  and School of Public Health
University of California Berkeley
Berkeley, CA

**Amélia Augusta de Lima Friche,
PhD, MPH**
Adjunct Professor of Epidemiology
  and Hearing, Speech and
  Language Sciences
Observatory for Urban Health—
  Belo Horizonte
Universidade Federal de
  Minas Gerais
Belo Horizonte, Brazil

Jannette Diaz
Vice President, Health Promotion &
  Wellness
Congreso de Latinos Unidos
Philadelphia, PA

Julia Díez, BSc, PhD
Postdoctoral Research Fellow
Universidad de Alcalá
Madrid, Spain

Bettye Ferguson
President
Belmont Alliance Civic Association,
  Community Development
  Corporation
Philadelphia, PA

Manuel Franco, MD, PhD
Assistant Professor, Epidemiology
  and Public Health
Universidad de Alcalá
Madrid, Spain

Marla Gold, MD
Professor and Dean Emerita
Health Management and Policy
Dornsife School of Public Health
Drexel University
Philadelphia, PA

Silvia A. González, MPH, PhD(c)
Healthy Active Living and Obesity
  Research Group
University of Ottawa
Ottawa, Canada

Marc N. Gourevitch, MD, MPH
Chair, Department of Public Health
Muriel G. and George W. Singer
  Professor Population Health,
  Department of Population Health
Professor, Department of Medicine
Professor, Department of Psychology
Grossman School of Medicine
New York University
New York, NY

Marcus Grant, BSc (Hons.), MA
Editor-in-Chief, Cities & Health
Advisor to WHO Healthy Cities
  Programme
Bristol, UK

Joseph S. Griffin, DrPH, MPH
School of Public Health
University of California, Berkeley
Berkeley, CA, USA

Pedro Gullón, MD, PhD, MPH
Postdoctoral Research Fellow
Universidad de Alcalá
Madrid, Spain

Rosie Mae Henson, MPH
UHC Doctoral Research Fellow
Urban Health Collaborative
Dornsife School of Public Health
Drexel University
Philadelphia, PA

Diana Rocio Higuera-Mendieta, MD, ScM
Scientific Researcher
Universidad de los Andes
Bogotá, Colombia

Jana A. Hirsch, MES, PhD
Assistant Research Professor
Epidemiology and Biostatistics,
    Urban Health Collaborative
Dornsife School of Public Health
Drexel University
Philadelphia, PA

Malo A. Hutson, PhD
Associate Professor of Architecture,
    Planning and Preservation
Director of the Urban Planning PhD
    Program
Graduate School of Architecture,
    Planning and Preservation
Columbia University
New York, NY

Katherine Indvik, Msc
Policy Engagement Specialist,
    SALURBAL Project
Urban Health Collaborative
Dornsife School of Public Health
Drexel University
Philadelphia, PA

Rennie Joshi, MPH
UHC Doctoral Research Fellow
Urban Health Collaborative
Dornsife School of Public Health
Drexel University
Philadelphia, PA

Abby C. King, PhD
Professor
Epidemiology & Population Health
    and Medicine
Stanford University
Stanford, CA

Neil Kleiman
Clinical Assistant Professor of Urban
    Planning and Public Service
Wagner Graduate School of Public
    Service
New York University
New York, NY

Jennifer Kolker, MPH
Associate Dean for Public Health
    Practice
Clinical Professor, Health
    Management and Policy
Policy and Community Engagement
    Core Lead, Urban Health
    Collaborative
Dornsife School of Public Health
Drexel University
Philadelphia, PA

Stephen E. Lankenau, PhD
Community Health and Prevention
Dornsife School of Public Health
Drexel University
Philadelphia, PA, USA

Adriana C. Lein, MSc
Master of Science in Global Health
Policy & Dissemination Coordinator
Drexel Urban Health Collaborative
Dornsife School of Public Health
    Drexel
Philadelphia, PA

Shoshanna Levine, DrPH
Program Director, City Health
    Dashboard
Grossman School of Medicine
New York University
New York, NY

Gina S. Lovasi, PhD, MPH
Dornsife Associate Professor of
    Urban Health, Epidemiology and
    Biostatistics
Co-Director, Urban Health
    Collaborative
Dornsife School of Public Health
Drexel University
Philadelphia, PA

Steve Melly, MS, MA
Geographic Information System
    Specialist
Urban Health Collaborative
Dornsife School of Public Health
Drexel University
Philadelphia, PA, USA

Stephen J. Mooney, MS, PhD
Assistant Professor, Epidemiology
School of Public Health
University of Washington
Seattle, WA, USA

Becky Ofrane, MPH
Manager of Partnerships, City
    Health Dashboard
Grossman School of Medicine
New York University
New York, NY

Jonathan Purtle, DrPH, MPH, MSc
Assistant Professor, Health
    Management and Policy
Center for Population Health and
    Community Impact
Dornsife School of Public Health
Drexel University
Philadelphia, PA

Harrison Quick, PhD
Assistant Professor
Epidemiology and Biostatistics
Dornsife School of Public Health
Drexel University
Philadelphia

Guy Robinson, PhD
Lecturer in Biology
Department of Natural Science
Fordham College at Lincoln Center,
    Fordham University
New York, NY

Ana V. Diez Roux, MD, PhD, MPH
Dean and Distinguished University
    Professor of Epidemiology,
    Epidemiology and Biostatistics,
Co-Director, Urban Health
    Collaborative
Dornsife School of Public Health
Drexel University
Philadelphia, PA

Andrew Rundle, MPH, DrPH
Associate Professor, Epidemiology
Co-Director, Obesity Prevention
    Initiative
Mailman School of Public Health
Columbia University
New York, NY

Olga L. Sarmiento, MD, PhD, MPH
Director, EpiAndes
Associate Professor, Public Health
Universidad de los Andes
Bogotá, Colombia

Faizan Shaikh, MPH, BDS
Research Assistant
Dornsife School of Public Health
Drexel University
Philadelphia, PA

José G. Siri, PhD, MPH
Research Fellow, Urban Health
International Institute for
    Global Health
United Nations University
Kuala Lumpur, Malaysia

Claire Slesinski, MSPH
Senior Program Manager for Global
    Urban Health
Urban Health Collaborative
Dornsife School of Public Health
Drexel University
Philadelphia, PA

Benjamin Spoer, PhD, MPH
Manager of Metrics and Analytics,
    City Health Dashboard
Grossman School of Medicine
New York University
New York, NY

Ivana Stankov, PhD
Senior Research Scientist
Urban Health Collaborate
Dornsife School of Public Health
Drexel University
Philadelphia, PA

Carolyn B. Swope, MPH, Well AP
Mailman School of Public Health
Columbia University
New York, NY

Lorna Thorpe, PhD, MPH
Professor
Director of the Division of
    Epidemiology
Department of Population Health
New York University
New York, NY

Vaishnavi Vaidya, MPH
Project Manager
Urban Health Collaborative
Dornsife School of Public Health
Drexel University
Philadelphia, PA

Kate Weinberger, PhD
Assistant Professor, Occupational
    and Environmental Health
School of Population and
    Public Health
University of British Columbia
Vancouver, Canada

FOREWORD

Mary T. Bassett

Any discussion about urban health will begin with the fact that most of humanity now lives in urban areas. About a decade into the 21st century, the urban portion of the global population surpassed 50%. This shift to majority urban will come last to Africa, where the rate of urban growth is the highest in the world. How has this centuries-long transformation in human settlement affected how we think about public health research and practice? The answer: not enough. Urban health has been a niche area, much as the climate crisis has been a niche area in environmental science. It is clear that this must change because urban is how people now live. *Urban Public Health: A Research Toolkit for Practice and Impact* is a valuable addition to the surprisingly slim number of books that investigate what urban health means and why its study is both distinct and important. Carefully crafted and thoughtful chapters grapple with the complexity of the urban setting as a physical and social space. The volume will appeal to a varied audience, including researchers, students, and practitioners alike.

Profoundly rooted in the idea of place, urban health must come to grips with definitional, conceptual, and methodological issues and draw on a range of disciplines. The volume brings this central challenge to the fore. Such emphasis on framing is especially helpful, given how broad the concept of place is as a central organizing idea. Each urban area has specific and unique features; each has shared characteristics. By using a place as a central unit of analysis, urban health stakes out its commitment to examining social, spatial, and physical characteristics of the urban setting as the pathway to the health of residents. By definition, urban health embraces the social determinants of health. Such big ideas require the careful thinking displayed in each chapter.

The modern city emerged with industrialization. The 19th-century imagination saw teeming cities as sources of pestilence and ill health. Beyond microbes, the disruption of rural social ties gave rise to social isolation, and low-wage factory work created greater misery among the displaced rural populations that created the emerging working class. Today, cities continue to capture the world's many challenges: escalating income inequality, racial and ethnic divisions, environmental pollution, and unsustainable growth that ignores the climate crisis. Cities are also hubs of excitement and transformation, nurturing innovation, creativity, and diversity.

Today, we know cities as places that can both threaten and promote health. Ebola transmission was amplified in the urban slums of Guinea, Libera, and Sierra Leone. Zika transmission in South America was associated with the densely populated urban favelas. More recently, a novel coronavirus took hold in Wuhan, a Chinese city of 11 million. Tuberculosis, long associated with poorly ventilated crowded housing, largely remains an urban scourge. But urban residence is also associated with longer, healthier lives. New York City has, for several years running, reported a longer average life expectancy at birth than the United States as a whole. Urban settings remain a magnet for many who seek a better life, and there are health data to support this promise.

This volume posits that we can do much better at understanding how the urban setting both creates and undermines opportunities for health. The many levels of urban life include residents, families, neighborhoods, social classes, races, ethnicities, nativity, governments, and the private sector. Further, cities include a whole ecology of infrastructure, institutions, and services that affect health. We do not have to resort to a modern-day miasma theory, which views cities as cauldrons that produce some amorphous brew. These many layers can be theorized, characterized, and measured. The understanding that emerges will help better ensure how cities promote and protect the health of all their residents beyond imploring individuals to make healthy choices.

Such understanding helps us see the risks posed as African urbanization has accelerated the growth of slums. These settlements typically lack infrastructure for water and sanitation, the foundation of 19th-century public health. Even as data from Africa suggested that cities had offered health advantages, pioneering work from the African Population & Health Research Center revealed the desperation of Nairobi slums. Researchers showed that key measures of population health, such as infant mortality rates, were higher in Nairobi slums than in rural areas. At the time, I found this observation incongruous. A visit to Mathare made it easy to understand how this might happen. Despite a landscape dotted with television antennas, a sign of affluence, this unincorporated settlement lacked rudimentary water and sanitation. Carts sold water in the alleyways. Government was reluctant to acknowledge these areas, offering no services, including health care. Drug shops and various largely unregulated private health care providers of uncertain training and quality filled this gap. Why would people migrate to worse conditions? How did human perception frame views of the slums and the decision to migrate? Connected to urban migration was the bleak prospects of life in the rural areas and the role of hope for a better future in propelling migration.

Urban areas are not islands. Any city is tied, in various ways, to surrounding areas. This example is illuminated by the chapters of this book, which address ways to approach such multilevel, multisectoral aspects of urban life.

A key insight in urban health is the observation that aggregate data can obscure areas of deprivation. There are many urban areas in the United States with a 25-year difference in life expectancy between neighborhoods. Typically, impoverished Black and Native American communities have the shortest lives. But how to disaggregate data? By income, by race, by neighborhood? What are appropriate boundaries of neighborhoods or communities? Among considerations are relationships to government structures, participation in political processes, and community views. Further, as diverse connections as kinship ties and political power may or may not be geographically contiguous. As an example, New York City, as many cities, is a city of neighborhoods. When the city health department decided to create more granular neighborhood summaries of community health, it used "community districts" as measuring units for the Community Health Profiles. These areas are the smallest units of city government, overseen by community boards. How much power these politically appointed boards wield is a matter of debate. Residents most likely have little awareness of the boundaries of these districts or even of the community boards. Their own views of what constitute the boundaries of their neighborhood may differ. But the selection of these units reflected the expectation that data would be used to advocate for resources and the Health Department's view that government is principally responsible for assuring resources for health.

Cities also have a role limiting risks for noncommunicable disease, which now comprises 80% of the global disease burden and accounts for most of the disease burden on all continents but Africa. Without cities, it is hard to imagine the growing dominance of processed and prepared food, the need for walkability and public transport, or the impact of buildings on energy consumption. Our urban world is indeed interconnected and complex. But complexity is never a synonym for inaction. This volume shines a light on how to understand, measure, and change the urban setting so that cities grow, people thrive, and no one is left behind.

PREFACE

Welcome to Urban Public Health: A Research Toolkit for Practice and Impact
An increasing majority of the human population resides in urban areas, and residents are affected in multiple ways by these settings. Our lives and our health are shaped by the design of buildings and transportation systems, access to improved sanitation and early childhood education, the availability of food stores and recreational spaces, and by a wide range of local policies from housing to health care access. As we begin, we hope to clarify the scope of this book and the goals that guide us in writing and structuring this book.

Urban health encompasses multiple population health outcomes shaped by urban settings
Similarly to related terms such as "population health" or "global health," urban health can be conceptualized as an object, a goal, and an area of scholarship and practice.[8] As an object of study, urban health refers to the current state of human health within, and in relationship to, urban environments. The object "urban health" is by definition multidimensional and multilevel, with individuals' health reflecting conditions in their household, neighborhood, and activity spaces, which in turn are shaped by the broader municipal or national setting. As a goal, urban health expresses the aspiration to shape urban environments in ways that support, rather than undermine, the health of all humans who spend time there, including those with the most precarious health status due to marginalized social position. Progress toward urban health can be measured by monitoring changes in population health in cities overall and through attention to geographic and socioeconomic disparities in health within and among cities. Finally, urban health as an area of scholarship and practice encompasses the knowledge, competencies, and activities particular to assessing and understanding and achieving urban health. In writing this book, we endeavor to orient readers to urban health, with attention to each of these ways of viewing urban health.

As with other topics with broad scope, there is a tension between "mainstreaming" urban health by highlighting commonalities with public health more broadly, and using it to bring focus to a more specialized "track" by articulating the specificity of urban health problems and solutions. Our text Urban Public Health seeks a middle ground, highlighting common aspects related to understanding population health generally while emphasizing the distinct challenges and opportunities encountered within urban health.

The Audience for Urban Public Health

Improving health in cities and other urban areas undoubtedly requires engaging many disciplines and sectors, including not only public health but also urban planning, social sciences, public policy, industry, education, and medicine, among others. Our hope is that trainees and researchers in public health, as well as those from other fields of study, will have new ideas on how to engage with each other and with urban health research after reading Urban Public Health. We include "public" in the book title not only to acknowledge that our vantage point is from public health research and practice, but also to position centrally the role of public decisions and public sector audiences as we discuss the foundational knowledge, techniques, and commitments that we see as crucially relevant to improving urban health.

The structure of Urban Public Health

Understanding and improving urban health requires a team with a range of skills and capabilities. We realize that the needed skills are highly varied, complex, and intertwined, and that any individual reader may only wish to fully engage with particular pieces of what Urban Public Health has to offer. To aid the reader in navigating this book, we divide our chapters into four parts. It is our hope that you will use those parts that are most applicable to your current work, and perhaps come back to other parts at a later time as necessary.

- **Part 1** lays the foundation of urban health, defining geographic and substantive scope, global trends, conceptual models and frameworks and discusses the inherent inequities faced in urban areas.
- **Part 2** Identifies data for urban health research, describing assessment and measurement, data collection, and mapping of urban health data.
- **Part 3** describes how to analyze and build evidence from the data identified in Part 2, including integration of data, use of data for descriptive analysis and causal explanation, synthesis of evidence, and systems thinking and tools.
- **Part 4** is devoted to the use of urban health research to inform action through partnerships and collaboration, including those which elevate community voices and capacities, use policy action to improve urban health, and support meaningful dissemination of research evidence to multiple audiences.

Across each of the four parts subheadings are used to aid readers in identifying the most pertinent information. Since many of the tools identified in this toolkit warrant their own book-length treatment, references are provided for interested readers who seek more depth.

While books are linear; urban health is not. If you read this book cover-to-cover you will see some topics discussed in multiple chapters, some foreshadowed early on and revisited in different ways across subsequent chapters. This redundancy is inevitable and deliberate, since often the same topic has new meaning depending on its context.

Why URBAN PUBLIC HEALTH: Our focus on both local and global urban health collaboration, research, and training

The authors of URBAN PUBLIC HEALTH are affiliated with the Drexel University Dornsife School of Public Health's Urban Health Collaborative, located in Philadelphia, the fifth largest and one of the oldest U.S. cities.

The idea to work together on this book arose from our own conversations about what urban health is, ways to prioritize our investment in projects and partnerships, and how our urban health training programs and fellowships should be designed. Our book draws on local and global examples of urban health work, both our own and from others. In doing so, we identify foundational knowledge, data sources, research approaches, and engagement strategies that will orient emerging urban health professionals to the roles and stages within urban health research which can have impact through partnership across disciplines, among sectors, and with communities. We are attentive to how our work in Philadelphia may be unique to our setting, embedded in the rich history of the region. However, we are also engaged in urban health research that characterizes variation across the US, throughout the Americas, and globally.

The chapters in this book were completed before the 2020 COVID pandemic struck, but in many ways the pandemic has served to highlight and make even more visible key themes emphasized in this book: the ways in which urban environments affect health, the critical role of data and evidence, the pervasive impact of social inequalities and racism on health in cities, and the fundamental role of public health practice and policy. The interconnectedness, vulnerability, and inequalities among global cities has perhaps never been as apparent as during the COVID-19 pandemic. In our work, especially in this unusual moment, we have an eye to what we can share with, and learn from, broader networks connecting cities and urban health research teams to each other.

Together, we hope to create and communicate information to guide cities toward better population health and health equity outcomes. Doing so requires attention to urban environment features that persist across years and decades, as well as population health crises (like the COVID-19 pandemic) that can unfold and change within months, weeks, or even days. Our understanding of the multiple ways that urban systems from multiple sectors affect residents' lives remains inevitably incomplete but continues to be rebuilt and elaborated with each generation of scholarship. Through URBAN PUBLIC HEALTH we share tools for charting a way forward and invite new voices to enrich the journey.

Let's begin.

PART I
Introduction to Urban Health

"The factors influencing urban health include urban governance; population characteristics; the natural and built environment; social and economic development; services and health emergency management; and food security."
—-The World Health Organization[1]

In this first part of the book, we define the scope of urban health and discuss key foundational concepts and approaches to health that are relevant to understanding and acting on health in cities. We review urbanization trends worldwide and discuss the implications of these trends for population heath. We consider the many ways in which urban areas may affect health and discuss different conceptualizations of the links between urban living and health. We illustrate the breadth of urban health research questions and the many options for policy and interventions to improve health and health equity in urban areas. The section concludes with a discussion of the fundamental importance of health inequities in urban places with a special focus on ways in which urban environments and urban policies affect health equity.

1. World Health Organization. Health topics: Urban health. http://origin.who.int/topics/urban_health/en/. Accessed June 28, 2020.

CHAPTER 1

What Is Urban Health?

Defining the Geographic and Substantive Scope

ANA V. DIEZ ROUX

WHY URBAN HEALTH?

Why a special focus on promoting health in cities or urban areas? How is the focus or approach of the field defined as urban health different from the focus or approach of public health (or population health) more broadly? Is there a specificity to etiologic understanding of the drivers of health in urban settings? Are there specific aspects of urban contexts that are important to maximizing the translation of knowledge into policies? Are there specific interventions or policies that are especially relevant in urban areas? These questions, which fundamentally refer to the specificity of the "urban" and how it may be relevant for both understanding and action in public health, must be at the core of any discussion of the field now referred to as "urban health." In this book, we will attempt to provide answers to these questions, or at least provide a rigorous and thoughtful discussion that will allow each reader to answer these questions for himself or herself.

To begin, there is broad agreement, as we will discuss in more detail in subsequent chapters, that the future of a large part of humanity will lie in cities. The proportion of the world's population that lives in urban areas, characterized primarily by high population density and its associated physical and social environmental features, has been increasing rapidly, even in regions of the world such as Africa and Asia that were traditionally less urbanized.[1] The obvious implication is that any effort to protect and promote human health in the future will require characterizing health in cities, understanding the drivers of health in cities, and identifying and implementing interventions or

Ana V. Diez Roux, *What Is Urban Health?* In: *Urban Public Health*. Edited by: Gina S. Lovasi, Ana V. Diez Roux, and Jennifer Kolker, Oxford University Press (2021). © Oxford University Press 2021.
DOI: 10.1093/oso/9780190885304.003.0001.

policies that are effective in urban contexts. This is the fundamental motivation that has driven the growing interest in urban health, as an object of study (i.e., the health of people living in urban areas and its determinants) and as an approach to guide action (i.e., the strategies than can be most effective at improving health in urban areas).

An important thing to remember as we embark on a study of urban health is that the impact of urban living on health is variable and malleable. As we will discuss in more detail in Chapter 2, there are examples where health outcomes are better in urban than in rural populations and examples where the opposite is true. This is because of the enormous heterogeneity in environmental factors (both social and physical) relevant to health that exist within both urban and rural areas. Recognizing and understanding this heterogeneity is critical to identifying effective policies. But, most important, it highlights the fact that there is no universal or unique impact of urban living on health: it is within our power to design, manage, and govern cities in ways that promote health and health equity.

Cities are characterized by population diversity and large social inequalities. These social inequalities have major implications for health and result in pronounced health inequities in cities by social class, race, and ethnic background, migration history, and other social factors. These inequities in health are often manifested spatially resulting in large and pronounced differences in health across neighborhoods (even adjacent neighborhoods) within a single city. These spatial differences are driven by residential segregation and its social and environmental consequences, a topic we will return to later in this book. A key point is that improving health in cities necessarily requires understanding and acting upon the causes of health inequities. Urban health inequities are not inevitable, and their malleability provides an opportunity for informed action. We will return to a discussion of urban health inequities (including what we mean by inequities) in Chapter 4.

Last but not least, cities are acting, via city governments, via the private sector, and via community organizations among other groups. These actions (expanding a public transportation system, rezoning a neighborhood to allow mixed use, changing the ways schools are financed, creating bike lanes, limiting advertising, imposing new taxes, etc.) can have major implications for health and health equity. These policies and interventions, often implemented for reasons completely unrelated to health promotion, can have major positive or negative impacts on health and health equity in cities. By evaluating the health impact of these actions, we can learn about the causes of health in cities and can also draw valuable lessons about what policies and interventions might work best to promote health. We will return to a discussion of practice and policy in urban settings in Chapter 14.

Having identified several key reasons to focus on urban health (Table 1.1), in the remainder of this chapter we will discuss the setting of urban health

Table 1.1 WHY FOCUS ON URBAN HEALTH?

Reason

1. Across the globe, populations are increasingly concentrated in urban areas.
2. Urban living can positively or negatively affect health.
3. Cities are characterized by large social and health inequities.
4. The actions of cities can have beneficial or adverse impacts on health and health equity.

(and what we mean exactly by "urban") and outline key conceptual elements relevant to understanding health in urban areas.

In the remainder of this chapter, we will discuss the setting of urban health (and what we mean exactly by "urban") and outline key conceptual elements relevant to understanding health in urban areas.

THE GEOGRAPHY OF URBAN HEALTH: URBAN AREAS, CITIES, AND NEIGHBORHOODS

A core defining element of the field of urban health is the focus on urban settings. This raises important questions about the definition of urban, of cities, and of neighborhoods within cities.

What Defines a Geographic Area as Urban?

Characterizing health in urban areas or contrasting health in urban (or more urban) areas to health in rural (or less urban) areas requires operationalization of what defines a geographic area as urban. This is no easy task. Because the term captures many interrelated dimensions, and because many of these dimensions can be characterized across a continuum, there is no universally used operational definition of "urban." Any dichotomous distinction between urban and rural is necessarily arbitrary given the large heterogeneity that is likely to be present within places classified as "urban" or "rural." Yet dichotomous definitions are commonly used to contrast health in urban and rural areas, and the definition used can impact the differences observed.[2]

Perhaps the cardinal feature of urban areas (and one that has implications for many physical and social environment features) is high population density. Accordingly, population density is often used by government agencies as a core metric in defining what qualifies as "urban." However, the ways in which high population density is used to classify an area as urban is highly variable. Urban areas can be defined based on a threshold of persons per geographic area (e.g., >x persons per square km).[3] Alternatively, areas of high population density can be identified based on the number of residents in a certain administrative jurisdiction (e.g., localities with at least x residents) with no specific reference to the geographic size of the jurisdiction. This measure can be thought of as a measure of population concentration rather than true density, as the geographic size of the jurisdiction is not considered explicitly.

An advantage of true density measures (i.e., people per square km) is that they can be directly compared across countries. However, they make no reference to the broader context in which a high population density area is located. For example, small geographic areas of very high density surrounded by areas of very low density (e.g., a small very dense town surrounded by rural areas) may be quite different from similarly dense areas that are surrounded by many other very high-density areas (dense neighborhoods that are part of a very dense metropolitan area spread out over a large geographic area). Definitions based on the population size of jurisdictions partly address this problem by defining what constitutes a contiguous urban unit of sorts (e.g., an urban "place" or city) and characterizing its population size. However, the ways in which jurisdictions are defined can lack comparability across countries. Moreover, areas defined as urban based on the population size of jurisdictions can differ substantially from each other in actual population density.

Globally, there is substantial variation in the definition of urban places. Some definitions combine thresholds of population density and population size. For example, the European Commission definition identifies as "urban centers" any contiguous stretch with at least 50,000 people and a population density of 1,500 per square kilometer.[4] The US Census also uses a combination of population concentration, density, and spatial contiguity in its definition of "urbanized area" (an area with population of at least 50,000 persons consisting of an urban nucleus with a population density of 1,000 persons per square mile together with adjoining territory with at least 500 persons per square mile).[5] Details of the definition have varied over time, and various government agencies use different definitions. The 2010 US Census and National Center for Health Statistics definitions of urban and rural areas are described in Box 1.1.

Beyond population-based definitions, definitions of urban used in international statistics may include employment characteristics as well as features of land use and access to services to varying extent, as illustrated in Table 1.2. These definitions create important challenges not only for comparability of levels of urbanization across countries or regions but also for estimating the pace of urbanization over time. Recognition of comparability challenges has resulted in calls for the creation of standardized measures. One example is the degree of urbanization (DEGURBA) classification[6] described in Box 1.2. When applied worldwide, the use of this approach has resulted in much higher estimates of urbanization including much higher estimates for regions of Africa and Asia than had been previously reported.[7] These high estimates, however, have been contested.

Box 1.1 US CENSUS AND NATIONAL CENTER FOR HEALTH STATISTICS CLASSIFICATION OF URBAN AND RURAL AREAS

US CENSUS

The 2010 US Census[8,9] defines urban areas as comprising "a densely settled core of census tracts and/or census blocks that meet minimum population density requirements, along with contiguous territory containing nonresidential urban land uses as well as territory with low population density included to link outlying densely settled territory with the densely settled core." Rural encompasses all territories not included within an urban area.

Two types of urban areas are defined: urbanized areas and urban clusters.

> An *urbanized area* is a statistical geographic entity consisting of a densely settled core created from census tracts or blocks and contiguous qualifying territory that together have a minimum population of at least 50,000 persons.

> An *urban cluster* is a statistical geographic entity consisting of a densely settled core created from census tracts or blocks and contiguous qualifying territory that together have at least 2,500 persons but fewer than 50,000 persons.

Urbanized areas and urban clusters are formed by aggregating census tracts or block groups and have minimum population and density requirements. Two population density thresholds are used in the delineation of urban areas (both urban areas and urban clusters): 1,000 persons per square mile (for the core) and 500 per square mile (for surrounding areas). A complex algorithm including contiguity as well as land cover and land use criteria are also used to define these areas.

Urbanized areas form the urban cores of metropolitan statistical areas. Urban clusters with at least 10,000 people form the urban cores of micropolitan statistical areas.

NATIONAL CENTER FOR HEALTH STATISTICS

The National Center for Health Statistics[10] defines six urbanization levels (four metropolitan and two nonmetropolitan). The scheme is based on the Office of Management and Budget's February 2013 delineation of MSAs and micropolitan statistical areas.

Six categories are defined ranging from most urban to least urban:

Large central metro—Counties in MSAs of 1 million or more population that
1. Contain the entire population of the largest principal city of the MSA, or
2. Have their entire population contained in the largest principal city of the MSA, or
3. Contain at least 250,000 inhabitants of any principal city of the MSA.

Large fringe metro—Counties in MSAs of 1 million or more population that did not qualify as large central metro counties

Medium metro—Counties in MSAs of populations of 250,000 to 999,999

Small metro—Counties in MSAs of populations less than 250,000

NONMETROPOLITAN CATEGORIES

Micropolitan—Counties in micropolitan statistical areas

Noncore—Nonmetropolitan counties that did not qualify as micropolitan

METROPOLITAN STATISTICAL AREA

An MSA is a county, or group of contiguous counties, that contains at least one urbanized area of 50,000 or more population. In addition to the county or counties that contain all or part of the urbanized area, a metropolitan statistical area may contain other counties if there are strong economic ties with the central county or counties, as measured by commuting.

MICROPOLITAN STATISTICAL AREA

A micropolitan statistical area is a county or group of continuous counties that contains an urban cluster of at least 10,000 population but no more than 49,999 population. In addition to the county or counties that contain all or part of the urban cluster, a micropolitan statistical area may contain other counties if there are strong economic ties with the central county or counties, as measured by commuting.

What Defines a Geographic Area as a "City"?

Aside from characterizing geographic areas as urban or not urban, urban health research and practice are often focused on discreet entities known as "cities." Defining cities is appealing because of the potential for linkage to structures

Table 1.2 COUNTRY-SPECIFIC DEFINITIONS OF URBAN USED BY THE
UNITED NATIONS IN THE 2018 WORLD URBANIZATION PROSPECTS REPORTS
(SELECTED COUNTRIES)

Country	Definition of Urban
Argentina	Localities with 2,000 inhabitants or more.
Australia	For 2001 and later, Significant Urban Centers representing concentrations of urban development with 10,000 inhabitants or more. Before 2001, urban centers with 1,000 inhabitants or more.
Bangladesh	Localities having a municipality (*pourashava*), town (*shahar*) committee, or cantonment board. In general, urban areas are a concentration of 5,000 inhabitants or more in a continuous collection of houses where the community sense is well developed and the community maintains public utilities, such as roads, street lighting, water supply, and sanitary arrangements. An area that has urban characteristics but has fewer than 5,000 inhabitants may, in special cases, be considered urban.
Bolivia	Localities with 2,000 inhabitants or more.
Botswana	Agglomerations of 5,000 inhabitants or more where at least 75% of the economic activity is nonagricultural.
Cambodia	For 1998 and later, communes that meet at least one of the following criteria: (i) population density exceeding 200 persons per square kilometer, (ii) male employment in agriculture below 50%, or (iii) 2,000 inhabitants or more.
Canada	For 1981 and later, areas with 1,000 inhabitants or more and at least 400 inhabitants per square kilometer.
China	For 2000, population of city districts with average population density of at least 1,500 persons per square kilometer and population of suburban-district units and township-level units meeting certain criteria, such as having contiguous built-up area, being the location of the local government, or being a street (*jiedao*) or having a resident committee. For 2010, the criteria used in the 2000 census plus residents living in villages or towns in outer urban and suburban areas that are directly connected to municipal infrastructure and that receive public services from urban municipalities.
Colombia	Administrative headquarters (*población cabecera*) with 2,000 inhabitants or more.
Democratic Republic of Congo	Places with 2,000 inhabitants or more where the predominant economic activity is nonagricultural; and places with fewer than 2,000 inhabitants that are considered urban because of their type of economic activity (predominantly nonagricultural).
Denmark	Localities with 200 inhabitants or more.
France	Based on the concept of urban unit, namely, communes with 2,000 inhabitants or more in dwellings separated by, at most, 200 meters.

(continued)

Country	Definition of Urban
India	Statutory places with a municipality, corporation, cantonment board, or notified town area committee and places satisfying all of the following three criteria: (i) 5,000 inhabitants or more; (i) at least 75% of male working population engaged in nonagricultural pursuits; and (iii) at least 400 inhabitants per square kilometer.
Italy	Communes with 10,000 inhabitants or more.
Mexico	Localities with 2,500 inhabitants or more.
Nigeria	Towns with 20,000 inhabitants or more.
Panama	Localities with 1,500 inhabitants or more, with all or most of the following urban characteristics: electricity, water supply and sewerage systems, paved roads and access to commercial establishments, secondary schools, and social and recreational centers. Some places with most of the aforementioned features were defined as urban even if they had fewer than 1,500 inhabitants.
Saudi Arabia	Cities with 5,000 inhabitants or more.
Spain	Municipalities (*municipios*) with 10,000 inhabitants or more.
United States	Densely settled territory that meets minimum population density requirements and with 2,500 inhabitants or more. A change in the definition for the 2000 census from place-based to density-based affects the comparability of estimates before and after this date.
Zimbabwe	Places officially designated as urban, as well as places with 2,500 inhabitants or more whose population resides in a compact settlement pattern and where more than 50% of the employed persons are engaged in non-agricultural occupations.

Source: United Nations[11]

of governance and political accountability. In addition, even though all cities may qualify as urban areas, they can show important heterogeneity in size, history, and economic characteristics, as well as in physical and social features that may be important to health. City boundaries need to be operationalized to precisely measure city characteristics, but there is no universal way to do so (Table 1.3).

While there is no unique or definitive way to delineate a city, there are at least three possible types of definitions: (i) administrative definitions based on political or administrative boundaries; (ii) functional definitions based on social or economic connections, such as country-defined metropolitan areas, that capture interconnectedness between a core city and nearby areas, and (iii) empirical definitions based on the geographic extent of physically built-up areas identified from satellite imagery using standardized criteria.[12-17]

Box 1.2 THE DEGREE OF URBANIZATION CLASSIFICATION OF URBAN AND RURAL AREAS

DEGURBA is used globally to classify local administrative units (such as municipalities or communes) into three types of areas: cities (densely populated areas), towns and suburbs (intermediate density areas), and rural areas (thinly populated areas).

The approach defines grid cells of one square kilometer across all populated global areas and uses population estimates to classify these cells as belonging to

- Urban centers (contiguous grid cells that each have a density of at least 1,500 inhabitants per square kilometer and that together have a population of at least 50,000 inhabitants)
- Urban clusters (contiguous grid cells with at least 300 inhabitants per square kilometer and at least 5,000 inhabitants in the cluster), or
- Rural cells (grid cells outside urban clusters and centers, many of which have a density below 300 inhabitants per square kilometer).

Local administrative units are then classified as cities if >50% of their population lies in urban centers; as towns and suburbs if >50% of the population lies in urban clusters and is not classified as a city; and rural otherwise (including areas where >50% of the population lives in rural grid cells).

Figure 1.1 shows population distributions in different regions of the world using the DEGURBA classification contrasted with estimates from the 2014 World Urban Prospects report.[18]

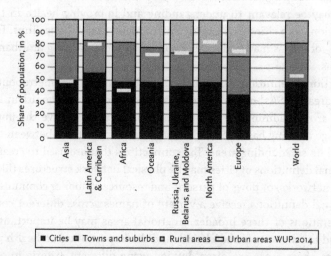

Figure 1.1 Population by degree of urbanization per major global region, 2015.
Source: European Commission, UN Habitat. *The State of European Cities 2016: Cities Leading the Way to a Better Future.* Brussels, Belgium: European Commission, Directorate-General For Regional and Urban Policy; 2016.[19]

Table 1.3 APPROACHES TO DEFINING AREAS AS URBAN AND DELINEATING CITY BOUNDARIES

Options to Classify Geographic Areas as Urban	Where to Draw the Boundaries for a City
Population density (residents/land area)	Administrative or municipal boundaries
Population concentration (no. of residents) in a specific jurisdiction or other geographic area	Functional urban agglomeration, tied together based on physical networks or flows such as commute patterns
Contiguity with and services in support of adjacent urban areas	Empirical urban footprint based on the extent of built-up area, often determined using remote sensing data
Land use and other features	
Employment not based primarily in agriculture	
Decision rule based on a combination of the previously listed options	

An advantage of administrative definitions of cities (e.g., city X governed by a mayor) is that they can be linked to administrative and political responsibility. An added advantage of focusing on administrative definitions of cities is that they are often easy to link to existing data on health and health-relevant aspects of the environment. A disadvantage is that, especially in large urban areas, administratively defined cities often only capture a core city. This may not fully represent the surrounding urban area (sometimes referred to as the urban agglomeration) that may encompass and affect the core city. Features of the entire urban agglomeration (including less urbanized areas linking urban cores) may be relevant to understanding and improving health in the city. In addition, core cities may impact surrounding populations. Thus, focusing only on core cities may lead to an incomplete understanding of urban health problems.

Functional definitions such as metropolitan areas (e.g., metropolitan statistical areas [MSAs] in the United States) better capture the urban agglomeration around administratively defined core cities and have the important advantage of being based on social and economic relations between the core city and its surrounding areas. The connections that are used to create these functional definitions of cities may be physical network structures (like water or road networks) or flows of persons and resources (labor or commute areas). Functional definitions receive a variety of names across different countries. Considerations of these broader functional areas may be important to understand the drivers of urban health and the impact of urban health policies. However, these areas are often defined using different criteria in different countries, making cross-country comparisons difficult.

Boundaries can also be drawn empirically based on the geographic extent of built-up areas, capturing the physical footprint of the city. The *Atlas of Urban Expansion* has used this approach on a global scale.[20] An advantage of this approach is that it can be applied systematically across countries and over time to track urban growth longitudinally. In addition, it captures the boundaries of urbanized areas in a systematic and data-driven fashion. Challenges may arise when linking such footprints to existing data such as population counts or health data because the boundaries identified do not necessarily correspond to geographic area identifiers available in census or health data. This can be overcome if finer georeferenced data are available, or if spatial overlay can be used to attribute data for other geographies to the built-up area (discussed further in Chapter 7).

With increasing availability of population and remote sensing data, there are emerging opportunities for harmonized definitions of cities or urban agglomerations for international comparisons. For example, the European Commission has proposed a standardized definition of a city and its commuting zone, which it refers to as a "functional urban area" (FUAs). FUAs consist of a densely inhabited city and a less densely populated commuting zone whose labor market is highly integrated with the city.[21] In this approach, cities are defined as local administrative units with >50% of the population living in urban centers defined using the DEGURBA approach (Box 1.2). Commuting zones are defined as local administrative areas where >15% of the working population commutes to the city. The combination of the city and its commuting area constitute the FUA. In Chapter 2, we review other ways in which cities have been defined, including strategies used by the United Nations[12] and the *Atlas of Urban Expansion*.[17] Box 1.3 describes the approach used by the SALURBAL Study, a large international collaboration to define cities for research purposes.

Defining Neighborhoods Within Cities

As we will discuss later in this book, many urban health questions pertain to differences in health across areas within a city. These areas are often referred to as neighborhoods. Much has been written on how neighborhoods can be defined. As in the case of cities, multiple types of definitions are possible. Each has advantages and disadvantages, and the appropriate definition depends on the both reason for defining neighborhoods and on practical considerations related to data availability.

Many cities have administratively defined neighborhoods such as planning districts, police precincts, or electoral subdivisions used for various governing or reporting purposes. As is the case for administratively defined cities, these smaller administrative units have the advantage that they can sometimes be linked to political responsibility and may also be easily linked to data relevant

Box 1.3 SALURBAL: DEFINING CITIES IN A LARGE INTERNATIONAL COLLABORATION ON URBAN HEALTH

Recognizing the complexity of defining cities and the need to be rigorous but practical to capitalize on easily available health data, SALURBAL used an approach that combines various criteria.[22] First, we identified the universe of cities of interest. Second, we operationalized cities and their component units so that various data sources could be linked to them. We used a three-level tiered system to define cities and their subunits. We labeled cities as Level 1, subcity components as Level 2, and neighborhoods as Level 3.

STEP 1: IDENTIFYING THE UNIVERSE OF SALURBAL CITIES

The project identified "cities" with ≥100,000 inhabitants as of 2010 in the 11 SALURBAL countries as the universe of interest (here we use the term "cities" in quotes broadly to refer to units that may be an urban agglomeration or some form of administratively defined cities). A cut-off population size of 100,000 inhabitants was selected because it is a threshold often used to define cities[23] and allows the inclusion of "cities" of varying size.

We created a draft list of "cities" with 100,000 inhabitants or more by combining information from two sources: The 2010 Atlas of Urban Expansion and a database of census data compiled on the City Population website.[24] Both data sources include complementary information, as one is based on the urban extent of each city and the other is based on administrative definitions. The consolidated draft list of "cities" was reviewed by each country team for face validity resulting in a few minor modifications to the list. A few additional modifications to the list were made while working to operationalize boundaries of these "cities" as clusters of smaller subcity units and as a result of comparisons with country defined metropolitan areas.

STEP 2: CREATING COMPLEMENTARY OPERATIONAL DEFINITIONS OF "CITIES" AND SUBUNITS WITHIN THEM

SALURBAL created three complementary ways to identify the boundaries of "cities" or Level 1 units:

1. L1AD: based on the built-up urban extent approximated through clusters of administratively defined areas
2. L1MA: based on country specific definitions of metropolitan areas
3. L1UX: based on the precise built up urban extent identified systematically using satellite imagery

In addition to defining "cities," SALURBAL also defined subcity units (Level 2) and neighborhoods within cities (Level 3).

Table 1.4 SALURBAL DEFINITIONS OF CITIES AND THEIR COMPONENT UNITS AT VARIOUS LEVELS

Level	Definition
Level 1 "city"	
L1AD (administrative)	"City" defined as a single administrative unit (e.g., *municipio*) or combination of adjacent administrative units (e.g., several *municipios*) that are part of the apparent urban extent as visually determined from satellite imagery. Each L1AD is defined based on its component Level 2 units.
L1MA (metropolitan areas)	"City" defined following the exact definition that each country provides for metropolitan areas (if available), as a combination of either Level 2 units or other units.
L1UX (urban extent)	"City" defined based on systematically identified urban extent based on built area; boundaries may not overlap exactly with administrative units.
Level 2 "subcity"	Administrative units (e.g., *municipios*) nested within L1AD. In some cases, this may be a single unit for each city; in other cases it will be multiple units. In some cases, Level 2 units may also be nested within L1MA.
Level 3 "neighborhood"	Smaller units such as census tracts that can be used as proxies for "neighborhoods" within a city. Level 3 units are nested within Level 2 units. They will also be approximately linked to L1UX so that census data can be linked to the L1UX for analyses. In some cases, Level 3 units may also be nested within L1MA.

A summary of the SALURBAL geographic definitions and "levels" is provided in Table 1.4. This multilevel and flexible data structure allows data to be linked at various levels depending on theoretical considerations and availability. By linking health outcomes to various levels, a variety of multilevel questions about urban health related to both between and within city variation can be explored.

to urban health. A disadvantage is that in many cases administrative areas may correspond poorly with the areas that residents think of as their neighborhoods, or with the areas within which they spend time and access various resources and services.

A second type of definition is based on the perceptions of residents. Although appealing in that these definitions may capture neighborhood social processes and interactions that may be relevant to health, they also have limitations. Residents may base how they define their neighborhood on different criteria (e.g., distance from their home, familiarity, social connections). Even when the criteria are specified, individual residents may apply criteria in different ways, resulting in varying definitions of neighborhood from resident to resident or even over time. In addition, residents' perceived neighborhoods may correlate only weakly with the spatial context affecting a specific behavior or health outcome. For example, food shopping may not be constrained only by perceived neighborhoods; rather, it may be influenced by resources within a given distance from the home (by areas much larger than what individuals may think of as their neighborhood).

A third type of definition that is uniformly created across locations is based on buffers of a fixed size around the home. This definition is based purely on spatial proximity. In addition, it is personalized in that each individual becomes the center of his or her "neighborhood." An advantage is standardization. In addition, the use of buffers of various sizes allows examination of sensitivity of results to the buffer size used. A disadvantage is that the sizes of the buffers used can appear arbitrary unless there is strong theory or prior research to suggest that a spatial context within a specific distance from the home is most relevant to the specific health outcome or behavior under investigation. Other personalized definitions somewhat akin to neighborhoods that can be used to characterize environmental exposures (such as activity spaces) are discussed in Chapter 6.

The definition of neighborhood that should be used in an urban health project depends on the purpose. Two common uses of neighborhood definitions in urban health are description and causal inference. When description of health differences across neighborhoods is the goal, and especially when the project is being carried out in partnership with local communities or with the goal of sharing with communities, alignment with politically meaningful or resident-accepted neighborhoods may be most useful. Sometimes administratively defined areas (such as census tracts or groups of continuous census tracts) may be an acceptable proxy for socially defined neighborhoods, which eases data acquisition including availability of appropriate denominator data to estimate rates and proportions.

When causal inference is the goal—that is, when we are interested in studying the effects of neighborhood context on health—the neighborhood definition should ideally be aligned with the hypothesized causal process. For example, examinations of the impact of the food environment on health may need to focus on an area within a relatively large radius of the home (because food shopping may occur within a relatively large area). In contrast, the impact of neighborhoods on mental health may operate through features of the immediate environment, perhaps even the block. We often lack the theory or prior empirical information needed to make specific predictions about the scale of the spatial context that is most relevant for causation of a particular health outcome. Thus, thoughtful sensitivity analyses using different definitions can be important. Even when the use of a specific neighborhood definition can be well justified, there may be utility in checking the robustness of results to the use of imperfect proxies such as census tracts to inform future efforts.

As in the case of defining cities, defining neighborhoods often requires making trade-offs and considering purpose and audience, theoretical validity, and the practicalities of operationalization and data availability (Table 1.5). There are also tradeoffs involving context specificity (e.g., using an approach that captures the social features of a particular city and the perceptions of its residents) versus a more uniform approach that is applicable across cities, making between-city comparisons of neighborhood-level drivers of health feasible. We will return to a discussion of neighborhood definitions and their implications in Chapters 5 and 12.

THE SUBSTANCE OF URBAN HEALTH: KEY ELEMENTS AND APPROACHES

The focus on health in urban areas or in comparison with nonurban areas is a distinguishing feature of urban health. But are there certain elements or approaches that are critical to understanding and improving health in urban areas? In this section, we describe some key elements that underlie many approaches to research and practice in urban health. These approaches are by no means specific to work in urban health and, in many ways, characterize the field of public health or interdisciplinary population health more broadly.[25] However, when applied to urban health, some of these elements or approaches develop a specific urban focus or become especially salient, as we describe in this section.

Table 1.5 CONSIDERATIONS IN CHOOSING A DEFINITION
OF "NEIGHBORHOOD"

Considerations

---

1. Purpose (description or causal inference)
2. Alignment with structures of administrative responsibility and decision-making
3. Resident and community recognition of the area as socially meaningful
4. Alignment with theory about the process by which health is affected
5. Data availability
6. Degree of tailoring to local contexts, versus uniform and generalizable methods

---

Place-Based

An emphasis on place-based approaches to understanding and intervening on health is perhaps one of the most defining features the urban health field. A focus on place as a critical context for health and on place-based features as causes of health outcomes emerges naturally from the urban focus. The place-based approach recognizes that the physical environments of places (be they cities themselves, neighborhoods within cities, or other spatial contexts such as parks and plazas) shape the social environment, and vice versa. These physical and social environments then play a critical role in influencing health and health equity, as we will discuss in more detail in Chapters 3 and 4. Thus, place is a critical dimension for describing urban health and understanding its determinants. An important corollary of this is that modification of places through intervention and policy becomes a critical avenue for health improvement in urban areas.

Multilevel

Beyond a focus on place generally, investigating or intervening on urban health problems often requires us to consider multiple levels of organization. Levels of organization can be defined in different ways and the relevance of different levels varies depending on the specific health outcome of interest. Examples of levels of organization that may be important to health include countries, states, cities, neighborhoods, families, workplaces, schools, and individuals, among others. In urban health, levels of interest are often linked to geographic contexts at various scales such as regions, metropolitan areas, core cities, and neighborhoods. These levels are meaningful to explanation because they have attributes specific to that level that may impact health or be amenable to action to improve urban health. For example, regions may be characterized by climate attributes, metropolitan areas may have economic features, cities may have specific city-level policies or transportation features, and neighborhoods may have specific social and built environment features (like pedestrian safety infrastructure and availability of healthy food stores). Thinking carefully about levels of organization, and investigating what features of these levels are relevant to a specific urban health issue, allows us to envision and identify opportunities for intervention at different levels.

Multisectoral

Identifying effective approaches to improve health in cities requires consideration of how multiple sectors may impact health. Sectors relevant to health in urban areas extend beyond the traditional health care services sector to also include urban planning and transportation, water and sanitation, education, social services, and the economy, among others. The role of multiple sectors is reflected in conceptual models of urban health (Chapter 3) and also influences the formulation of research questions and the policy actions that are considered. The "health in all policies" approach, reviewed in more detail in Chapters 3 and 14, explicitly recognizes how policies in multiple areas often thought to be unrelated to health can have major health impacts. This approach helps draw attention to the multiple sectors and systems that may have a role in improving urban health.

Multi-Outcome

As we will discuss in chapter 2, urban living can be beneficial or harmful for health. Simply as a consequence of high population density, multiple health problems can become concentrated and coexist in cities. Urban environments can affect multiple different health-related processes, each of which can simultaneously impact many different health conditions. Sometimes a common process (e.g., built environment effects on physical activity) can impact a set of related conditions (e.g., obesity, diabetes, and cardiovascular outcomes). Sometimes correlated environmental features (e.g., high traffic and high levels of violence) can result in correlated health outcomes (e.g., neighborhoods with high motor vehicle–related injuries linked to traffic and high homicide rates linked to violence). Sometimes health outcomes can also influence each other. For example, high neighborhood homicide rates (indicating high levels of violence) can serve as stressors that influence stress-related outcomes like asthma exacerbations or mental health. Although some urban health studies or policies may be narrowly focused on a specific health outcome, often multiple health outcomes need to be considered simultaneously. The focus on cities as systems (a topic we will return to in Chapter 11) can be especially useful in understanding how urban environments generate health and disease across multiple types of outcomes.

Equity-Focused

Urban areas are home to large social and health inequities, as discussed further in Chapter 4. They are also home to important diversity in race, ethnicity, country of origin, gender expression, and sexual preference. Many cities have large populations of immigrants. Differences in health by social class and across social groups stem from history and life course processes involving differential access to resources, education, and work, as well as chronic and acute experiences of racism and discrimination. In addition, inequities are magnified and reinforced by place-based differences generated as a result of residential segregation and consequent differences in power and resources across urban neighborhoods. Advantaged and disadvantaged neighborhoods are often in very close proximity to each other resulting in large inequities manifested across relatively small geographic areas. Urban policies can increase or reduce social and health inequities, as discussed further in Chapter 14. Maximizing health equity in cities is not only important for social justice reasons; it is also critical to improving overall population health.

Community and Policy Maker Engagement

Improving health and health equity in cities requires community and policy maker engagement across the range of urban health activities, from identifying the most pressing problems, to conducting research, to developing policies and interventions, to implementing and evaluating these policies and interventions. This engagement can take many forms, ranging from full community-based participatory research to purposive dissemination and translation of traditional research. It can involve local community partners, practitioners, and policy makers. A typology of community engagement is discussed in Chapter 14, and communication and partnership strategies are further highlighted in Part IV of this book.

Interdisciplinary

As we describe in more detail in Chapter 12, understanding and improving urban health requires an interdisciplinary approach. This results from the multilevel and multisectoral drivers of urban health. Understanding these drivers and effectively acting on them requires input from many disciplines. A prominent feature of urban health has been the collaboration between health and urban planning professionals. But other disciplines including sociology, anthropology, political science, economics, environmental science, toxicology, and even the arts are important to urban health research and action. The clinical and medical professionals involved in urban health also include a broad range of disciplines beyond public health, including medicine, nursing, dentistry, and the health professions more broadly.

Environmentally Conscious

By definition, urban health focuses on the impact of the environment on the health of urban populations. But it also considers the impact of urban living on regional and planetary ecosystems. It seeks to identify ways to design and

Box 1.4 URBAN SUSTAINABILITY AND URBAN HEALTH

By Marcus Grant

Public health evolves—as a discipline and a practice, the nature of its definition, its focus, and its execution changes.[26] At its heart is the eternal human ambition of reshaping the conditions for better health.[27] We now need public health to embrace urban sustainability and urban health and to bind these two fields of applied science tightly together.

The concept of sustainability highlights the physical limitations of global ecosystems and emphasizes the need to use science, technology, and policy to tackle today's great challenges. The sustainability-related concepts of "safe operating space for humanity,"[28] "planetary boundaries,"[29] and "ecosystem services"[30] are important additions to our public health toolbox. We now need these as we face complex and pressing public health challenges closely linked to environmental concerns. Key examples include threats posed by climate change[31] and loss of biodiversity.[32]

The potency of adding the precursor "urban" to both sustainability and health reflects the unprecedented and seemingly continual process of urbanization at the global level. Much of the predicted urban population growth in the coming decades will be informal in nature. Most urban population growth will be accommodated in the fringes and interstices of small- and medium-sized cities in middle- and low-income countries.[33]

The impact of urban areas on resource use and waste has always extended outside the urban limits. The land-take for food and water for people in the urban areas and the transport and communications infrastructure needed to move supplies and information into and out of the urban area all impact the surrounding landscape. The disposal of urban wastes contributes to toxic accumulations by air (incineration), land, and water, affecting areas well beyond the city limits. Globalization of trade, finance, capital, and labor has led to urban areas becoming closely networked with other cities but more detached from their impact footprints locally. This is having dire consequences[34] and is exacerbating inequities in health and access to healthy environments.[35] Negative consequences to the surrounding areas are often overlooked in local urban governance and decision-making.

At a global policy level, the creation of 17 Sustainable Development Goals[36] reflects grave concern with the sustainability of urban places and has important implications for addressing public health in urban areas. At the UN Conference on Housing and Sustainable Urban Development in Quito 2016 (referred to as Habitat III), all member states adopted the New Urban Agenda. This is an action-oriented series of commitments to support the achievement of a range of Sustainable Development Goals targets through rethinking the way we build, manage, and live in cities.

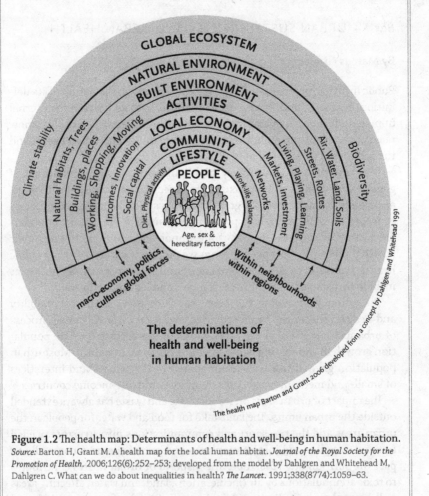

Figure 1.2 The health map: Determinants of health and well-being in human habitation.
Source: Barton H, Grant M. A health map for the local human habitat. *Journal of the Royal Society for the Promotion of Health.* 2006;126(6):252–253; developed from the model by Dahlgren and Whitehead M, Dahlgren C. What can we do about inequalities in health? *The Lancet.* 1991;338(8774):1059–63.

The Health Map model (Figure 1.2) provides a schematic diagram of the determinants of health from the point of view of settlement planning and design.[37] It has been created to help public health engage with the activities of the many built environment professions who together shape our urban environments. These include those trained as town planners, urban designers, landscape architects, and transport planners as well as the decision makers engaged in investment, development, and management of land.

The scene is set for public health to focus on urban development as it impacts both health and environmental sustainability[37,38] by

- Linking sustainable development and population health, through promoting local solutions for people's health that also have planetary health co-benefits, and visa versa[39];

- Addressing both communicable disease and noncommunicable disease, through identifying elements of urban form, pattern, and design that can benefit health and health equity[40]; and
- Advocating for policies and urban environments that support health by working closely with city planners, transport planners, urban designers, architects, and landscape architects[41]

Health needs to be at the center of the global urban agenda.[42] The public health profession can only do this in close partnership with those who govern, invest in, develop, and design our human settlements.[43]

govern cities so that they are simultaneously healthy and environmentally sustainable. We discuss the interrelatedness of health and environmental systems and how they are manifested in cities when we review the planetary health approach in Chapter 3. Box 1.4 reflects on the important theme of urban sustainability and its links to urban health. Attention to the environment is key not only to urban health today but also to the health and survival of future generations.

Bridging Local to Global

The global impact of urbanization, and the consequent increasing relevance of urban environments to health across the globe, implies that promotion of urban health must include a global focus. The ability to compare and contrast the experience of cities all over the world can generate enormous opportunities for learning. Local experiences thus acquire global relevance, and global experiences and trends can inform local decisions. The large and growing numbers of national and global networks of cities, many of them with a growing health focus, is a testament to the recognition of the interrelatedness of local and global experiences and actions. Urban health research has also increasingly become more global, as reflected in international organizations centered on urban health[44] and emerging research collaborations such as SALURBAL,[45] MINDMAP,[46] and RICHE Africa.[47]

REFERENCES

1. United Nations Department of Economic and Social Affairs Population Division. World urbanization prospects: The 2014 revision. 2014; https://www.un.org/en/development/desa/publications/2014-revision-world-urbanization-prospects.html.

2. Hall SA, Kaufman JS, Ricketts TC. Defining urban and rural areas in U.S. epidemiologic studies. *Journal of Urban Health*. 2006;83(2):162–175.

3. National Center for Health Statistics. NCHS urban–rural classification scheme for counties. 2017; https://www.cdc.gov/nchs/data_access/urban_rural.htm.

4. Dijkstra L, Poelman H. A harmonised definition of cities and rural areas: The new degree of urbanization. European Commission. January 2014; https://ec.europa.eu/regional_policy/sources/docgener/work/2014_01_new_urban.pdf.

5. Urban area criteria for the 2010 Census. 76 Fed. Reg. 53029 (August 24, 2011).

6. European Commission. Degree of urbanisation methodology. 2018. https://ec.europa.eu/eurostat/web/degree-of-urbanisation/methodology.

7. Angel S, Lamson-Hall P, Guerra B, Liu Y, Galarza N, Blei AM. *Our Not-So-Urban World*. New York: New York University; 2018.

8. Department of Commerce. Urban area criteria for the 2010 Census. *Federal Register*. 2011;76:53029.

9. US Census Bureau. 2010 Census urban and rural classification and urban area criteria. 2010; https://www.census.gov/programs-surveys/geography/guidance/geo-areas/urban-rural/2010-urban-rural.html.

10. Ingram DD, Franco SJ. NCHS urban-rural classification scheme for counties. *Vital and Health Statistics Series 2, Data Evaluation and Methods Research*. 2012(154):1–65.

11. United Nations Department of Economic and Social Affairs Population Division. World urbanization prospects: The 2018 revision. 2018; https://population.un.org/wup/Download/.

12. United Nations Department of Economic and Social Affairs Population Division. The world's cities in 2016—data booklet. 2016. https://www.un.org/en/development/desa/population/publications/pdf/urbanization/the_worlds_cities_in_2016_data_booklet.pdf.

13. Parr JB. Spatial definitions of the city: Four perspectives. *Urban Studies*. 2007;44(2):381–392.

14. Frey WH, Zimmer Z. Defining the city. In: Paddison R, ed. *Handbook of Urban Studies*. London: SAGE; 2001:14–35.

15. Fang C, Yu D. Urban agglomeration: An evolving concept of an emerging phenomenon. *Landscape and Urban Planning*. 2017;162:126–136.

16. European Environment Agency. Urban atlas. 2010. https://www.eea.europa.eu/data-and-maps/data/copernicus-land-monitoring-service-urban-atlas.

17. Angel S, Blei AM, Parent J, et al. *Atlas of Urban Expansion—2016 Edition*. Cambridge, MA: NYU Urban Expansion Program at New York University, UN-Habitat, and the Lincoln Institute of Land Policy; 2016.

18. Dijkstra L. Everything you heard about urbanisation is wrong. World Bank. 2018; https://olc.worldbank.org/system/files/Everything%20you%20heard%20about%20urbanisation%20is%20wrong.pdf.

19. European Commission, UN Habitat. *The State of European Cities 2016: Cities Leading the Way to a Better Future*. Brussels, Belgium: European Commission; 2016.

20. Angel S, Blei AM, Civco DL, Parent J. *Atlas of Urban Expansion*. Cambridge, MA: Lincoln Institute of Land Policy; 2012.

21. Organisation for Economic Co-operation and Development. *Redefining Urban: A New Way to Measure Metropolitan Areas*. Paris: OECD; 2012.

22. Quistberg DA, Diez Roux AV, Bilal U, et al. Building a data platform for cross-country urban health studies: The SALURBAL study. *Journal of Urban Health*. 201996(2):311–337.

23. Angel S, Blei AM, Parent J, et al. *Atlas of Urban Expansion—2016 Edition: Areas and Densities*. Cambridge, MA: NYU Urban Expansion Program at New York University, UN-Habitat, and the Lincoln Institute of Land Policy; 2016.

24. City Population. City population: Population statistics for countries, administrative divisions, cities, urban areas and agglomerations—interactive maps and charts. 2020; http://citypopulation.de/. Accessed June 28, 2020.

25. Diez Roux AV. On the distinction—or lack of distinction—between population health and public health. *American Journal of Public Health*. 2016;106(4):619–620.

26. Tulchinsky TH, Varavikova EA. *The New Public Health*. London: Academic Press; 2014.

27. Lang T, Rayner G. Ecological public health: The 21st century's big idea? *BMJ*. 2012;345(1):e5466–e5466.

28. Rockström J, Steffen W, Noone K, et al. A safe operating space for humanity. *Nature*. 2009;461(7263):472.

29. Steffen W, Richardson K, Rockstrom J, et al. Planetary boundaries: Guiding human development on a changing planet. *Science*. 2015;347(6223):1259855.

30. Millennium Ecosystem Assessment. *Ecosystems and Human Well-Being: Health Synthesis*. Washington, DC: World Resources Institute; 2005.

31. United Nations, World Health Organization. *Climate and Health Country Profiles—2015: A Global Overview*. 2015.

32. Romanelli C, Cooper D, Campbell-Lendrum D, et al. Connecting global priorities: Biodiversity and human health: A state of knowledge review. 2015. https://www.cbd.int/health/SOK-biodiversity-en.pdf.

33. Laros M, Jones F. *The State of African Cities 2014: Re-Imagining Sustainable Urban Transitions*. Nairobi, Kenya: United Nations Human Settlement Programme; 2014.

34. World Economic Forum. The global risks report 2017: 12th edition. 2017; http://www3.weforum.org/docs/GRR17_Report_web.pdf.

35. Raworth K. A doughnut for the anthropocene: Humanity's compass in the 21st century. *Lancet Planetary Health*. 2017;1(2):e48–e49.

36. United Nations General Assembly. Transforming our world: The 2030 Agenda for Sustainable Development. 2015; https://sustainabledevelopment.un.org/post2015/transformingourworld/publication.

37. Barton H, Grant M. A health map for the local human habitat. *Journal of the Royal Society for the Promotion of Health*. 2006;126(6):252–253.

38. Barton H, Thomspson S, Burgess S, Grant M. *The Routledge Handbook of Planning for Health and Well-Being*. London: Routledge; 2015.

39. de Leeuw E. Global health disruptors: The urban planet. *The BMJ Opinion*. November 30, 2018; https://blogs.bmj.com/bmj/2018/11/30/global-health-disruptors-the-urban-planet/.

40. Grant M, Braubach M. Evidence review on the spatial determinants of health in urban settings. In. *Urban Planning, Environment and Health: From Evidence to Policy Action*. Copenhagen, Denmark: WHO Regional Office for Europe; 2010:22–97.

41. Grant M, Barton H. No weighting for healthy sustainable local planning: Evaluation of a participatory appraisal tool for rationality and inclusivity. *Journal of Environmental Planning and Management*. 2013;56(9):1267–1289.

42. World Health Organization. Health as the pulse of the new urban agenda. Paper presented at the United Nations Conference on Housing and Sustainable Urban Development. Quito, Ecuador; 2016.

43. Grant M, Brown C, Caiaffa WT, et al. Cities and health: An evolving global conversation. *Cities & Health*. 2017;1(1):1–9.

44. International Society for Urban Health. [Home page]. 2019; https://isuh.org/.

45. Diez Roux AV, Slesinski SC, Alazraqui M, et al. A novel international partnership for actionable evidence on urban health in Latin America: LAC-urban health and SALURBAL. *Global Challenges*. 2019;3(4):1800013.

46. Beenackers MA, Doiron D, Fortier I, et al. MINDMAP: Establishing an integrated database infrastructure for research in ageing, mental well-being, and the urban environment. *BMC Public Health*. 2018;18(1):158.

47. Vearey J, Luginaah I, Magitta NwF, Shilla DJ, Oni T. Urban health in Africa: A critical global public health priority. *BMC Public Health*. 2019;19(1):340.

CHAPTER 2
Global Urbanization and Health Trends

ANA V. DIEZ ROUX

In this chapter we review the features of urbanization worldwide and its many consequences. We then highlight major health challenges in urban areas and briefly discuss how the urban context may shape various types of health outcomes. We conclude with an overview of the place of urban health in the agenda of international organizations and initiatives.

URBANIZATION PATTERNS WORLDWIDE

The term *urbanization* refers to the growth of populations living in urban areas. As we noted in Chapter 1, defining urban areas is complex and the definitions used often vary across countries. However, despite limitations of existing data, several features of urbanization and of trends over time in urbanization across the globe can be clearly identified.

Urban Living as a Key Characteristic of the Future of Humanity

Levels of urbanization are already very high in many regions of the world and are rapidly increasing in regions that were historically less urbanized. According United Nations (UN) data[1] in 2018, 55.3% of the world population lived in urban areas (using country-specific definitions). However, there is quite a bit of heterogeneity across regions: rates of urbanization were highest in North America (82.2%) and in Latin America and the Caribbean

Ana V. Diez Roux, *Global Urbanization and Health Trends* In: *Urban Public Health*. Edited by: Gina S. Lovasi, Ana V. Diez Roux, and Jennifer Kolker, Oxford University Press (2021). © Oxford University Press 2021.
DOI: 10.1093/oso/9780190885304.003.0002.

(80.7%) followed by Europe (74.5%) and Oceania (68.2%). Lower rates of urbanization were reported in Africa and Asia (42.5% and 49.9%, respectively), but they are rapidly increasing over time (Figure 2.1). New estimates using recently proposed systematic definitions of urban areas suggest that worldwide urbanization may be as high as 84% and 80% in Asia and Africa, respectively,[2] although these estimates have been debated.[3] Notably, regional estimates hide important variation among countries within a region (Figure 2.2). Regardless of the method used to identify urban areas, projections suggest that by 2050 over two-thirds of the world's population will live in urban areas.[1]

A notable fact is that increases in population overall coupled with the increasing proportion of the population living in urban areas results in dramatic increases in the absolute number of urban residents: for example, the global urban population increased from 2.87 billion in 2000 to 4.22 billion in 2018, an increase of 1.35 billion new urban residents in just 18 years.[1] It is estimated that by 2050 6.68 billion people will live in urban areas across the globe.

Increasing Importance of Urbanization in Lower- and Middle-Income Countries

Another key feature of urbanization is that a large and growing proportion of the world's urban population is concentrated in lower- and middle-income countries (LMICs). In 2018, of the 4.22 billion urban residents, 975 million were in high-income countries, 3.017 billion were in middle-income countries, and 224 million were in low-income countries.[1] Between 2018 and 2050 the urban population is expected to increase by 2.46 billion with 93% of this growth occurring in LMICs. Cities in high-income countries will add only 163 million people to their urban populations during this period. In contrast, cities in middle- and lower-income countries will need to absorb 2.3 billion people.[1]

By 2050, it is estimated that 83% of the urban population worldwide, or approximately 5.54 billion people, will live in the urban areas of LMICs (Figure 2.3).[1] This rapid and profound transformation has major implications for the governance and management of rapidly expanding urban areas of the developing world. Urbanization in the context of limited resources to establish the necessary infrastructure creates many challenges for growing urban populations across the globe as exemplified by the growth in the absolute numbers of residents of urban slums. On the other hand, as we will discuss later in this chapter, well-managed urbanization also creates opportunities to promote health and environmental sustainability.

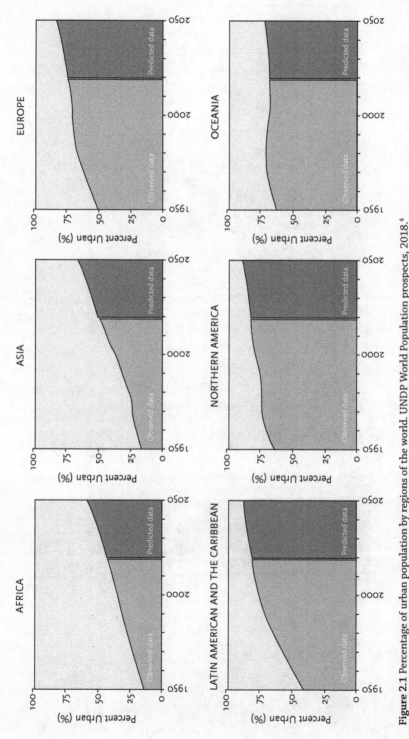

Figure 2.1 Percentage of urban population by regions of the world. UNDP World Population prospects, 2018.[4]

Source: United Nations Department of Economic and Social Affairs Population Division. World urbanization prospects: The 2018 revision, online edition. 2018; https://population. un.org/wup/Download/; adapted from United Nations Department of Economic and Social Affairs Population Division. World urbanization prospects: The 2014 revision 2014; https:// www.un.org/development/desa/publications/2014-revision-world-urbanization-prospects.html.

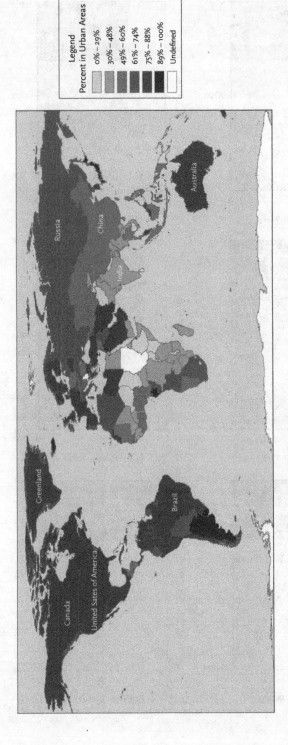

Figure 2.2 Percentage of population in urban areas for different countries.
Source: United Nations Department of Economic and Social Affairs Population Division. World urbanization prospects: The 2018 revision, online edition. 2018; https://population.un.org/wup/Download/.

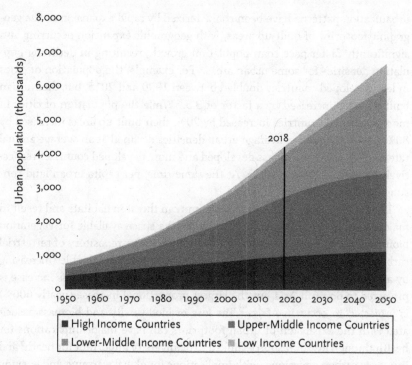

Figure 2.3 Increases in the urban population of higher-, middle-, and lower-income countries, 1950–2050.[5]

Source: United Nations Department of Economic and Social Affairs Population Division. World urbanization prospects: The 2018 revision, online edition. 2018; https://population.un.org/wup/Download/; Adapted from Aerni P. Coping with migration-induced urban growth: Addressing the blind spot of UN Habitat. *Sustainability.* 2016;8(8):800.

Environmental Impacts of Urbanization

A third important feature of urbanization is its environmental impact. The growth of urban areas not only creates multiple environmental challenges but also creates opportunities. It has been estimated that cities are responsible for approximately 70% of global energy consumption and 75% of global CO_2 emissions, with transport and buildings being among the largest contributors to emissions.[6] Although urbanization can have many adverse environmental consequences (resulting in more energy use, more pollution, and encroachment on natural environments), the relationship between urbanization and the environment is complex and depends on the nature of urbanization itself. Urbanization can be managed so that it actually results in more efficient use of resources and minimizes emissions, pollution, and the impact of human settlements on the natural environment.

A major driver of the environmental consequence of urbanization is the size of the geographic footprint of urban areas. Urban areas have traditionally been characterized by compactness and high population densities. However, recent urbanization patterns have been characterized by rapid expansion of the geographic footprint of built-up areas, with geographic expansion occurring at a significantly faster pace than population growth, resulting in declining population densities for some urban areas.[7] For example, the population of cities in less developed countries doubled between 1990 and 2015, but their urban built-up areas increased by a factor of 3.5.[8] While the population of cities in more developed countries increased by 20%, their built-up areas increased by 80%. As a consequence, average urban densities declined at an average annual rate of 2.1% and 1.5% in less developed and more developed countries respectively between 1990 and 2015. At the same time, per capita urban land consumption increased.

This rapid expansion of urban footprints can threaten habitats and result in major losses of biodiversity. It also reduces the space available for vegetation biomass (e.g., through deforestation), which is a major repository of terrestrial carbon.[7] By some estimates, urban landcover could nearly double (increasing by as much as 185%) between 2000 and 2030.[7] Nearly half of this increase is projected to occur in Asia but the largest proportional increase (nearly 600%) is projected to occur in Africa.[7] The loss of biodiversity and biomass associated with the expansion of urban footprints can have major implications for health through loss of resources linked to biodiversity important for heath[9] and increased carbon emissions (with implications for global warming and ensuing health consequences). The increase in impervious surfaces also affects the land available for agricultural production (which is necessary to sustain urban population growth) and, depending on how the expansion of urban areas occurs (i.e. via densification or urban sprawl), could affect exposure to floods.[10]

Analyses conducted by the Atlas of Urban Expansion suggest that

urban growth is mostly taking place in an unplanned and disorderly manner, informality is becoming more common over time, cities are expanding their territories faster than their populations, residential densities are decreasing dramatically, and public spaces and the lands allocated to streets and arterial roads are in decline suggesting that the contemporary model of urbanization is becoming highly unsustainable.[11]

However, well-managed urbanization can have multiple environmental benefits. For example, high-density urban areas tend to have lower per capita energy use and greenhouse emissions than low-density suburban development.[12] Higher density development can also minimize the impacts of population growth on loss of biomass, biodiversity, and land available for agricultural production.[7,10] High population density coupled with mixed land use can reduce the use of motor vehicles and concomitant energy use and emissions.[7] Cities can be designed in ways that encourage walking and cycling with multiple environmental (and health) benefits. Public green spaces in cities can both buffer heat and provide opportunities for recreation. Cities can also be designed to reduce waste and to eliminate wastewater in environmentally sustainable ways.

Heterogeneity of Urban Areas

A fourth important feature of urbanization is the presence of important heterogeneity across urban areas. Cities differ in population size as well as in other features including density, street network, transportation features, land use patterns, and governance characteristics, among others. The UN estimated that in 2018 two billion people, or close to one half of the world's urban population, lived in cities with fewer than 500,000 inhabitants, and another 400 million, or 10%, lived in settlements between 500,000 and 1 million (cities are defined as urban agglomerations or contiguous built-up areas with a population of 300,000 or more, although in some cases metropolitan areas or other administrative definitions are used instead of urban agglomerations).[13] Thus, nearly 60% of the world's urban population resided in cities of less than 1 million residents. An additional 20% of urban dwellers worldwide lived in a medium-sized cities of 1 million to 5 million inhabitants, 8% lived in cities of 5 to 10 million, and only about 13% of the world's urban dwellers lived in 33 megacities of >10 million inhabitants.[1] It is estimated that by 2030 there will be 43 megacities with more than 10 million inhabitants, most of them in developing countries. However, many of the fastest-growing urban agglomerations are cities with fewer than 1 million inhabitants, many of them in Asia and Africa.[1] Figure 2.4 shows the marked heterogeneity in city size across regions of the world and how this distribution is expected to change over time.

Box 2.1 illustrates how populations are distributed across cities of various size using another approach to systematically define cities across the world. *The Atlas of Urban Expansion* defined cities based on built up area and a population size of 100,000 or more identifying a universe of 4,231 cities with populations of 100,000 or more worldwide in 2010.[8] Despite differences resulting from different ways of defining cities the patterns observed clearly suggest that it is critical to focus not only on the large megacities but also on the many smaller cities that include significant portions of urban populations. These smaller but often growing cities provide unique opportunities for planning and building cities that are healthier and more environmentally sustainable.

URBAN LIVING AND HEALTH

Research on differences in health between urban and rural areas has shown varied results depending on the outcome, the country context, and the time

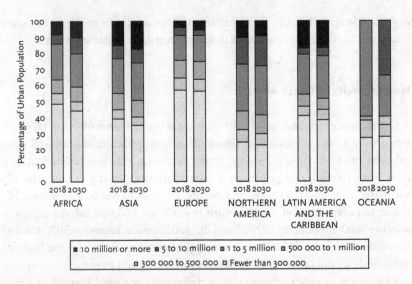

Figure 2.4 Percentage of urban population by city size across regions.
Source: United Nations Department of Economic and Social Affairs Population Division. World urbanization prospects: The 2018 revision, online edition. 2018; Adapted from United Nations Department of Economic and Social Affairs Population Division. The world's cities in 2016—data booklet. 2016; https://www.un.org/en/development/desa/population/publications/pdf/urbanization/the_worlds_cities_in_2016_data_booklet.pdf.

period in question. During the industrial revolution, the health of city dwellers was affected by the dismal living and working conditions in growing cities. Box 2.2 draws on literature to describe a picture of 19th-century London, a city that was growing exponentially at the time. These conditions motivated many public health crusaders of the time and spurred the development of water and sanitation systems (an excellent example is Edwin Chadwick's "sanitation revolution") and the identification and control of infectious diseases.

Despite adverse health conditions in many early cities, broader trends show that historically and over time urbanization was associated with declining death rates.[14] There are many examples today of cases where health in urban areas is better than in less developed rural areas,[15] possibly do in part to differences in resources and material living conditions. But even today it is difficult to draw generalizable and simple conclusions about whether urban living is good or bad for health. For example, current US data shows that obesity rates tend to be higher in more rural than in more urban areas.[16] In contrast, in many other countries the opposite pattern is observed, with obesity rates being higher in more urban as compared with rural places.[17] Adding complexity to such urban–rural contrasts, both rural and urban areas can be very heterogeneous, and urban areas in particular are home to very large

Box 2.1 POPULATION IN CITIES OF DIFFERENT SIZE: *THE ATLAS OF URBAN EXPANSION*

The Atlas of Urban Expansion (AUE) used a systematic process to identify a universe of cities of 100,000 residents or more. Cities are defined based on the extent of their built-up area rather than by their administrative or jurisdictional boundaries. The AUE defines cities as "agglomerations of contiguous built-up areas (and the open spaces in and around them) that may contain a large number of municipalities but, more often than not, constitute a single labor market."[1] Thus, in principle, a city may be composed of one municipality, a portion of a municipality, many municipalities, or portions of many municipalities.

To identify these cities and estimate their population, the AUE followed the following steps:

1. Identify all cities with ≥100,000 population in several reference databases, including UN Population Division database, the City Population website,[19] consultations with the Chinese Academy of Sciences, and other sources as needed.

Table 2.1 CHARACTERISTICS OF CITIES ACCORDING TO THE ATLAS OF URBAN EXPANSION

	Cities		Population	
	n	%	*n*	%
Region				
East Asia and the Pacific	1,081	26	652,310,754	26
Southeast Asia	229	5	143,551,770	6
South and Central Asia	693	16	387,180,823	16
Western Asia and North Africa	301	7	176,496,133	7
Sub-Saharan Africa	329	8	186,702,647	8
Latin America and the Caribbean	483	11	310,444,386	12
Europe and Japan	781	18	389,298,026	16
United States, Canada, Australia, and New Zealand	334	8	242,563,694	10
City population				
100,000–427,000	3,143	74	622,020,086	25
427,001000–1,570,000	811	19	621,981,767	25
1,570,001000–5,715,000	225	5	617,006,284	25
5,715,001+	52	1	627,540,096	25
TOTAL (all categories)	4231	100	2,488,548,233	100

Source: Adapted from *Atlas of Urban Expansion*, Volume 1.[1]

2. Visually examine these cities on Google Earth to determine whether any of these cities were part of a larger urban agglomeration.
3. Combine cities if they were part of an urban agglomeration and use the name of the core city (with exceptions for cities with multiple cores) to identify an agglomeration in their database.
4. For each city on this list, estimate a population total of the built-up area (or urban extent) by combining local census counts for enumeration districts when available or using other approximations based on available population data from various sources.

Of the 4,231 cities, 3,143 (74% of total cities) had populations of 100,000 to 427,000 and included 25% of the total population of cities. An additional 811 cities (19% of total cities) had populations of more than 427,000 and less than 1,570,000 and included an additional 25% of the total city population. A total of 277 cities had populations of >1,570,000 and included the remaining 50% of the city population (with half of this or 25% living in 52 cities with populations over 5,715,000).[20] As part of the project the AUE is conducting a more detailed assessment of the characteristics and changes over time in a global sample of 200 cities selected from the full universe stratified by region, population size, and number of cities in each country.

Source: Adapted from Angel et al. 2016.[8]

inequalities in social conditions and in health, as we will discuss further in Chapter 4.[18] As a result, overall comparisons of urban to rural areas may hide important variations. Even among urban areas, the relation between city size (or population density) and health is complex as illustrated by the research on urban scaling reviewed in Box 2.3.

The precise implications of urban living for health are highly context and outcome dependent. This is because there is no unique way of "being urban": what urban living means for health can vary significantly based on how cities are organized and governed. Table 2.2 outlines the many different ways in which urban living can be good or bad for health. The mixture of these factors, and their effects on different health pathways, will ultimately determine how and whether urban living is beneficial for health. In addition, the impact of urban living on health may also differ depending on other factors such as socioeconomic position. For example, some research has found that living in more urban areas may be associated

Box 2.2 URBAN LIVING IN 19TH-CENTURY ENGLAND

In 1800 the population of London was around a million but had qua-
drupled by 1880. Coal smoke was everywhere, and raw sewage poured
into the Thames. The streets were often littered with garbage and manure.
Cholera outbreaks were frequent (in 1854 Snow conducted his famous investigation of the cholera outbreak in Soho). Child labor was common and
poverty was rampant but also coexisted with great wealth. The coming of
the railroad in 1830 displaced many residents and facilitated the expansion of the city.

In *Sketches by Boz* published in 1836 Charles Dickens, sometimes referred to as the first and the greatest of urban novelists, presents a vivid
picture of life in early 19th-century London.

Here he describes the streets of London in the morning:

> Covent garden market, and the avenues leading to it, are thronged with
> arts of all sorts, sizes, and descriptions, from the heavy lumbering wagon,
> with its four stout horses, to the jingling costermonger's cart with its
> consumptive donkey. The pavement is already strewed with decayed
> cabbage-leaves, broken haybands, and all the indescribable litter of a veg-
> etable market; men are shouting, carts are backing, horses neighing, boys
> fighting, basket-women talking, piemen expatiating on the excellence of
> their pastry, and donkeys braying.

And in the evening:

> But the stress of London to be beheld in the very height of their glory,
> should be seen on a dark, dull, murky winter's night, when there is just
> enough damp gently stealing down to make the pavement greasy, without
> cleansing it of any of its impurities; and when the heavy lazy mist, which
> hangs over every object, makes the gas-lamps look brighter and the
> brilliantly-lighted shops more splendid, from the contrast they present to
> the darkness around.

In an article for *Household Words* written in 1851, Dickens describes
what it was like to have live cattle markets and slaughterhouses in the city:

> In half a quarter of a mile's length of Whitechapel, at one time, there shall
> be six hundred newly slaughtered oxen hanging up, and seven hundred
> sheep but, the more the merrier proof of prosperity. Hard by Snow Hill and
> Warwick Lane, you shall see the little children, inured to sights of brutality

from their birth, trotting along the alleys, mingled with troops of horribly busy pigs, up to their ankles in blood but it makes the young rascals hardy. Into the imperfect sewers of this overgrown city, you shall have the immense mass of corruption, engendered by these practices, lazily thrown out of sight, to rise, in poisonous gases, into your house at night, when your sleeping children will most readily absorb them, and to find its languid way, at last, into the river that you drink.

Many other novelists have been keen observers of 19th-century city life with all its energy and creativity but also its inequality and sordidness.

Box 2.3 CITY SIZE AND HEALTH

By Usama Bilal

Around 150 years ago, Farr observed that "as a rule, the greater this [population] density, the shorter the duration of life; and this life-duration is seen to follow a ratio appreciable by simple arithmetic."[21,22] It is likely that, had there not been a revolutionary amount of hygiene reforms in the 19th century, cities would not have been able to grow to become as dense as they are now. Cities pose special challenges for public health, as they represent areas of increased crowding and social and economic interactions.[23,24] With the increase in chronic diseases and the re-emergence of infectious diseases in urban cores in the developing world, there is an urgent need to understand the health consequences of this expanded urbanization process and how it can be managed to promote health. The Lancet Commission on Planetary Health has identified rapid population growth and urbanization as an especially complex problem for the following decades, both in terms of their role as increasing susceptibility to health hazards from climate change and as a driver of accumulating environmental hazards.[25]

To understand the health consequences of urbanization and population growth, cities must be understood as highly complex systems where emergent phenomena give rise to patterns of health and disease not present in other areas.[23,24] Understanding the urban scaling of health outcomes can provide the building blocks to understand the dynamics and processes that link urban growth to population health. The emerging literature on urban scaling has shown how understanding the ways that urban factors grow with city size can help create a theory of city living.[24,26–28]

The idea of studying scaling traces back to the study of metabolic outcomes in mammals that has shown how some features such as the basal metabolic rate grow less than expected with animal size.[26,29] This empirical finding led to the realization that fractal structures in living systems (such as the capillary or pulmonary systems) optimize energy delivery and thus reduce the required rate of energy expenditure per unit of size.[26] Applying the same techniques to cities can lead to analogous insights regarding how the functioning of urban systems generates population health. For example, we can study how energy expenditures, residue production (trash, pollution), and other outputs (wealth, crime)[24] change with city growth and link to health.

Figure 2.5 shows an example of known scaling patterns (social contacts and road network length) and their possible health scaling implications (infectious disease and transport injuries). When city size increases, social contacts[30] and infectious diseases may become relatively more common (increasing at a rate that is more than proportional to the population increase), while the length of the road network[31] and (hypothetically) transport injuries may become less common.

So far, only the scaling properties of outcomes like the number of AIDS cases, accidents or violent crime have been studied systematically across metropolitan areas in different countries.[28,32,33] A few studies have looked at the scaling patterns in some types of mortality or infectious disease incidence. For example, a study in US metropolitan areas has found a

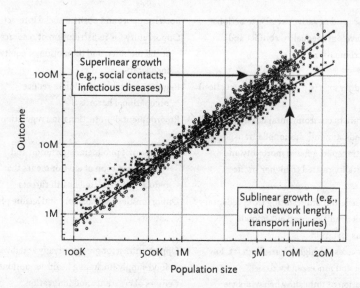

Figure 2.5 Potential association between city size, urban features and health outcomes.

superlinear scaling phenomenon for sexually transmitted infections[34] (they are more common in larger cities), while a study in US counties, and Swedish and Brazilian municipalities, has examined a wider variety of outcomes,[35] finding that infectious diseases show superlinear scaling (more common in larger cities) and noncommunicable diseases show sublinear scaling (more common in smaller cities).

with higher cardiovascular risk in persons of low education but with lower cardiovascular risk in those of higher education.[36] Thus the health impact of living in urban areas may be dependent on other conditions making it difficult to identify a single "effect" of urban living on health. We review conceptual models of how urban contexts can affect health in more detail in Chapter 3.

Table 2.2 IS URBAN LIVING GOOD OR BAD FOR HEALTH?

Negative impacts of urban living on health	Positive impacts of urban living on health
High population density and overcrowding, services not appropriately resourced or adapted for population density	Better access to services such as health care, water and sanitation, social services etc, opportunities for more accessible public services
Violence and negative social interactions	Social support and positive social interactions
High levels of inequality, conflict and discrimination	Opportunity for redistribution of resources, social mobility, and promotion of equity and inclusion
Hazardous jobs (e.g. industry, construction)	Regulation and monitoring to reduce occupational hazards
Exposure to environmental hazards related to industry and automobile transportation	Environmental protections and regulations
More transport-related morbidity and mortality related to higher traffic	Promotion of public transportation and walking, creation of environments that reduce traffic-related health threats
More sedentarism resulting from sedentary work conditions and automobile transportation	Opportunities for transport and leisure physical activity
Easier access to high calorie, high fat, low fiber and processed foods	Opportunities for greater, steady and diverse food supply (including healthier options)
Promotion of unhealthy behaviors via advertising and social norms	Centers of creativity and innovation, opportunity for promotion of healthy social norms

Despite some differences in health between urban and rural areas, the major causes of mortality and morbidity are often very similar (although their levels and distributions may differ). Nevertheless, understanding how the urban context can create, magnify, or reduce health threats and how it can be intervened on to enhance health is critical given the large and growing proportion of the world's population that lives in urban areas. In this section we provide illustrative examples of how urban living may influence a variety of health conditions. In Chapter 3 we step back discuss conceptual models linking features of urban areas to health and consider the implications of these models for research and policy.

Noncommunicable Diseases

Noncommunicable diseases (NCDs) are the leading cause of morbidity and mortality worldwide. A high burden of NCD morbidity and mortality also characterizes urban populations. Research has shown that greater urbanization rates are associated with higher levels of NCD risk factors in LMIC,[37] although it is not universally true that urban populations have higher NCD risk than rural populations.[38] Urban environments can be conducive to the development of NCD through environmental exposures such as air pollution (often high in urban areas because of concentration of industry and traffic) as well as through the creation of physical and social environments that promote sedentary lifestyles and unhealthy consumption.

Several features of city living, and city environments, can contribute to a high prevalence of the NCD risk factors of obesity, hypertension, and diabetes. Urban living is associated with greater consumption of processed, packaged, and convenience foods, often high in calories, sugar, and salt content, and with lower consumption of fruits and vegetables.[39] Factors driving these patterns include food availability and advertising, changes in cultural norms, and long work hours and commute times, leaving less time to prepare foods in the home.[40]

City living may also discourage active lifestyles and promote sedentary behaviors. City residents may be more likely to have sedentary jobs and to have less time for leisure or recreational physical activity.[41] This is particularly true in settings characterized by urban sprawl, as increased reliance on motorized transportation and associated reductions in walking and use of public transportation (which often involves some walking) can reduce physical activity from transportation.[42] Long commute times have been linked to greater stress and adverse mental health impacts,[43,44] an important health consequence in its own right, but also a possible contributor to NCDs.

Greater use of motorized transportation, especially cars and buses, can lead to higher levels of air pollution,[45] which, in turn, increases cardiovascular and respiratory morbidity and mortality.[46] The use of biomass for indoor cooking remains an important health challenge in both rural and urban areas of some LMIC.[47] Other unhealthy environmental exposures linked to industry or other sources that may affect cancer risk or other outcomes can also be more common in urban areas.[48] Asthma prevalence is high in urban environments and has been linked to exposures more common in urban areas, including indoor allergens such as dust mites and mold and ambient exposure due to traffic emissions.[49] Exposures in early life, including adverse environmental and lifestyle factors associated with disadvantaged urban environments, may modify immune development and result in increased risk for allergic diseases and asthma.[50]

Infectious Disease

Cities face major infectious disease challenges from both old and emerging infectious agents. Migration patterns, crowded housing, intense social interactions, cultural norms, inadequate water and sanitation access, and temperature and other climate-linked changes can facilitate infectious disease transmission. Urban sprawl can disrupt ecosystems and cause increased contact with vectors. Examples of infectious diseases that contribute to mortality and morbidity in cities include those transmitted through contaminated water (e.g., cholera, giardia), by mosquito (e.g., Dengue, Zika) and person-to-person (e.g., tuberculosis, HIV/AIDS). It has been estimated that 18% of the world's urban population lacked access to improved sanitation as of 2015, with increased residency in slums and informal settlements exacerbating risks and inequalities in water- or sanitation-related infectious illnesses.[51] Changing ecological conditions likely influenced the emergence of Zika and Dengue as major urban health problems.[52,53] In many countries, driven in part by migration and displacement, poverty, transactional sex, and gender-based violence, HIV/AIDS prevalence is higher in urban settings.[34,54] Higher incidence of sexually transmitted infections has been linked to urbanization and specifically to larger city population size.[55] Crowding, high population density, and social interactions as well as influx of immunologically vulnerable groups can facilitate the transmission of diseases like influenza in certain urban settings.[56] Urban areas may be especially conducive to the emergence of antibiotic resistant organisms because of the high use of antibiotics in areas of high population density.[57,58]

Injuries and Violence

Injuries are a major cause of death in urban areas. Worldwide, traffic crashes account for 1.25 million deaths annually, with 90% of these deaths in LMIC.[59] Fatal collisions involving pedestrians are especially prevalent in urban areas.[60] Many features of cities including inadequate road infrastructure, poor traffic management, limited enforcement of traffic laws, and low vehicle safety standards contribute to a high burden of mortality and morbidity.[59] Increases in personal vehicle ownership and widespread use of motorcycles, particularly in urban areas of LMICs, are also important drivers of increased crashes and crash-related fatalities.[59,61]

Urban areas in many countries experience a high burden of violence.[62,63] Urban violence results from many interacting factors including political factors (i.e., state violence and social conflict), institutional factors (i.e., extrajudicial violence and police brutality), economic factors (i.e., poverty and inequality, unemployment, organized crime, and human and drug trafficking), and social factors (i.e., discrimination, gangs, ethnic violence, and physical and sexual abuse).[64] Built environment features, such as spatial diffusion and low street connectivity (i.e., isolated streets), can also make urban environments prone to violence.[65,66] Neighborhood interventions on the built environment have been effective in reducing violence.[66] Gun access and ownership is also a strong predictor of firearm-related homicide.[67] Beyond the direct effect on victims, exposure to violence can have many other health consequences.

Substance Use

Smoking remains important health challenge in many urban areas,[68] although in some cases smoking levels are lower in large cities than in smaller towns.[69] The prevalence of smoking is enhanced by many interrelated processes occurring in urban areas including advertising, easy access to tobacco outlets and products, and social norms promoting or facilitating the use of tobacco products. Yet city-level implementation of smoke-free policies, such as those used in Mexico City, have documented impacts on norms, behaviors, and tobacco exposure.[70] Alcohol intake presents a complex pattern. Studies have found that rural residence appears to be protective against any alcohol consumption, but a risk factor for the development of an alcohol disorder[71] although this pattern may itself be highly variable by regional or country context. Access and social norm factors that can vary across urban and rural areas are likely to be important drivers of alcohol abuse.

Both urban and rural areas experience substance abuse and its many health consequences as illustrated by the recent opioid epidemic in the United States.[72] Features of the urban context that influence drug abuse include drug prescriptions and marketing, socioeconomic disadvantage, discrimination, and lack of opportunities, as well as accessibility to illegal drug markets and the creation of norms that facilitate and promote drug abuse in its many forms.

Mental Health

There is a long tradition of research on the mental health consequences of urban living. Urban environments could in theory protect mental health through availability of greater support and services. But urban living can be a source of stress when linked to overcrowding, social isolation and social or economic disadvantage. Urban environments may contribute to depression and other adverse mental health outcomes including through features of social environments (such as chronic exposure to social stressors linked to violence or poverty) as well as features of built environments (including physical attributes such as physical disorder or housing features) that may operate through stress pathways.[73–75]

Health Impacts of Heat and Climate Change

City dwellers are especially vulnerable to the adverse health implications of climate change. The urban heat island effect magnifies the impact of rising temperatures. Climate change can have adverse impacts on air pollution. Rising temperatures can also interact with higher air pollution levels in cities, resulting in even greater adverse health impacts. The sheer population density of cities enhances the adverse effects of storms and unpredictable weather patterns. Climate change will have major impacts on the basic infrastructure and resources of many cities including buildings, water access, transportation, and roads, among others,[6] all of which have major implications for health. Cities are often located in coastal areas making them vulnerable to flooding. Climate changes including temperature rises, changes in rainfall, and floods can affect the transmission of infectious diseases via direct transmission or ecologic changes that facilitate vector-borne infections. The rapid growth of cities especially in LMICs has been accompanied by the rapid growth informal settlements, many of which are highly vulnerable to extreme weather events as a result of their location or structures.[6] Heat can also interact with social conditions in cities affecting the most vulnerable and magnifying health inequities.

Cities are highly vulnerable to the adverse consequences of environmental disasters including flooding, storms and fires. For example, the UN estimates that of the 1,692 cities with at least 300,000 inhabitants in 2014, 944 (56% of cities) were at high risk of exposure to at least one of six types of natural disaster (cyclones, floods, droughts, earthquakes, landslides, and volcano eruptions).[13] These cities were home to 1.4 billion people. In addition, around 15% of cities were at high risk of exposure to two or more types of natural disaster. Nearly 30 cities—including the megacities of Tokyo, Osaka, and Manila—faced high risk of exposure to three or more types of disaster. Overall, it was estimated that 82% of cities, home to nearly 2 billion people, were located in areas that faced high risk of mortality associated with at least one type of environmental disaster, and 89% of cities were located in areas that were highly vulnerable to economic losses associated with environmental disasters.[76] Table 2.3 summarizes the conclusions of the Intergovernmental Panel on Climate Change on the implications of climate change for cities.

Table 2.3 IMPLICATIONS OF CLIMATE CHANGE FOR CITIES: SELECTED CONCLUSIONS OF THE INTERGOVERNMENTAL PANEL ON CLIMATE CHANGE

Selected conclusions about cities and climate change

- Action in urban centers is essential to successful global climate change adaptation. Urban areas hold more than half the world's population and most of its built assets and economic activities. They also house a high proportion of the population and economic activities most at risk from climate change, and a high proportion of global greenhouse gas emissions are generated by urban-based activities and residents.

- Much of key and emerging global climate risks are concentrated in urban areas. Rapid urbanization and rapid growth of large cities in low- and middle-income countries have been accompanied by the rapid growth of highly vulnerable urban communities living in informal settlements, many of which are on land at high risk from extreme weather.

- Urban climate change risks, vulnerabilities, and impacts are increasing across the world in urban centers of all sizes, economic conditions, and site characteristics.

- Cities are composed of complex interdependent systems that can be leveraged to support climate change adaptation via effective city governments supported by cooperative multilevel governance.

- Urban adaptation action that delivers mitigation co-benefits is a powerful, resource-efficient means to address climate change and to realize sustainable development goals.

- Urban adaptation provides opportunities for incremental and transformative adjustments to development trajectories toward resilience and sustainable development via effective multilevel urban risk governance, alignment of policies and incentives, strengthened local government and community adaptation capacity, synergies with the private sector, and appropriate financing and institutional development.

Source: Revi et al.[6]

The demographic trends discussed in this chapter, as well as growing recognition of the challenges and opportunities that urbanization presents for both population health and the environmental sustainability of our planet, have spurred multiple international initiatives relevant to urban health. The need to promote urban health is increasingly being recognized as critical to the achievement of other social goals, including the sustainable development goals and the new urban agenda.[77] Here we highlight a few of these initiatives.

United Nations Agencies and the New Urban Agenda

A number of UN initiatives have had an important urban focus. Key among these has been UN Habitat (the UN Human Settlements program) through organization of the World Urban Forum and the HABITAT conferences. The World Urban Forum was established in 2001 and brings together multiple urban stakeholders every two years to examine pressing global issues related to the impact of urbanization on people and the environment. The UN Conference on Housing and Sustainable Urban Development (HABITAT) has met every 20 years since 1976. HABITAT III held in Quito in 2016 engaged a broad range of stakeholders with the goals of securing renewed political commitment for sustainable urban development. It resulted in the adoption of the New Urban Agenda,[78] an ambitious document highlighting actionable priorities for urban areas across the globe. The Agenda reflects a vision of urban areas as "cities for all" and encourages countries and other stakeholders to commit to building and managing cities so that they are just, safe, healthy, accessible, affordable, resilient, and sustainable.

Another major UN initiative with important connections to urban health is the adoption of the 2030 Sustainable Development Goals (SDGs).[79] The SDGs, adopted by world leaders in 2015, provide a framework for ending poverty, building economic growth, improving education, and increasing job opportunities while protecting and enhancing human health and well-being, tackling climate change, and promoting environmental sustainability. Box 2.4 reviews the relevance of the SDGs for urban health. Discussions of urban health in the context of the New Urban Agenda and the SDGs have focused primarily on access to health care and to some extent on traditional public health issues of water and sanitation and infant mortality, with limited discussion of the impact of urban environments on the epidemics of chronic disease and injuries, which are major sources of morbidity and mortality in urban areas. Thus, there continues to be important opportunity to broaden the view of urban health in these international initiatives.

Box 2.4 URBAN HEALTH AND THE SUSTAINABLE DEVELOPMENT GOALS

The SDGs are a set of 17 global goals set by the UN General Assembly in 2015 for the year 2030.[80] Each of the goals has a set of targets that are measured with indicators. The goals are

1. No poverty: End poverty in all its forms everywhere.
2. Zero hunger: End hunger, achieve food security and improved nutrition and promote sustainable agriculture.
3. Good health and well-being: Ensure healthy lives and promote well-being for all at all ages.
4. Quality education: Ensure inclusive and equitable quality education and promote lifelong learning opportunities for all.
5. Gender equality: Achieve gender equality and empower all women and girls.
6. Water and sanitation: Ensure availability and sustainable management of water and sanitation for all.
7. Affordable and clean energy: Ensure access to affordable, reliable, sustainable and modern energy for all.
8. Decent work and economic growth: Promote sustained, inclusive and sustainable economic growth, full and productive employment and decent work for all.
9. Industry, innovation, and infrastructure: Build resilient infrastructure, promote inclusive and sustainable industrialization and foster innovation.
10. Reducing inequality: Reduce inequality within and among countries.
11. Sustainable cities and communities: Make cities and human settlements inclusive, safe, resilient and sustainable.
12. Responsible consumption and production: Ensure sustainable consumption and production patterns.
13. Climate action: Take urgent action to combat climate change and its impacts.
14. Life below water: Conserve and sustainably use the oceans, seas and marine resources for sustainable development.
15. Life on land: Protect, restore and promote sustainable use of terrestrial ecosystems, sustainably manage forests, combat desertification, and halt and reverse land degradation and halt biodiversity loss.
16. Peace, justice, and strong institutions: Promote peaceful and inclusive societies for sustainable development, provide access to justice for all and build effective, accountable and inclusive institutions at all levels.
17. Partnerships for the goals. Strengthen the means of implementation and revitalize the Global Partnership for Sustainable Development.

The 17 goals are interdependent, and many have implications for health in cities. However, two of the 17 goals: goal 3 and goal 11 are of special relevance to urban health. Each goal has a set of specific targets associated with them. More information is at https://sustainabledevelopment.un.org/. Although the goals are not binding, it is expected that countries that ratified the SDGs will work toward developing plans to achieve the goals and monitor indicators for each target. The goals provide a framework for advancing health and environmental sustainability. Given urbanization trends worldwide, urban health is critical to achievement of many of the SDGs.

Several other UN agencies have had an urban health focus. For example, in 2016, the World Health Organization launched its first Global Report on Urban Health, calling for the creation of healthier cities by shaping healthier urban environments.[81] The Pan American Health Organization launched its own urban health initiative in 2011.[82]

Networks of Cities

Cities are increasingly coming together in networks to promote various urban agendas. The C40 Cities, a network of the world's megacities,[83] and Local Governments for Sustainability (ICLEI), a global network of over 1500 cities, towns, and regions,[84] convene city-level actors to meet the challenges of climate change mitigation, urban resilience and adaptation, and sustainable development. Regional city networks focused on urban governance and various social, economic, environmental, and data infrastructure issues facing cities include the EUROCITIES network (which convenes government officials from Europe's largest cities),[85] the Centro Iberoamericano de Desarrollo Estratégico Urbano, which includes cities in Spanish- and Portuguese-speaking countries,[86] as well as Open Cities Africa[87] and Open Cities Asia.[88] Although these initiatives are not health focused, they are increasingly recognizing the need to integrate urban health promotion with efforts to improve the environmental sustainability of cities. A few health focused networks also exist. Examples include the Big Cities Health coalition in the United States,[89] the WHO European Healthy Cities Network,[90] and the Pan American Health Organization Movement of Healthy Cities, Municipalities and Communities of the Americas.[91]

Academic and Scientific Networks and Programs

Scientists and academics have also led important collaborative initiatives to generate, exchange, and disseminate knowledge of place-based drivers of urban health and environmental sustainability. Examples include the International Society for Urban Health,[92] which focuses on the links between urban environments and health, and the Urban Health Network for Latin America and the Caribbean,[93] which promotes exchange to enhance urban health and environmental sustainability throughout the region. The Research Initiative for Cities and Health Equity focused on countries throughout Africa, also works to support interdisciplinary research collaboration and shape an urban health research agenda region-wide.[94] In Asia, the South East Asia Sustainability Network brings together higher education institutions and sustainability organizations to further the integration of sustainability perspectives in teaching, research, and practice.[95] Through its program on systems approaches to urban health and well-being, the International Science Council also promotes place-based approaches to health and environmental sustainability.[96]

Foundations and Development Agencies

Foundation-driven initiatives including the Wellcome Trust's Our Planet, Our Health,[97] Rockefeller's 100 Resilient Cities,[98] and Bloomberg's What Works Cities program[99] are also key players in agenda-setting, investments, and capacity-building. In the private sector, the Carbon Disclosure Project, a not-for-profit organization engages businesses and investors around monitoring and disclosure of environmental impacts.[100]

Multilateral organizations are also involved in various networks focused on urban issues. These include among others the World Bank's Sustainable Cities Initiative in Central Asia and Europe,[101] the African Development Bank's numerous initiatives and partnerships (i.e., African Carbon Support Program, Green Growth Initiative, and Sustainable Energy for All),[102] and the Inter-American Development Bank's programs in urban development and housing.[103] Cities Alliance, a global partnership focused on urban poverty coordinated by the World Bank and the UN Centre for Human Settlements, works with a range of governmental, international, and private sector actors on issues of urban settlement upgrading, funding and investments, and supporting policies, planning, and capacity development.[104]

REFERENCES

1. United Nations Department of Economic and Social Affairs Population Division. World urbanization prospects: The 2018 revision, online edition. 2018; https://population.un.org/wup/Download/.

2. Pesaresi M, Melchiorri M, Siragusa A, Kemper T. Atlas of the human planet—Mapping human presence on earth with the global human settlement layer. Publications Office of the European Union. 2016; https://ghsl.jrc.ec.europa.eu/documents/Atlas_2016.pdf?t=1476360675.

3. Angel S, Lamson-Hall P, Guerra B, Liu Y, Galarza N, Blei AM. *Our Not-So-Urban World*. New York: New York University;2018.

4. United Nations Department of Economic and Social Affairs Population Division. World urbanization prospects: The 2014 revision. 2014; https://www.un.org/en/development/desa/publications/2014-revision-world-urbanization-prospects.html.

5. Aerni P. Coping with migration-induced urban growth: Addressing the blind spot of UN Habitat. *Sustainability*. 2016;8(8):800.

6. Revi A, Satterthwaite D, Aragón-Durand F, et al. Urban areas. In: *Climate Change 2014: Impacts, Adaptation, and Vulnerability: Part A: Global and Sectoral Aspects. Contribution of Working Group II to the Fifth Assessment Report of the Intergovernmental Panel on Climate Change*. Cambridge, UK: Cambridge University Press; 2014:535–612.

7. Seto KC, Güneralp B, Hutyra LR. Global forecasts of urban expansion to 2030 and direct impacts on biodiversity and carbon pools. *Proceedings of the National Academy of Sciences*. 2012;109(40):16083–16088.

8. Angel S, Blei AM, Parent J, et al. *Atlas of Urban Expansion—2016 Edition: Areas and Densities*. Cambridge, MA: NYU Urban Expansion Program at New York University, UN-Habitat, and the Lincoln Institute of Land Policy. 2016.

9. Millennium Ecosystem Assessment. *Ecosystems and Human Well-Being: Health Synthesis*. Washington, DC: World Resources Institute; 2005.

10. Eigenbrod F, Bell V, Davies H, Heinemeyer A, Armsworth P, Gaston K. The impact of projected increases in urbanization on ecosystem services. *Proceedings of the Royal Society B: Biological Sciences*. 2011;278(1722):3201–3208.

11. Clos J. Foreword. In: Angel S, Blei AM, Parent J, et al., eds. *Atlas of Urban Expansion. Vol 1: Areas and Densities*. New York: New York University; 2016.

12. Norman J, MacLean HL, Kennedy CA. Comparing high and low residential density: Life-cycle analysis of energy use and greenhouse gas emissions. *Journal of Urban Planning and Development*. 2006;132(1):10–21.

13. United Nations Department of Economic and Social Affairs Population Division. The world's cities in 2016—data booklet. 2016; https://www.un.org/en/development/desa/population/publications/pdf/urbanization/the_worlds_cities_in_2016_data_booklet.pdf.

14. Dye C. Health and urban living. *Science*. 2008;319(5864):766–769.

15. Galea S. Urban built environment and depression: A multilevel analysis. *Journal of Epidemiology & Community Health*. 2005;59(10):822–827.

16. Lundeen EA, Park S, Pan L, O'Toole T, Matthews K, Blanck HM. Obesity prevalence among adults living in metropolitan and nonmetropolitan counties--United States, 2016. *Morbidity and Mortality Weekly Report*. 2018;67(23):653.

17. Prasad A, Gray CB, Ross A, Kano M. Metrics in urban health: Current developments and future prospects. *Annual Review of Public Health*. 2016;37: 113–133.

18. World Health Organization Centre for Health Development. *Hidden Cities: Unmasking and Overcoming Health Inequities in Urban Settings.* Geneva, Switzerland: World Health Organization; 2010.

19. City Population. City Population: Population statistics for countries, administrative divisions, cities, urban areas and agglomerations—interactive maps and charts. 2020; http://citypopulation.de/. Accessed June 25, 2020.

20. Angel S, Blei AM, Civco DL, Parent J. *Atlas of Urban Expansion.* Cambridge, MA: Lincoln Institute of Land Policy; 2012.

21. Farr W. Density or proximity of population: Its advantages and disadvantages. In: *Transactions of the National Association for the Promotion of Social Science, Cheltenham Meeting, 1878.* London, Longman, Green; 1879:530–535.

22. Anonymous. Over-density of population in cities. *Scientific American.* 1879;40(3):32.

23. Franco M, Bilal U, Diez-Roux AV. Preventing non-communicable diseases through structural changes in urban environments. *Journal of Epidemiology and Community Health.* 2015;69(6):509–511.

24. Bettencourt LM. The origins of scaling in cities. *Science.* 2013;340(6139): 1438–1441.

25. Whitmee S, Haines A, Beyrer C, et al. Safeguarding human health in the Anthropocene epoch: Report of the Rockefeller Foundation–Lancet Commission on planetary health. *The Lancet.* 2015;386(10007):1973–2028.

26. West G. *Scale: The Universal Laws of Growth, Innovation, Sustainability, and the Pace of Life in Organisms, Cities, Economies, and Companies.* New York: Penguin; 2017.

27. Bettencourt L, West G. A unified theory of urban living. *Nature.* 2010;467(7318): 912–913.

28. Bettencourt LMA, Lobo J, Helbing D, Kühnert C, West GB. Growth, innovation, scaling, and the pace of life in cities. *Proceedings of the National Academy of Sciences.* 2007;104(17):7301–7306.

29. West GB, Brown JH, Enquist BJ. A general model for the origin of allometric scaling laws in biology. *Science.* 1997;276(5309):122–126.

30. Meyer S, Held L. Power-law models for infectious disease spread. *Annals of Applied Statistics.* 2014;8(3):1612–1639.

31. Samaniego H, Moses ME. Cities as organisms: Allometric scaling of urban road networks. *Journal of Transport and Land Use.* 2008;1(1). doi:10.5198/jtlu. v1i1.29

32. Gomez-Lievano A, Youn H, Bettencourt LMA. The statistics of urban scaling and their connection to Zipf's Law. *PLoS ONE.* 2012;7(7):e40393.

33. Alves LGA, Ribeiro HV, Lenzi EK, Mendes RS. Distance to the scaling law: A useful approach for unveiling relationships between crime and urban metrics. *PLoS ONE.* 2013;8(8):e69580.

34. Patterson-Lomba O, Goldstein E, Gómez-Liévano A, Castillo-Chavez C, Towers S. Per capita incidence of sexually transmitted infections increases systematically with urban population size: A cross-sectional study. *Sexually Transmitted Infections.* 2015;91(8):610–614.

35. Rocha LE, Thorson AE, Lambiotte R. The non-linear health consequences of living in larger cities. *Journal of Urban Health.* 2015;92(5):785–799.

36. Fleischer NL, Diez Roux AV, Alazraqui M, Spinelli H, De Maio F. Socioeconomic gradients in chronic disease risk factors in middle-income countries: Evidence of effect modification by urbanicity in Argentina. *American Journal of Public Health.* 2011;101(2):294–301.

37. Goryakin Y, Rocco L, Suhrcke M. The contribution of urbanization to non-communicable diseases: Evidence from 173 countries from 1980 to 2008. *Economics & Human Biology.* 2017;26:151–163.

38. Rural Health Research Gateway. Rural Communities: Age, Income, and Health Status. *Rural Health Research Recap* 2018; https://www.ruralhealthresearch.org/assets/2200-8536/rural-communities-age-income-health-status-recap.pdf. Accessed June 25, 2020.

39. Seto KC, Ramankutty N. Hidden linkages between urbanization and food systems. *Science.* 2016;352(6288):943-945.

40. Kearney J. Food consumption trends and drivers. *Philosophical Transactions of the Royal Society B: Biological Sciences.* 2010;365(1554):2793–2807.

41. Ojiambo RM, Easton C, Casajús JA, Konstabel K, Reilly JJ, Pitsiladis Y. Effect of urbanization on objectively measured physical activity levels, sedentary time, and indices of adiposity in Kenyan adolescents. *Journal of Physical Activity and Health.* 2012;9(1):115–123.

42. Stevenson M, Thompson J, de Sá TH, et al. Land use, transport, and population health: Estimating the health benefits of compact cities. *The Lancet.* 2016;388(10062):2925–2935.

43. Milner A, Badland H, Kavanagh A, LaMontagne AD. Time spent commuting to work and mental health: Evidence from 13 waves of an Australian cohort study. *American Journal of Epidemiology.* 2017;186(6):659–667.

44. Wang X, Rodríguez DA, Sarmiento OL, Guaje O. Commute patterns and depression: Evidence from eleven Latin American cities. *Journal of Transport & Health.* 2019;14:100607.

45. Cepeda M, Schoufour J, Freak-Poli R, et al. Levels of ambient air pollution according to mode of transport: A systematic review. *Lancet Public Health.* 2017;2(1):e23–e34.

46. Hoek G, Krishnan RM, Beelen R, et al. Long-term air pollution exposure and cardio-respiratory mortality: A review. *Environmental Health.* 2013;12(1).

47. Wiedinmyer C, Dickinson K, Piedrahita R, et al. Rural–urban differences in cooking practices and exposures in northern Ghana. *Environmental Research Letters.* 2017;12(6):065009.

48. Environmental Protection Agency. *Air Toxics Emissions: EPA's Strategy for Reducing Health Risks in Urban Areas.* Research Triangle Park, NC: Office of Air Quality Planning and Standards;1999.

49. Jie Y, Isa ZM, Jie X, Ju ZL, Ismail NH. Urban vs. rural factors that affect adult asthma. In: Whitacre DM, ed. *Reviews of Environmental Contamination and Toxicology, Volume 226.* New York, NY: Springer; 2013:33–63.

50. Gern JE. The Urban Environment and Childhood Asthma study. *Journal of Allergy & Clinical Immunology.* 2010;125(3):545–549.

51. UN-Habitat. *World Cities Report* 2016: *Urbanization and Development -Emerging Futures.* Nairoboi, Kenya: United Nations Human Settlements Programme; 2016.

52. Asad H, Carpenter DO. Effects of climate change on the spread of zika virus: A public health threat. *Reviews on Environmental Health.* 2018;33(1):31–42.

53. Matysiak A, Roess A. Interrelationship between climatic, ecologic, social, and cultural determinants affecting Dengue emergence and transmission in Puerto Rico and their implications for Zika response. *Journal of Tropical Medicine.* 2017;2017:1–14.

54. Garcia-Calleja JM. National population based HIV prevalence surveys in sub-Saharan Africa: Results and implications for HIV and AIDS estimates. *Sexually Transmitted Infections.* 2006;82(Suppl 3):iii64–iii70.

55. Van Donk M. "Positive" urban futures in sub-Saharan Africa: HIV/AIDS and the need for ABC (a broader conceptualization). *Environment and Urbanization.* 2006;18(1):155–175.

56. Adiga A, Chu S, Eubank S, et al. Disparities in spread and control of influenza in slums of Delhi: Findings from an agent-based modelling study. *BMJ Open.* 2018;8(1):e017353.

57. Li J, Cao J, Zhu Y-g, et al. Global survey of antibiotic resistance genes in air. *Environmental Science & Technology.* 2018;52(19):10975–10984.

58. Almakki A, Jumas-Bilak E, Marchandin H, Licznar-Fajardo P. Antibiotic resistance in urban runoff. *Science of the Total Environment.* 2019;667:64–76.

59. World Health Organization. Global status report on road safety 2015. Geneva, Switzerland: World Health Organization; 2015.

60. de Andrade L, Vissoci JRN, Rodrigues CG, et al. Brazilian road traffic fatalities: A spatial and environmental analysis. *PLoS ONE.* 2014;9(1):e87244.

61. Patel A, Krebs E, Andrade L, Rulisa S, Vissoci JRN, Staton CA. The epidemiology of road traffic injury hotspots in Kigali, Rwanda from police data. *BMC Public Health.* 2016;16(1):697.

62. Briceño-León R. Urban violence and public health in Latin America: A sociological explanatory framework. *Cadernos de Saúde Pública.* 2005;21(6): 1629–1648.

63. Muggah R, Tobón KA. *Citizen Security in Latin America: Facts and Figures.* Rio de Janeiro, Brazil: Igrape Institute;2018.

64. Moser CON. Urban violence and insecurity: An introductory roadmap. *Environment and Urbanization.* 2004;16(2):3–16.

65. Graif C, Gladfelter AS, Matthews SA. Urban poverty and neighborhood effects on crime: Incorporating spatial and network perspectives. *Sociology Compass.* 2014;8(9):1140–1155.

66. Kondo MC, Andreyeva E, South EC, MacDonald JM, Branas CC. Neighborhood interventions to reduce violence. *Annual Review of Public Health.* 2018;39(1):253–271.

67. Siegel M, Ross CS, King C. The relationship between gun ownership and firearm homicide rates in the United States, 1981–2010. *American Journal of Public Health.* 2013;103(11):2098–2105.

68. Idris BI, Giskes K, Borrell C, et al. Higher smoking prevalence in urban compared to non-urban areas: Time trends in six European countries. *Health & Place.* 2007;13(3):702–712.

69. Liu L, Edland S, Myers MG, Hofstetter CR, Al-Delaimy WK. Smoking prevalence in urban and rural populations: Findings from California between 2001 and 2012. *American Journal of Drug & Alcohol Abuse.* 2016;42(2):152–161.

70. Thrasher JF, Pérez-Hernández R, Swayampakala K, Arillo-Santillán E, Bottai M. Policy support, norms, and secondhand smoke exposure before and after implementation of a comprehensive smoke-free law in Mexico City. *American Journal of Public Health.* 2010;100(9):1789–1798.

71. Borders TF, Booth BM. Rural, suburban, and urban variations in alcohol consumption in the United States: Findings from the National Epidemiologic Survey on Alcohol and Related Conditions. *Journal of Rural Health.* 2007;23(4):314–321.

72. Monnat SM. The contributions of socioeconomic and opioid supply factors to US drug mortality rates: Urban–rural and within-rural differences. *Journal of Rural Studies*. 2019;68:319–335.

73. Gruebner O, Rapp MA, Adli M, Kluge U, Galea S, Heinz A. Cities and mental health. *Deutsches Ärzteblatt International*. 2017;114(8):121.

74. Purtle J, Nelson KL, Yang Y, Langellier B, Stankov I, Diez Roux AV. Urban–rural differences in older adult depression: A systematic review and meta-analysis of comparative studies. *American Journal of Preventive Medicine*. 2019;56(4):603–613.

75. Cantor-Graae E. The contribution of social factors to the development of schizophrenia: A review of recent findings. *The Canadian Journal of Psychiatry*. 2007;52(5):277–286.

76. Gu D, Gerland P, Pelletier F, Cohen B. Risks of exposure and vulnerability to natural disasters at the city level: A global overview. *United Nations Technical Paper*. 2015;2.

77. Singh S, Beagley J. Health and the new urban agenda: A mandate for action. *The Lancet*. 2017;389(10071):801–802.

78. United Nations General Assembly. *New Urban Agenda*. New York: United Nations; 2017. 978-92-1-132731-1.

79. United Nations. Transforming our world: The 2030 agenda for sustainable development. 2015; https://sustainabledevelopment.un.org/post2015/transformingourworld/publication.

80. United Nations. Sustainable Development Goals knowledge platform. https://sustainabledevelopment.un.org/. Accessed June 25, 2020.

81. World Health Organization. *Global Report on Urban Health: Equitable, Healthier Cities for Sustainable Development*. Geneva, Switzerland: World Health Organization; 2016.

82. Pan American Health Organization. Integration of background documents for the strategy and plan of action on urban health in the Americas. 2011; https://www.paho.org/en/documents/integration-background-documents-strategy-and-plan-action-urban-health-americas.

83. C40 Cities. About C40. https://c40.org/about. Accessed July 25, 2019.

84. ICLEI. About us. http://iclei.org/en/About_ICLEI_2.html. Accessed July 25, 2019.

85. EUROCITIES. About EUROCITIES. Accessed July 25, 2019; https://cities4europe.eurocities.eu/eurocities/about_us.

86. Secretaría General Iberoamericana (SEGIB). Cohesión social/CIDEU, Centro Iberoamericano de desarrollo estratégico urbano. 2018; https://www.segib.org/cumbres-iberoamericanas/

87. Open Cities Project. About. https://opencitiesproject.org/about/. Accessed June 1, 2019.

88. Open Cities Asia. About. http://opencitiesproject.github.io/about/. Accessed June 1, 2019.

89. deBeaumont. Big Cities Health Coalition. https://www.debeaumont.org/programs/big-cities-health-coalition/. Accessed June 25, 2020.

90. World Health Organization. WHO European Healthy Cities Network. http://www.euro.who.int/en/health-topics/environment-and-health/urban-health/who-european-healthy-cities-network. Accessed June 25, 2020.

91. Pan American Health Organization. Healthy municipality initiative. https://www.paho.org/hq/index.php?option=com_content&view=article&id=10706:about-healthy-municipalities&Itemid=820&lang=en. Accessed June 25, 2020.

92. International Society for Urban Health. Mission Vision & Guidance. 2020; https://isuh.org/about/mission-vision/. Accessed June 25, 2020.

93. Diez Roux AV, Slesinski SC, Alazraqui M, et al. A novel international partnership for actionable evidence on urban health in Latin America: LAC-Urban health and SALURBAL. *Global Challenges*. 2018;3(4):1800013.

94. Oni T, Smit W, Matzopoulos R, et al. Urban health research in Africa: Themes and priority research questions. *Journal of Urban Health*. 2016;93(4):722–730.

95. South East Asia Sustainability Network. Introduction. 2018; http://www.seasn.usm.my/index.php/ms/about-us/introduction. Accessed July 25, 2019.

96. International Science Council. Overview. https://council.science/about-us. Accessed July 25, 2019.

97. Wellcome Trust. Our planet, our health: Responding to a changing world. https://wellcome.ac.uk/what-we-do/our-work/our-planet-our-health. Accessed July 25, 2019.

98. 100 Resilient Cities. About us. https://100resilientcities.org/about-us/. Accessed July 25, 2019.

99. Bloomberg Philathropies. About What Works Cities. https://whatworkscities.bloomberg.org/about/. Accessed July 25, 2019.

100. Carbon Disclosure Project. Our work. https://www.cdp.net/en/info/about-us. Accessed July 25, 2019.

101. World Bank. Sustainable Cities Initiative. http://worldbank.org/en/region/eca/brief/sustainable-cities-initiative. Accessed July 25, 2019.

102. African Development Bank Group. Topics. https://afdb.org/en/topics-and-sectors/topics/. Accessed July 25, 2019.

103. Inter-American Development Bank. Projects. https://iadb.org/en/projects. Accessed July 25, 2019.

104. Cities Alliance. About Cities Alliance. http://citiesalliance.org/about-cities-alliance. Accessed July 25, 2019.

CHAPTER 3

Conceptual Models and Frameworks for Understanding the Links Between Urban Environments and Health

ANA V. DIEZ ROUX

In Chapter 1 we outlined the foundations of the urban health approach. In Chapter 2 we reviewed urbanization trends worldwide and discussed what we know about health in urban areas. In this chapter we step back to review different conceptualizations of the links between places and health with a special emphasis on urban places. We also discuss the links between urban health and two important and increasingly influential approaches to population health: the health in all policies approach and the planetary health approach. Building on prior chapters, we conclude with a review and typology of urban health research questions and urban health policies.

CONCEPTUALIZING THE LINKS BETWEEN PLACES AND HEALTH

As we noted in Chapter 1, a focus on the impact of places on health is a key characteristic of the urban health approach. Overall there are four fundamental ways to conceptualize the links between places and health: (i) places as contexts for health; (ii) places as causes or determinants of health; (iii) places as reinforcers or moderators of interindividual health differences; and (iv) places as integral components of the systems that give rise to health. These four conceptualizations are not mutually exclusive. Rather, they can be thought of as complementary and nested within each other (Figure 3.1) reflecting increasing complexity.

Ana V. Diez Roux, *Conceptual Models and Frameworks for Understanding the Links Between Urban Environments and Health* In: *Urban Public Health.* Edited by: Gina S. Lovasi, Ana V. Diez Roux, and Jennifer Kolker, Oxford University Press (2021). © Oxford University Press 2021. DOI: 10.1093/oso/9780190885304.003.0003.

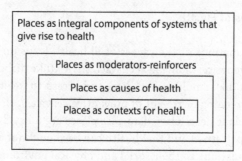

Figure 3.1 Nested conceptualizations of the link between places and health.

Places as Contexts for Health

There is a long tradition in public health of describing the places within which population health manifests itself. This is clearly reflected in the famous epidemiologic triad of person, time, and place. Contrasting levels of health and disease across places is a fundamental component of descriptive epidemiology and key to the core public health function of disease surveillance. The common focus on agent–host–environment (with the environment often serving as a stand in for places) is also a key component of the epidemiologic approach. In urban health, the conceptualization of places as contexts for health is reflected in work that profiles health in a specific urban community or work that contrasts levels of health in urban and rural areas, across cities, or across neighborhoods within a city.

Much work has gone into using existing data to create reliable and valid estimates of the state of various health outcomes (e.g., prevalence, incidence or mortality rates, and life expectancy) across places.[1,2] In addition to traditional sources, recent approaches have increasingly leveraged novel data such as geographically linked electronic health records[3,4] or even social media data.[5,6] Sophisticated statistical methods including a variety of small area estimation methods have increasingly been used to derive more detailed and more precise descriptions of heterogeneity in health across places.[7,8] In Chapter 7 we review some of these methods in more detail.

Descriptions can yield powerful insight and can also motivate action. For example, the documentation of place differences in health immediately raises questions about whether targeting of interventions or policies to certain places is warranted. More fundamentally, the description of place differences raises critical questions about why health is spatially patterned the way it is and, consequently, about the role of places and place-linked factors in the causation of health and disease. Place-based differences or the examination of places as contexts for health can thus provide important clues regarding etiology.

Places as Causes of Health

Traditional explanations of the causes of ill health focus on individual-level factors such as genetics, biomedical characteristics (like diabetes, blood pressure), behaviors (like smoking and diet) and access to health care (such as availability of screening or receipt of preventive services). However, it is also clear from abundant descriptive data that places are a key dimension across which health is patterned and that health can be thought of as the patterned response of populations to their social and physical environments. These social and physical environments are linked to the places where individuals live, work, go to school, and socialize. This recognition has spurred a large body of work on the causal links between features of places and health.

An example of a conceptual model linking features of places (in this case urban neighborhoods) to health is shown in Figure 3.2. An important principle of this conceptual model is that urban places (neighborhoods) have both physical and social features that are important to health and that these physical and social features are interrelated. Another important component is the delineation of individual-level pathways through which these factors affect health, along with the recognition that factors along these pathways may influence each other (e.g., stress may affect behaviors and behaviors can be used to cope with stress). This model also emphasizes how neighborhood factors contribute to health equity by noting the role of residential segregation in

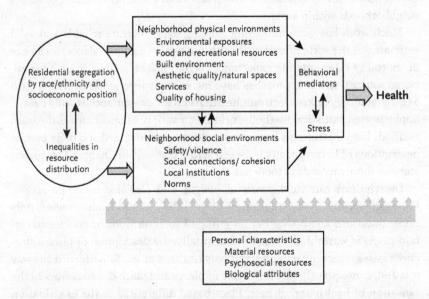

Figure 3.2 Conceptual model of the hypothesized links between neighborhood environments and health.[9]

Source: Diez Roux AV, Mair C. Neighborhoods and health. *Annals of the New York Academy of Sciences.* 2010;1186(1):125–145.

shaping the health-relevant features of neighborhoods.[10] It thus places differences in neighborhood environments in the context of broader structural factors, such as residential segregation and the unequal distribution of power and resources across social groups.

Figure 3.3 shows a more expansive model linking features of cities and neighborhoods to health and placing these levels in the context of global and national trends. This model expands on the model shown in Figure 3.2 in various ways. It recognizes the presence of determinants at multiple levels of organization, ranging from global trends to city-level processes to local neighborhood environments and individual characteristics; it specifically notes the role of different stakeholders—civil society, government, nonprofits, businesses, and international organizations in affecting these determinants, and it emphasizes the role of place-based policies and practices within and outside the traditional health sector.[11]

Another key difference from the model illustrated in Figure 3.2 is that it explicitly highlights environmental outcomes as primary outcomes of interest (not only as determinants) and also notes the interrelated and reinforcing nature of human health and environmental sustainability. A central focus of the model is the fact that policies or other actions may have important co-benefits in both domains.

An important dimension that is not explicitly represented in either model is the life course. The time lags through which place-based factors affect health can vary substantially. Some may operate with relatively short lags (e.g., changes to pedestrian infrastructure promoting walking and therefore increasing physical activity almost immediately), but others may operate over much longer time frames, even over the life course. Thus, the impact of places depends on the life-course history of exposures rather than only on exposure at a particular point in time.

Isolating the causal effects of places on health presents numerous analytical challenges. These are related to the fact that places may affect health through long causal chains that can sometimes extend over long periods of time. Some aspects of where we live have immediate consequences for our health, while others have more subtle influences that can be difficult to detect but that have the potential to become prominent as they accumulate over time. In addition, the impact of specific features of places can be difficult to disentangle from the impact of other place-based features or individual characteristics. A first key challenge is, of course, defining and measuring the relevant place-based constructs (often specific social or physical features of cities or neighborhoods). A second challenge is isolating the impact of any specific place-based factor from other factors, especially individual characteristics that are associated with place of residence (i.e., separating context from composition). A third key challenge is leveraging and properly accounting for changes over time in place-based features of interest, other relevant place and individual-level

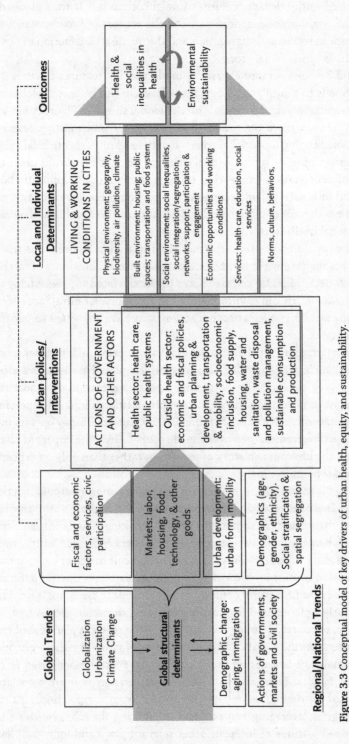

Figure 3.3 Conceptual model of key drivers of urban health, equity, and sustainability.
Source: Diez Roux AV, Slesinski SC, Alazraqui M, et al. A novel international partnership for actionable evidence on urban health in Latin America: LAC-Urban Health and SALURBAL. *Global Challenges.* 2018;3(4):1800013.

health determinants, and health outcomes to derive more robust estimates of causal effects. We will return to these methodologic challenges in Chapter 9.

Places as Moderators or Reinforcers of Inter-Individual Health Differences

In thinking about the role of places in the causation of health, it is important to recognize that place-based features must necessarily operate through individual-level processes. Sometimes places can affect the health of individuals by directly shaping exposures to environmental toxins or by influencing behaviors and psychosocial stress, as discussed in the prior sections. But at other times places may operate by enhancing or buffering the impact of individual-level attributes. For example, city or neighborhood features, such the availability and pricing of sugar-sweetened beverages, can moderate the impact of obesity genes on the development of obesity: the impact of genes on obesity may be stronger in a context where sugar sweetened beverages are easily available and therefore more easily consumed by individuals. In another example, stressful neighborhoods may interact with heart disease-related genes.[12] Residential proximity to unhealthy fast foods may interact with stress at work to promote the consumption of unhealthy foods, and food environments may influence adherence to dietary guidelines.[13]

Places may also serve to reinforce the impact of individual level characteristics through reinforcing mechanisms or feedbacks. For example, dietary preferences of residents may partly shape foods offered for sale in neighborhoods, and the foods offered for sale may, in turn, promote and reinforce certain dietary preferences. Walkable neighborhoods may encourage walking, which promotes additional walkable destinations, further promoting walking behaviors.

Another example is the reinforcing role of individual-level socioeconomic characteristics and residential segregation in driving health inequities. Individuals are sorted into different neighborhoods based at least in part on their income (which affects their ability to purchase or rent housing). Residential segregation by income creates differences in the power and resources of neighborhoods, leading to very different neighborhood environments. These environmental differences reinforce residential segregation as those with more income are able to choose to live in neighborhoods with better environments. This creates a vicious cycle by which neighborhood segregation by income creates and reinforces neighborhood environmental differences, which, in turn, reinforce and magnify income inequities in health. The presence of feedbacks highlights the importance of systems thinking as we consider conceptual frameworks for urban health.

Places as Integral Components of the Systems That Give Rise to Health

Although useful as simplified representations to guide research and action, common conceptual models of the links between places and health do not fully capture the dynamic processes within and across levels of organization that drive health and environmental outcomes. These dynamic processes involve feedback (via reinforcing or balancing feedback loops) and dependencies across units (i.e., processes by which actions or outcomes in one neighborhood or city affect another). To fully capture these processes, we need to characterize the systems that give rise to health and environmental outcomes at multiple levels. Understanding the functioning of the system as a whole can be important to draw inferences about causes of observed outcomes under varying conditions and to understand the plausible impacts of interventions or policies.[14]

Most fundamentally, complex systems are characterized by four features. The first is the presence of factors operating at various levels of organization (i.e., cities, neighborhoods, homes, and individuals). A second feature is the presence of heterogeneous units (e.g., different kinds of people or neighborhoods). A third feature is the presence of dependencies (i.e., the behavior of one person influences the behavior of others through social networks and norms; neighborhoods and cities are interconnected and influence each other via flows of people and resources). A fourth feature is the presence of reinforcing or balancing feedbacks (i.e., greater mixed land use promotes more walking, which, in turn, promotes greater land use mix). These features give rise to the observed outcomes of system functioning which often cannot be accurately predicted without considering the functioning of the system as a whole. The features of complex systems are reviewed in more detail in Chapter 11 (see Box 11.1).

The dynamic relations that characterize systems explain why the impact of a given perturbation of a system (i.e., through a policy or intervention) may vary depending on the condition of the other parameters of the system (sensitivity to initial conditions or context dependency). For example, the impact of increased use of public transportation on health may depend in part on the extent to which other initiatives reduce traffic congestion. In the context of reduced congestion, the overall benefit may be positive because of increased physical activity. But, in the context of high congestion, physical activity–related benefits may be overshadowed by adverse health effects related to exposure to air pollution.

Systems can be schematically captured using causal loop diagrams.[15] In addition to making explicit the relations that are believed to be fundamental to system functioning these causal loop diagrams can be used to identify new interventions or consider the plausible effects of interventions under varying conditions.[16] Figure 3.4 shows an example of a causal loop diagram reflecting the plausible relations between a city's transportation system, select policies,

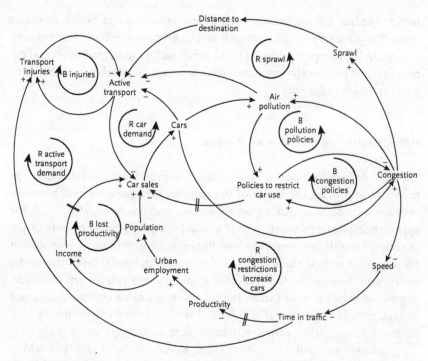

Figure 3.4 A causal loop diagram developed by the Salud Urbana en América Latina (SALURBAL) Project.

Source: Diez Roux AV, Slesinski SC, Alazraqui M, et al. A novel international partnership for actionable evidence on urban health in Latin America: LAC-Urban Health and SALURBAL. *Global Challenges.* 2018;3(4):1800013.

and health-related outcomes such as car use, active transport, and air pollution levels.

Once an evidence-based conceptual model of the system is developed, approaches such as agent-based models, systems dynamics models or network analyses can be used to quantitatively interrogate how perturbations (i.e., via policies or interventions, unexpected events, or changes in population or other conditions) impact the system under varying conditions.[17] Systems thinking underlies the planetary health approach to urban health reviewed later in this chapter as it explicitly accounts for feedbacks between health and the environment. We discuss the use of systems methodologies for urban health in more detail in Chapter 11.

MULTISECTORAL APPROACHES TO URBAN HEALTH

In this section we briefly describe two multisectoral approaches to health that are closely tied to the conceptualizations that we previously described. The health in all policies approach explicitly recognizes the many ways in which factors outside the traditional health -care system affect health in urban areas. The planetary health approach emphasizes how policies that promote health can have important benefits for other sectors (e.g., environmental co-benefits) and policies that promote environmental sustainability can have important health co benefits.

Urban Health and Health in All Policies

The CDC defines the "health in all policies" approach as "a collaborative approach to improving the health of all people by incorporating health considerations into decision-making across sectors and policy areas (p. 5)."[18] The approach implies a recognition that a broad range of policies outside of the traditional health-care sector can have important health impacts. Examples of these policies include those that affect resources and social inequities: social policy, economic policy, and educational policy. These policies are, of course, of great relevance to urban areas. In urban settings, other critically important policies include those that affect physical structures and environments: sanitation, housing, urban planning policies (such as zoning), street design, cycling policies, and mobility policies (such as congestion pricing and vehicle use restrictions). The potential impact of these policies on urban health can be inferred from the conceptual models of the drivers of urban health previously reviewed in this chapter. A health in all policies approach requires collaborations across sectors and fields. Box 3.1 reviews the history and goals of collaborations between urban planning and public health.

A key element of the health in all policies approach is the need to recognize and evaluate the potential health impact of policies before they are enacted. Sometimes this can draw attention to the ways the health impact can be beneficial but other times it can alert us to detrimental effects. Health impact assessment (HIA)[19,20] has emerged as an approach that can be used to estimate the plausible health impact of policies and programs before they are implemented. In HIA, it is also important to evaluate the health equity impact of policies, recognizing that some policies that promote health can sometimes also increase health inequities. The information obtained can be used to make decisions about programs or policies or to implement strategies that can buffer any adverse health impacts.

An important challenge in doing HIAs is the availability of evidence that can be used to reliably predict the health impacts of a specific policy or program. There is continuing need to rigorously evaluate the health impact of urban policies to learn what urban policies have the greatest potential for promoting health and reducing health inequities. The results of policy evaluations can enhance scientific knowledge about health determinants, be used

Box 3.1 URBAN PLANNING AND URBAN HEALTH

By Jana A. Hirsch

Urban planning, like public health, is a varied field. Two of the largest domains are land-use planning and transportation planning. Land-use planning focuses on how spaces are used and on the ways in which different uses (residential, commercial, industrial, and other uses) are distributed. Transportation planning focuses on the movement of people within the city, including by car, transit, bicycle, or on foot.

Urban planners identify existing problems within cities, gather and analyze information on the problems, design alternatives or solutions to the problems, and then synthesize these solutions through iterative public meetings to best represent public choices.[21] Planning can happen at a number of scales, with land uses often planned through a network of small jurisdictions and transportation often planned using a cohesive, regional approach.

Implementation of plans often requires government tools such as regulation (e.g. zoning) and taxation. Local public health agencies participate in some of these processes; for example, during site plan review or zoning compliance public health agencies may analyze the environmental health impacts of the project under review (effects on air, water, and land). Newer tools, including health impact assessments, help public health agencies to quantify other health impacts beyond those traditionally considered and allow examination of the health impacts of policies and decisions whose health impacts were previously ignored.

Collaboration between urban planning and public health is critical for meeting health challenges of urban environments and facilitating promotion of urban health. In considering today's efforts to reconnect these two fields it is helpful to consider the history of the relation between these two fields.

In the late 19th century, urban neighborhoods were often blamed for poor health. The popular notion of *miasma*, or "bad air," was the concept that unpleasant atmospheres could cause sickness and urban unrest. Many practices to address this concern, including sanitary surveys and park planning, can be viewed as joint efforts by the fields of planning and public health.[22] In the name of health, planners comprehensively planned sewer and water systems and worked to alleviate crowded living conditions with outdoor recreation spaces. Indeed, "by the end of the nineteenth century, modern American urban planning emerged as a field that used physical interventions to respond to urban public health crises."[22p691]

However, throughout most of the 20th century, these two fields diverged, heading in drastically different directions. With the arrival of germ theory (the notion that specific agents caused specific infectious diseases), public health moved away from miasma and environmental determinants. Treatments focused on specific interventions, including immunizations and chlorination of drinking water. This new public health shifted toward different types of professionals, specifically biologists, chemists, and physicians. Similarly, under pressures from industry and private landowners, planning shifted toward automobile-centric planning and the separation of different land uses. During this same time, both fields experienced increases in specialization and professionalization reflected in different languages and standards that created distance between the fields, reducing opportunities for collaboration.

By the end of the 20th century, the two fields began to reconnect. On the public health side, this reunion is often credited to the emergence of social epidemiology and an awareness of the growing inequalities in health across population groups and geographies. On the planning side, this recoupling is sometimes attributed to a growing interest in sustainable, walkable cities with the density and amenities to enhance human and environmental health. Underlying both processes is a renewed emphasis on equity.

Public health professionals can help encourage the incorporation of public health and safety into planning and planning implementation by remaining involved in the full planning process. Challenges remain, including assessment techniques, confronting health disparities, democratizing planning practices, and developing a clearly articulated urban health agenda.[23] Nonetheless, many cities across North America have formalized connections between urban or regional planning and public health departments. Several early examples include Ingham County Health Department in Michigan, the Tri-County Health Department in Denver, and the San Francisco Department of Public Health.[21] Many schools now offer dual degrees in public health and planning or architecture and numerous resources exist for training a generation of interdisciplinary urban health practitioners (http://healthyplaces.gatech.edu/). With concerted, cohesive effort, these two fields will continue to support each other as they build a healthy urban future for all.

by policymakers to identify and prioritize programs and policies, and provide critical inputs into future HIAs. Adopting a health in all policies approach requires significant partnership between health and other policy actors. Citizen engagement should also be a key component of the process. We discuss the health in all policies approach in Chapter 14.

Urban Health and Planetary Heath: The Interrelatedness of Health and Environmental Sustainability

The planetary health movement that emerged in recent years has emphasized the tight interrelatedness of population health and the environment.[24,25] It goes beyond traditional environmental health approaches in explicitly recognizing and highlighting environmental outcomes linked to sustainability in their own right. A key principle of the planetary health approach is that many policies that promote heath can have significant environmental co-benefits, and similarly many policies that protect the environment can have significant health co-benefits. For example, policies that reduce consumption of meat or promote active transportation via walking or cycling may help reduce greenhouse gas emissions and air pollution. On the other hand, policies aimed at reducing energy use and greenhouse gas emissions (via for example increase public transportation and bike use) can reduce heat-related deaths and promote physical activity. Thus, in considering the benefits of urban policies, both health and environmental benefits need to be considered together.

The growing relevance of urbanization means that cities and urban areas generally can have a significant impact on the ecology of the planet. Just as cities can be designed and managed so that they are healthier and more equitable, they can also be designed and managed so that their adverse environmental impacts are minimized. This includes reducing the size of physical urban footprints (to minimize land use and threats to biodiversity), reducing energy consumption and waste (to reduce greenhouse gas emissions and other environmental consequences such as water and soil contamination), promoting active transportation (to reduce emissions and promote high-density areas that reduce urban footprints), and promoting dietary patterns rich in local fruits and vegetables (to reduce adverse environmental consequences of meat consumption and transportation of foods). Many of these strategies can have favorable population health impacts as well.

A planetary health approach to urban health implies thinking systemically in ways that explicitly consider the dependencies and feedbacks between health and the environment broadly understood.[26] It also implies placing cities within their broader contexts and considering the links between core cities, peripheral suburban areas, and rural areas. Understanding how mobility and food production and distribution systems function across urban and less urban areas is fundamental to a planetary health approach and to promoting urban health. Box 3.2 provides examples of the health and environmental co-benefits of selected urban policies.

Box 3.2 A PLANETARY HEALTH APPROACH TO URBAN
HEALTH: HEALTH AND ENVIRONMENTAL CO-BENEFITS
OF SELECTED URBAN POLICIES

Building high density, compact cities can

• promote health via increased walkability and lower traffic-related mortality.
• protect the environment via less car use and lower greenhouse gas (GHG) and air pollution emissions and via smaller urban footprints with less disruption of natural habitats.

Reducing reliance on fossil fuels in cities can

• promote health via lower air pollution.
• protect the environment via lower GHG emissions.

Promoting consumption of less meats and processed foods can

• promote health through greater intake of fresh fruits and vegetables and whole grains.
• protect the environment through lower GHG emissions and more efficient land use, reducing habitat and biodiversity threats.

Greening of cities can

• promote health through increased physical activity, better mental health, and temperature reduction.
• protect the environment through promotion of biodiversity and reductions in water run-off.

URBAN HEALTH RESEARCH QUESTIONS AND POLICY OPTIONS

In this section, we build on prior discussions of the principles of urban health (Chapter 1), recent trends in urbanization (Chapter 2), and conceptual frameworks for urban health (earlier in this chapter) to propose a typology of research questions in urban health. We also propose a typology of the policies and interventions that may be relevant to health in urban areas. These typologies serve to highlight key concepts and will be useful as we advance in more detailed discussions of research approaches and policy actions in later chapters of this book.

A Typology of Urban Health Research Studies

A myriad of research studies (and associated questions) relevant to urban health are possible, and many different typologies can be constructed. Here we describe one possible typology that emphasizes three dimensions: the contrasts of interest, the types health outcomes examined, and the goals of the research.

One dimension across which urban health research studies can be classified pertains to contrasts of interest. Two types of studies are possible: studies focused on comparing urban to rural areas and studies contrasting different urban areas to each other. Studies focused on urban to rural comparisons often rely on the urban–rural classifications we have reviewed earlier in this book. An important limitation of these studies is that often heterogeneous urban areas as well as heterogeneous rural areas are lumped together. Nevertheless, by broadly characterizing the associations of urban living with various health outcomes, studies of urban–rural comparisons can provide a useful starting point to understand how urban places are linked to health.

Studies comparing different urban areas with each other can, in turn, be classified into two types: studies of health across different cities and studies of health across different neighborhoods within a city. The growth of cities worldwide has generated interest in studies contrasting multiple cities. An important strength of these studies is that they capitalize on between city variation to identify what city-level factors may be most strongly related to health outcomes. Purely city-level analyses, however, ignore within city variation. Studies of differences in health within cities, (i.e. studies of neighborhood health effects) have received much attention in the public health literature over the past 20 years.[27] By capitalizing on important neighborhood differences in health within cities, these studies can help identify the specific mechanism through which urban physical and social environments affect health. However, they are limited if within-city heterogeneity in the factor of interest is low or difficult to disentangle from other correlated characteristics of place.

A second dimension across which studies can be classified pertains to the main health outcomes of interest. Health outcomes can be broadly classified into risk factors (e.g., behaviors and biomarkers of interest due to known health consequences), levels of health (e.g. mortality, morbidity, and prevalence/incidence), differences in health (by age, gender, race or ethnicity, social class etc.), and trajectories of health over time. Thus, for example, research questions about differences between cities can be about why some cities have higher mortality than others (levels of health), why some cities have greater inequities in mortality by education than others (differences or inequities in health), or why some cities have more rapidly decreasing mortality than others (trajectories of health).

A third dimension across which research studies can be classified pertains to the main goal of the study, specifically whether the goals of the study are primarily descriptive of a specific context or time period, advancing our understanding of generalizable causes (or etiology), or whether the main goal is to evaluate the health impacts of a policy or intervention. Of course, this distinction is somewhat artificial because description can generate hypotheses about etiology, etiologic understanding is important to the identification of effective policies, and evaluations of interventions or policies can shed light on underlying causes. Nevertheless, it is possible to classify studies broadly in terms of their main goals, recognizing that there is a continuum across all three goals of description, causal inference, and policy evaluation.

Table 3.1 summarizes the typology, with rows representing contrasts, columns representing study goals, and distinctions among outcome types noted within some cells. Examples of research questions and sample studies that fall into different categories and that refer to different outcomes (levels of health, inequities, or trajectories) are shown in the cells. It is possible for studies to span multiple categories. For example, a given multilevel study with data on neighborhoods across multiple cities could examine both city and neighborhood differences in health. This study would therefore simultaneously focus on within and between city differences. Likewise, a study can simultaneously examine how neighborhood factors are related to health risk factors (e.g., hypertension prevalence) and differences in health (e.g., inequities by race within and across neighborhoods). Such a study would therefore simultaneously examine factors related to both levels and inequities in health.

A Typology of Urban Health Policies and Interventions: Mechanisms and Strategies

Given that the ultimate goal of urban health research is to inform urban interventions and policies to improve health and promote health equity in urban areas, it is helpful to briefly consider the broad categories of urban policies and interventions that could be relevant to health. Part IV of this book will discuss dissemination and policy translation for urban health in more detail.

Many urban policies and interventions have the potential to affect health. These policies and interventions can be classified based on the specific mechanisms through which they can promote health and based on the policy strategy used. Mechanisms can include reductions of environmental hazards (like reductions in air pollution levels or lead), supporting behavior change (increasing physical activity or reducing tobacco consumption), increasing access to health promoting services (increasing access to primary care), or increasing social inclusion (reducing poverty and discrimination). A number of strategies can be used to affect these mechanisms, which, in turn, affect

Table 3.1 A TYPOLOGY OF URBAN HEALTH RESEARCH QUESTIONS AND ILLUSTRATIVE EXAMPLES

		Goal	
Contrast	Description	Causal Understanding	Policy Evaluation
Urban–rural	Charts of urban–rural differences in asthma prevalence (levels), race differences in asthma (differences), or changes in asthma prevalence over time (trajectories)	How does migration from a rural to an urban area affect health? Do these effects differ by income?	Is the impact of a policy to make public transportation free for older adults on mental health of older adults similar in urban and rural areas (levels)?
Between city	Rankings of cities based on life expectancy (levels) or based on health inequities (differences)	What factors are associated with higher city-level life expectancy (levels), smaller income inequalities in life expectancy (differences), or with greater increases in life expectancy over time (trajectories)?	Do cities that actively subsidize public transportation have more physically active residents (levels)? Do they have smaller income inequities physical activity and obesity (differences)?
Within city	Maps of differences in life expectancy within cities (levels); focus groups on main health problems in different neighborhoods (levels); maps of race differences in life expectancy in different neighborhoods (differences)	What neighborhood factors are associated with more obesity (levels)? What neighborhood factors are associated with smaller race differences in obesity (differences)? Or with smaller increases in obesity over time (trajectories)	Does the opening of a neighborhood fruit and vegetable market improve diet of residents (levels)? Does lead abatement in low-income neighborhoods reduce inequities by race in lead poisoning (differences)?

Table 3.2 A TYPOLOGY OF URBAN POLICIES OR INTERVENTIONS THAT MAY AFFECT HEALTH BASED ON THE MECHANISM THEY OPERATE ON AND THE STRATEGY USED, WITH ILLUSTRATIVE EXAMPLES

Strategy	Health-Related Mechanism			
	Reduction of Environmental and Physical Hazards	Changing Behaviors	Increasing Access to Services	Increasing Social Inclusion
Laws and regulations	Air pollution standards; lead standards	Caps on tobacco or alcohol outlet densities; advertising prohibitions; menu labeling	Health insurance requirement	Housing antidiscrimination laws; minimum wage laws
Economic incentives	Carbon tax Congestion pricing	Tobacco and beverage taxes		
Physical environment and infrastructure	Traffic bumps Creation of green spaces	Improved public transportation; bike lanes; subsidies for healthy food stores	Creation of health centers Improving access to sanitation	Mixed-income housing
Social and health care-policy		Health education campaigns	Free screening	Conditional cash transfer programs; income tax exemptions

health. Strategies include laws and regulations (e.g., restricting tobacco sales to minors), creating economic incentives or disincentives (e.g., tobacco taxes), improving physical environments and infrastructure (e.g., new transportation projects or neighborhood greening), and changing social and health-care policy (e.g., welfare policy, tax policy). Table 3.2 shows examples of policies and interventions that fall into these categories.

Building the evidence base for the health effects of these policies is an important priority for urban health. It is important to recognize that these policies may operate through multiple mechanisms to affect multiple health outcomes. For example, street enhancements can both reduce injury risk and encourage physical activity,[28] and public transportation initiatives that reduce air pollution can facilitate active lifestyles.[29] In some cases, there may be unintended adverse health consequences as well. For example, urban tree planting projects may provide environmental benefits (e.g., cooling) and psychological benefits but may increase exposure to pollen allergens.[30] In evaluating the health impact of these policies, it is important to evaluate not only their impact on overall health levels but also their impact on health inequities as many well-intentioned interventions can have the unintended consequence of increasing health inequities. As noted in the section on planetary health, it is also important to consider (and evaluate) the environmental co-benefits of policies.

REFERENCES

1. Givens M, Gennuso K, Jovaag A, Dijk JWV, Johnson S. County health rankings key findings. University of Wisconsin Population Health Institute. 2019; https://www.countyhealthrankings.org/reports/2019-county-health-rankings-key-findings-report.

2. US Centers for Disease Control and Prevention. Small-Area Life Expectancy Estimates Project (USALEEP). National Center for Health Statistics. 2018; https://www.cdc.gov/nchs/nvss/usaleep/usaleep.html.

3. Schinasi LH, Auchincloss AH, Forrest CB, Diez Roux AV. Using electronic health record data for environmental and place based population health research: A systematic review. *Annals of Epidemiology*. 2018;28(7):493–502.

4. Casey JA, Schwartz BS, Stewart WF, Adler NE. Using electronic health records for population health research: A review of methods and applications. *Annual Review of Public Health*. 2016;37:61–81.

5. Sinnenberg L, Buttenheim AM, Padrez K, Mancheno C, Ungar L, Merchant RM. Twitter as a tool for health research: A systematic review. *American Journal of Public Health*. 2017;107(1):e1–e8.

6. Huang X, Smith MC, Jamison AM, et al. Can online self-reports assist in real-time identification of influenza vaccination uptake? A cross-sectional study of influenza vaccine-related tweets in the USA, 2013–2017. *BMJ Open*. 2019;9(1):e024018.

7. Arias E, Escobedo LA, Kennedy J, Fu C, Cisewski JA. US small-area life expectancy estimates project: Methodology and results summary. National Center for Health Statistics. 2018; https://www.cdc.gov/nchs/nvss/usaleep/usaleep.html.

8. Quick H, Terloyeva D, Wu Y, Moore K, Diez Roux AV. Trends in tract-level prevalence of obesity in Philadelphia by race-ethnicity, space, and time. *Epidemiology.* 2020;31(1):15–21.

9. Diez Roux AV, Mair C. Neighborhoods and health. *Annals of the New York Academy of Sciences.* 2010;1186(1):125–145.

10. Diez Roux AV, Mair C. Neighborhoods and health. *Annals of the New York Academy of Sciences.* 2010;1186:125–145.

11. Diez Roux AV, Slesinski SC, Alazraqui M, et al. A novel international partnership for actionable evidence on urban health in Latin America: LAC-Urban Health and SALURBAL. *Global Challenges.* 2019;3(4):1800013.

12. Mooney SJ, Grady ST, Sotoodehnia N, et al. In the wrong place with the wrong SNP: The association between stressful neighborhoods and cardiac arrest within beta-2-adrenergic receptor variants. *Epidemiology.* 2016;27(5):656–662.

13. Feathers A, Aycinena AC, Lovasi GS, et al. Food environments are relevant to recruitment and adherence in dietary modification trials. *Nutrition Research.* 2015;35(6):480–488.

14. Diez Roux AV. Complex systems thinking and current impasses in health disparities research. *American Journal of Public Health.* 2011;101(9):1627–1634.

15. Sterman J. *Business Dynamics: Systems Thinking and Modeling for a Complex World.* Boston: Irwin/McGraw-Hill; 2000.

16. Trani J-F, Ballard E, Bakhshi P, Hovmand P. Community based system dynamic as an approach for understanding and acting on messy problems: A case study for global mental health intervention in Afghanistan. *Conflict and Health.* 2016;10(1):25.

17. Cerda M, Keyes KM. Systems modeling to advance the promise of data science in epidemiology. *American Journal of Epidemiology.* 2019;188(5):862–865.

18. Rudolph L, Caplan J, Ben-Moshe K, Dillon L. *Health in All Policies: A Guide for State and Local Governments.* Washington, DC: American Public Health Association; 2013.

19. Pennington A, Dreaves H, Scott-Samuel A, et al. Development of an urban health impact assessment methodology: Indicating the health equity impacts of urban policies. *European Journal of Public Health.* 2017;27(Suppl 2):56–61.

20. National Research Council. *Improving Health in the United States: The Role of Health Impact Assessment.* Washington, DC: National Academies Press; 2011.

21. Malizia EE. City and regional planning: A primer for public health officials. *American Journal of Health Promotion.* 2005;19(5 Suppl):1–13.

22. Corburn J. Reconnecting with our roots: American urban planning and public health in the twenty-first century. *Urban Affairs Review.* 2007;42(5):688–713.

23. Corburn J. Confronting the challenges in reconnecting urban planning and public health. *American Journal of Public Health.* 2004;94(4):541–546.

24. Myers SS. Planetary health: Protecting human health on a rapidly changing planet. *The Lancet.* 2018;390(10114):2860–2868.

25. Whitmee S, Haines A, Beyrer C, et al. Safeguarding human health in the Anthropocene epoch: Report of the Rockefeller Foundation–Lancet Commission on planetary health. *The Lancet.* 2015;386(10007):1973–2028.

26. Pongsiri MJ, Gatzweiler FW, Bassi AM, Haines A, Demassieux F. The need for a systems approach to planetary health. *The Lancet: Planetary Health*. 2017;1(7):e257–e259.

27. Duncan DT, Kawachi I. *Neighborhoods and Health*. Oxford: Oxford University Press Oxford; 2018.

28. Heath GW, Parra DC, Sarmiento OL, et al. Evidence-based intervention in physical activity: Lessons from around the world. *The Lancet*. 2012;380(9838):272–281.

29. Frank L, Sallis JF, Conway JM, Chapman JE, Saelens BE, Bachman W. Many pathways from land use to health: Associations between neighborhood walkability and active transportation, body mass index, and air quality. *JAPA*. 2006;72(1):75–87.

30. Davern M, Farrar A, Kendal D, Giles-Corti B. *Quality Green Space Supporting Health, Wellbeing and Biodiversity: A Literature Review*. Victoria: University of Melbourne; 2016.

CHAPTER 4

Urban Health Inequities

ANA V. DIEZ ROUX

WHAT ARE URBAN HEALTH INEQUITIES?

Nearly 30 years ago, Whitehead defined health inequities as differences in health that are unnecessary, avoidable, unfair, and unjust.[1] More recently, Braveman and colleagues[2p2] defined health equity to mean that

> everyone has a fair and just opportunity to be healthier. This requires removing obstacles to health such as poverty, discrimination, and their consequences, including powerlessness and lack of access to good jobs with fair pay, quality education and housing, safe environments, and health care.

When we refer to health inequities, we are therefore referring to differences in health that stem from social conditions. These social conditions shape the environments that individuals live in; the types of jobs they have; and the resources they have access to, including money, education, and social connections as well as the power and control that they have over their lives and environments. All these things, in turn, affect health through many interrelated pathways such as environmental exposures, behaviors, stress, and access to quality health care. Most important, health inequities are avoidable through action on their fundamental causes and sometimes also through intervening on the pathways linking social determinants to health.

Urban areas are characterized by diversity in race, ethnicity, gender and sexual orientation, country of origin, migration history, and socioeconomic position. Because these factors are often closely linked to social conditions, urban areas are also the site of large health inequities linked to these factors. Figure 4.1 shows differences in race and ethnic composition across the urban–rural continuum in

Ana V. Diez Roux, *Urban Health Inequities* In: *Urban Public Health.* Edited by: Gina S. Lovasi, Ana V. Diez Roux, and Jennifer Kolker, Oxford University Press (2021). © Oxford University Press 2021.
DOI: 10.1093/oso/9780190885304.003.0004.

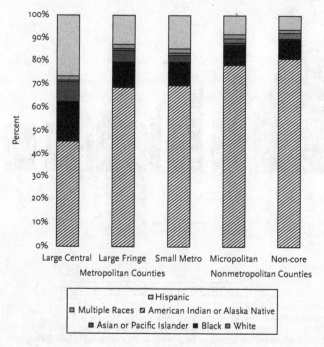

Figure 4.1 Differences in race and ethnic composition across levels of urbanicity in the United States, 2011. Definition of urbanicity based on NCHS categories[3] (see Chapter 1, Box 1.1, for details). Level of urbanization decreases from left to right.[4]

Source: Adapted from Meit M, Knudson A, Gilbert T, et al. *The 2014 Update of the Rural–Urban Chartbook.* Bethesda, MD: Rural Health Research and Policy Centers; 2014, Data Table 4.

the United States. There is substantially greater race and ethnic diversity in more urban areas. Urban areas are also often characterized by high income inequalities.[5] As shown in Figure 4.2, a significant proportion of urban populations of LMIC live in slums. Although the percentages of urban residents in slums is lower now than it was two decades ago, the absolute numbers are higher as a result of urbanization and population growth.[6] These social characteristics of urban areas (race and ethnic diversity, high income inequality, and poor neighborhood conditions such as inadequate housing and service) have significant implications for health and lead to large health inequities in cities. Thus, a focus on characterizing, understanding and acting to reduce health inequities by race, social class, or other factors is a key focus of research and action in urban health.

DESCRIBING URBAN HEALTH INEQUITIES

Describing health inequities is a key first step in motivating actions to reduce inequities. Broadly speaking, descriptions of health inequities can focus on differences across individuals, differences across neighborhoods, or even differences across cities themselves. As is the case for the description of health

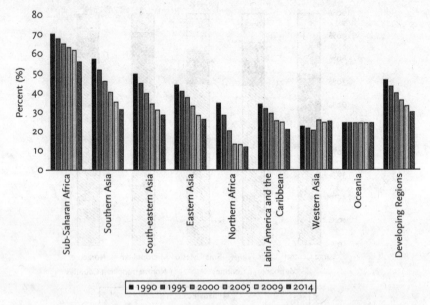

Figure 4.2 Percentage of urban population living in slums (1990–2014). UN-Habitat defines slums as a contiguous settlement that lacks one or more of the following five conditions: access to clean water, access to improved sanitation, sufficient living area that is not overcrowded, durable housing and secure tenure.

Source: UN Habitat. *World Cities Report 2016: Urbanization and Development: Emerging Futures.* Nairobi, Kenya: United Nations Human Settlements Programme; 2016.

inequities more generally, the quantification of the magnitude of inequities can be done using absolute differences (e.g., rate differences) or relative differences (e.g., rate ratios). Both approaches have their advantages and disadvantages and provide complementary information.[7]

Differences Across Individuals

Health inequities across individuals can be described using a range of individual-level indicators that capture differences in social circumstances. These include categories based on race, ethnicity, gender identity, sexual orientation, and immigration status. They can also include indicators of socioeconomic position such as income, wealth, education, or occupation. Each of these measures has strengths and limitations.[8,9] Examples of the use of these measures to quantify health inequities in urban settings are shown in Box 4.1. Exploring why health inequities are larger in some areas than in others can provide important clues to the causes of health inequities or point to the urban policies that may most effectively reduce health inequities.

Box 4.1 also shows an example of the quantification of inequities by race and ethnicity. Measures of socioeconomic position and race/ethnicity often

Box 4.1 EXAMPLES OF INEQUITIES IN HEALTH BY INCOME AND RACE IN URBAN AREAS

Researchers have used a variety of data sources to quantify health inequities by education, income, and race or ethnicity within urban areas. Fleischer and colleagues[10] have used individual-level indicators of education and survey data to quantify health inequities by socioeconomic position in the prevalence cardiovascular risks factors in urban areas of Argentina (Figure 4.3). Chetty and colleagues[11] have used detailed income data derived from social security data linked to mortality records to quantify inequities in life expectancy by income in US cities. Both Fleischer and Chetty also investigated heterogeneity in the magnitude of inequities. For example, Fleischer showed that the size and even sometimes the directionality of inequities in urban areas was modified by the level of

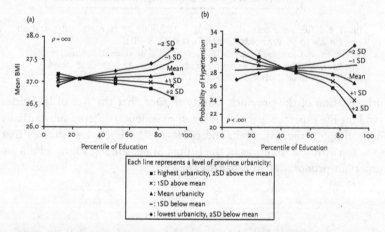

Figure 4.3 Predicted mean body mass index (BMI) and probability of hypertension by individual-level education in men stratified by province-level urbanicity. Each line represents a level of province urbanicity:

• highest urbanicity, 2 standard deviations (SD) above the mean

x 1 SD above mean

▲ Mean urbanicity

– 1 SD below mean

♦ lowest urbanicity, 2 SD below mean

Source: Fleischer NL, Diez Roux AV, Alazraqui M, Spinelli H, De Maio F. Socioeconomic gradients in chronic disease risk factors in middle-income countries: Evidence of effect modification by urbanicity in Argentina. *American Journal of Public Health*. 2011;101(2):294–301. Data from National Survey of Risk Factors for Non-Communicable Diseases Argentina, 2005.

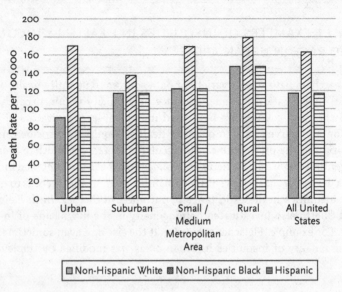

Figure 4.4 All-cause mortality rate (per 100,000) by race and urbanization Level for 25- to 34-year-olds, United States, 2013–2015.

Source: Stein EM, Gennuso KP, Ugboaja DC, Remington PL. The epidemic of despair among White Americans: Trends in the leading causes of premature death, 1999–2015. *American Journal of Public Health.* 2017;107(10):1541–1547.

urbanization of the province. Chetty showed that the size of inequities (and the life expectancy for lower income residents) differed substantially depending on the city. Stein and colleagues[12] (Figure 4.4) showed that race and ethnic differences in the United States among young adults are especially pronounced in urban areas.

capture not only interrelated but also distinct aspects of social circumstances. For example, health inequities by race may partly reflect differences in income and wealth, but they may also reflect the adverse effects of racism. Racism can affect health by truncating economic opportunities (and thereby affecting income, wealth, and residential location) but may also operate through the stress-related effects of discrimination itself. The diversity of urban areas in terms of race and ethnic background makes inequities by race/ethnicity an important challenge in urban settings.

Differences Across Neighborhoods

A focus on health inequities across neighborhoods is especially prominent in urban health because of the inherent place-based nature of the urban health approach. Many descriptions of urban health inequities therefore focus on differences across places (often loosely defined neighborhoods) that differ in features such as economic characteristics or race/ethnic composition. A prime example of this approach is the creation of maps of cities that show life expectancy differences across neighborhoods (often in close proximity to each other) within a city. Figure 4.5 shows examples of such maps. These maps can be powerful advocacy tools that can help highlight the magnitude of urban health inequities in ways that are easy to understand. They can be used to support and inform debate and discussion on the social, economic, and political causes of inequities more broadly.

An important methodologic challenge in describing urban health inequities across neighborhoods is the creation of reliable estimates of health levels for small areas. The measures used can be means (such as mean body mass index), proportions (such as percentage with diabetes), rates (such as mortality rates), or other summary measures (such as life expectancy). The reliability of these measures is strongly influenced by the sample size (in case of surveys) or the population and numbers of events (in case of rates). A variety of statistical methods (described in more detail in Chapter 7) can be used to leverage sparse data to derive reliable estimates, even for small areas. One such approach was recently used to estimate life expectancy for census tracts in US cities.[13] These methods often require important assumptions that should be considered when the data are used.

Differences Across Cities

Although less frequently studied, cities themselves can also differ in levels of health and these differences are often linked to the social and economic characteristics of cities. For example, the SALURBAL study has documented important differences in life expectancy across cities. City-level health differences are associated with differences in the city-level measured of education (Box 4.2). Documenting differences in health across cities can provide important clues regarding the role of urban health policies. As shown in Box 4.1., cities also differ in the levels of health inequities by other factors like income. Thus, city-level factors can generate inequities across cities and can also modify the magnitude of inequities by individual or neighborhood characteristics.

CAUSES OF URBAN HEALTH INEQUITIES: THE ROLE OF RESIDENTIAL SEGREGATION

As we reviewed in Chapter 3, many interrelated features of urban social and physical environments operating through a multiplicity of pathways and

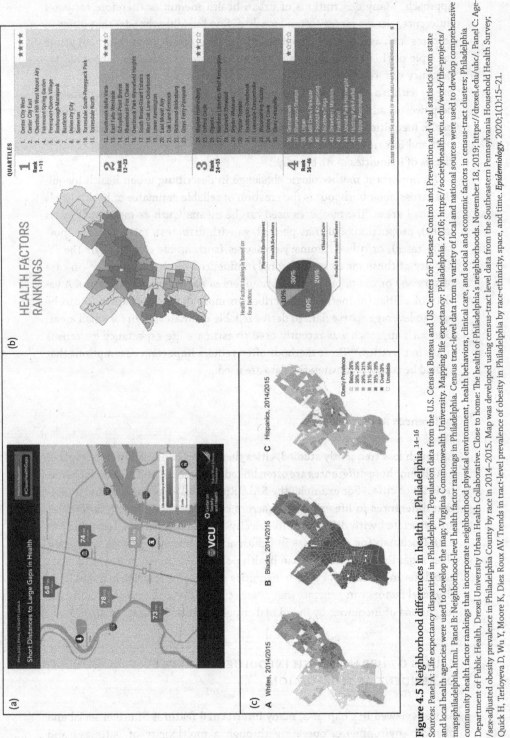

Figure 4.5 Neighborhood differences in health in Philadelphia.[14-16]

Sources: Panel A: Life expectancy disparities in Philadelphia. Population data from the U.S. Census Bureau and US Centers for Disease Control and Prevention and vital statistics from state and local health agencies were used to develop the map; Virginia Commonwealth University. Mapping life expectancy. Philadelphia. 2016; https://societyhealth.vcu.edu/work/the-projects/mapsphiladelphia.html. Panel B: Neighborhood-level health factor rankings in Philadelphia. Census tract-level data from a variety of local and national sources were used to develop comprehensive community health factor rankings that incorporate neighborhood physical environment, health behaviors, clinical care, and social and economic factors in census-tract clusters; Philadelphia Department of Public Health, Drexel University Urban Health Collaborative. Close to home: The health of Philadelphia's neighborhoods. November 18, 2019; https://drexel.edu/uhc/. Panel C: Age-/sex-adjusted obesity prevalence in Philadelphia County by race in 2014–2015. Map was developed using census-tract level data from the Southeastern Pennsylvania Household Health Survey; Quick H, Terloyeva D, Wu Y, Moore K, Diez Roux AV. Trends in tract-level prevalence of obesity in Philadelphia by race-ethnicity, space, and time. *Epidemiology*. 2020;1(1):15–21.

Box 4.2 INEQUITIES IN HEALTH ACROSS CITIES IN LATIN AMERICA: THE SALURBAL STUDY

Claire Slesinski

THE SALURBAL PROJECT

Since April 2017, the Dornsife School of Public Health at Drexel University and partners throughout Latin America and in the United States have been working together to study how urban environments and urban policies impact the health of city residents throughout Latin America and the environmental sustainability of cities. This research aims to inform policies and interventions to create healthier, more equitable, and more sustainable cities world-wide. The five-year project, called SALURBAL, or Salud Urbana en América Latina (Urban Health in Latin America), is funded by Wellcome Trust as part of its Our Planet, Our Health initiative, which focuses on research examining the connections between the environment and human health.

LIFE EXPECTANCY IN LATIN AMERICAN CITIES

There is a high level of variation in life expectancy and causes of death across urban areas in Latin America.[17] Global and regional summaries of life expectancy and causes of death can hide significant variability across cities.[18] Studies that characterize mortality across heterogeneous cities are needed to inform urban policies. Urban environments that differ across neighborhoods, cities, and countries can have a major impact on life expectancy and causes of death. The SALURBAL project is working to address these gaps in research within the Latin American context.

LIFE EXPECTANCY AND INEQUITY

Health inequities can manifest in a variety of ways, including life expectancy in different groups of people. To understand patterns of mortality and life expectancy in Latin American cities, SALURBAL has compiled mortality records for all recorded deaths in 366 cities across 10 countries for 2012 to 2014.[19] In Figure 4.6, each circle represents one city whose placement on the graph demonstrates the city's overall life expectancy, with separate panels for men and women. The figure shows large variations in life expectancy among cities within each country. When average life expectancy in these cities is then compared to the average number of years of educational attainment among men and women in that city, we can see that cities with higher levels of education also experience higher levels of life expectancy.

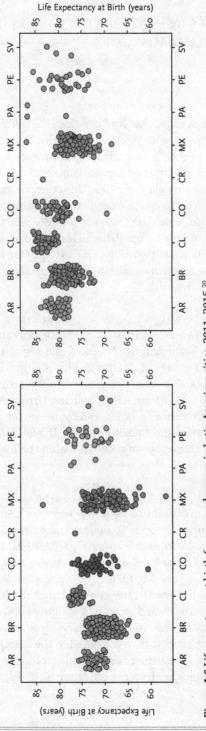

Figure 4.6 Life expectancy at birth for men and women in Latin American cities, 2011–2015.[20]

Source: Lein A, Slesinski C, Bilal U, Indvik K, Melly S, Diez Roux AV. Mortality and life expectancy in Latin American cities: Data from the SALURBAL project. Urban Health Network for Latin American and the Carribean, Data Brief. 2019.

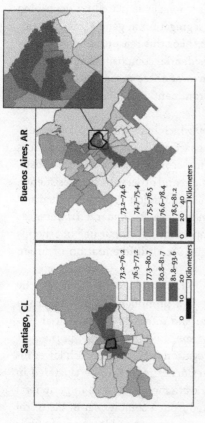

Figure 4.7 Life expectancy at birth (in years) in areas within Santiago, Chile and Buenos Aires, Argentina.

Source: Mortality and life expectancy in Latin American cities: Data from the SALURBAL project. Urban Health Network for Latin American and the Carribean, Data Brief. 2019;2; and Bilal U, Alazraqui M, Caiaffa WT, et al. Inequalities in life expectancy in six large Latin American cities from the SALURBAL study: An ecological analysis. *The Lancet: Planetary Health.* 2019;3(12):e503–e510.

SALURBAL has also identified striking disparities in life expectancy within individual cities.[21] Some of the cities with the highest life expectancy in the region also have the widest disparities in life expectancy across different sectors of the city. For example, differences in life expectancy can be seen across smaller sections of Santiago de Chile and Buenos Aires, Argentina (Figure 4.7). While some residents of Santiago de Chile experience an average life expectancy of over 90 years, people living in other parts of the city may live on average only to 73 years of age. A similar but smaller gap in life expectancy can be seen in Buenos Aires, where life expectancy ranges from 73 years to just over 81 years.

These analyses of differences in life expectancy only begin to reveal the inequities that exist in Latin American cities. SALURBAL researchers are implementing dozens of studies to examine how social inequities and built environment factors may be influencing a whole range of health outcomes and environmental impacts in cities.

interacting with personal and family circumstances (including individual social circumstances as well as behavioral and biologic factors operating over the life course) shape health in cities. Many of the same factors create and reinforce health inequities.

There is a large literature documenting the causes of health inequities by socioeconomic position and race/ethnicity.[22] The processes described in this literature, which involve life course exposures operating through behaviors, stress-related process, and environmental exposures, certainly apply to urban areas. However, in urban health, a special emphasis is placed on describing and understanding the role of residential segregation in generating, sustaining, and even reinforcing health inequities.[23] For this reason, residential segregation, which results in differences in residential composition of areas, has implications for the environmental features of these areas and for health. Thus, residential segregation features prominently in discussions of the causes of urban health inequities.

Residential segregation is the process by which individuals are sorted into neighborhoods in a nonrandom manner based on a complex set of factors often operating over long periods involving economic resources and costs, personal preferences, decisions by government and others about investments, and social processes linked to racism and discrimination at the individual and institutional levels. Residential segregation thus results in marked differences in the socioeconomic, race, and ethnic composition of various neighborhoods within cities, sometimes referred to as the social differentiation of urban space.[24]

Residential segregation by socioeconomic position, and often also by race, ethnicity, and immigration history, is a prominent feature of urban areas across the world, although the form and intensity of residential segregation varies across countries and over time.[25-27] For example, in the past many US cities were characterized by segregation patterns in which lower income and often Black, Latino, or Asian residents tended to be clustered in the central areas of cities, whereas whites were more clustered in peripheral and suburban areas. These patterns resulted from a complex set of historical processes including redlining, differential investments and location of public housing, and racism, among others. More recently these patterns have started to change, resulting in greater concentrations of wealthy Whites in central areas and displacement of lower-income and Black and Latino residents to suburban cores.[25] This change is closely linked to the process of gentrification of previously poor central urban areas. We will discuss gentrification and its implications for health later in this chapter.

Figure 4.8 illustrates some of the dynamic processes linking residential segregation to health and health inequities, and the measurement of residential segregation is discussed in Box 4.3.

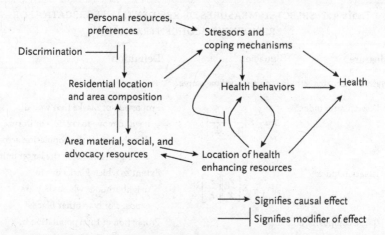

Figure 4.8 Dynamic relations linking residential segregation to health.[28]
Source: Diez Roux AV. Complex systems thinking and current impasses in health disparities research. *American Journal of Public Health.* 2011;101(9):1627–1634.

As shown in Figure 4.8, persons are sorted into neighborhoods on the basis of preferences and resources, which can be modified by the impact of discrimination via contemporary or historic processes. Area composition (such as the percent of low-income residents) affects the material and advocacy power of residents, which, in turn, reinforces segregation and differences in area composition. The advocacy power of residents affects the location of services and other health related factors (e.g., stores offering high-quality healthy food tend to locate in wealthier neighborhoods and hazardous industries tend to locate in lower-income areas). The presence of these amenities and hazards, in turn, reinforces differences in area housing cost (and composition). This link between the composition of an area and its environmental features—be they exposures to toxic substances or availability of health promoting resources—is at the core of the demands of the environmental justice movement.[29]

The location of services in certain areas shapes and, in turn, is reinforced by the behaviors of residents (e.g., proximity of healthy foods affects food purchasing patterns, and the purchasing behaviors of residents affect what is sold). Stress related to disadvantage, discrimination, or neighborhood factors

Box 4.3 MEASURING RESIDENTIAL SEGREGATION

Sharrelle Barber

Residential segregation is a complex construct that can be measured in several different ways. There has been significant debate on various ways to conceptualize and measure segregation.[24,30] Table 4.1 describes

Table 4.1 SELECTED MEASURES OF RESIDENTIAL SEGREGATION OR RESIDENTIAL CONCENTRATION

Measure	Equation	Definition
Metropolitan area- city- or county-level measures		
Dissimilarity index[a]	$D = \dfrac{1}{2} \sum\limits_{i=1}^{n} \left\| \dfrac{w_i}{W_T} - \dfrac{b_i}{B_T} \right\|$	Proportion of Blacks that would need to move to create a uniform distribution of the population across all neighborhoods in the larger unit
Isolation index[b]	$_xP^*_x = \sum\limits_{i=1}^{n} \left[\dfrac{x_i}{X} \right]\left[\dfrac{x_i}{t_i} \right]$	Extent to which Blacks live in neighborhoods where they are exposed only to other Blacks
Racial composition	X/T	Proportion of total population in county (T) that is Black (X)
Neighborhood-level measures		
G_i^* statistic[c]	$G_i^* = \dfrac{\sum\limits_{j=1}^{n} w_{ij}x_j - \bar{x}\sum\limits_{j=1}^{n} w_{ij}}{S\sqrt{\dfrac{[N\sum\limits_{j=1}^{n} w_{ij}^2 - (\sum\limits_{j=1}^{n} w_{ij})^2]}{N-1}}}$	Extent to which racial composition of a neighborhood and its surrounding neighborhoods deviates from composition of larger surrounding metropolitan area, city, or county
Index of concentration at the extremes	$(w-b)/t$	Extent to which Blacks (b) are concentrated into the most extreme demographic distributions, that is, mostly White (w) or mostly/all Black
Racial composition	x/t	Proportion of total population in neighborhood (t) that is Black (x)

Note: All examples in the table focus on segregation of non-Hispanic Blacks, but they can be applied to segregation of other race/ethnic groups as well as different socioeconomic groups. Note that racial composition and the index of concentration of the extremes refer to the composition of specific areas (e.g. neighborhoods). Although they are sometimes referred to as measures of segregation, they do not directly measure the presence of nonrandom distributions across broader geographic areas (like the dissimilarity index or the G statistic). Hence, they can also be more precisely referred to as measures of concentration.
[a]In equation, w = number of Whites living in neighborhood i (typically census tract), W = number of Whites living in the metropolitan area (or city or county), b = number of Blacks living in neighborhood i, and B = number of blacks living in the metropolitan area (or city or county). n is number of neighborhoods.
[b]In equation, x = number of Blacks living in neighborhood i, X = number of Blacks living in the metropolitan area, t = number of people living in neighborhood i, and N = total number of neighborhoods.
[c]In equation, w_{ij} = spatial weight linking focal neighborhood i and neighborhood j (indicates how much weight is given to spatially proximal neighborhoods when calculating the measure), x_j is the number of Blacks living in neighborhood j, $\bar{x}$ s the mean number of Blacks in the neighborhoods within the metropolitan area, and $S = \sqrt{\dfrac{\sum_{j=1}^{n} x_j^2}{N} - \bar{x}^2}$

a few selected measures of segregation that have been used in urban health studies. The measure chosen should be driven by the purpose. All examples in the table focus on segregation of non-Hispanic Blacks, but measures are also available to capture segregation of multiple race/ethnic groups as well as different socioeconomic groups.

can lead to coping behaviors, such as increasing calorie intake, that help reduce levels of stress. Although they may help reduce stress, these behaviors may also have adverse physical health effects through other mechanisms. The extent to which residents adopt certain coping behaviors in response to stress may also be modified by the environmental context. For example, residents may cope with stressors by increasing their calorie intake especially if high-calorie foods (such as fast foods) are easily available in the neighborhood. In a different neighborhood context with walkable streets and parks, more healthful coping strategies may involve physical activity and social engagement.

Other larger reinforcing loops are also possible. For example, neighborhood socioeconomic deprivation may result in greater stress, greater stress may lead to greater calorie intake, greater calorie intake may promote availability of fast-food stores, which, in turn, may drive down property prices, further increasing area deprivation. Spatial and nonspatial social networks may also create dependencies in behaviors that reinforce or buffer the impact of environmental factors. Environmental features may also interact dynamically with each other. For example, poor areas may have less accessible destinations and may also be less safe, factors that detract from walking and reinforce each other. These features may magnify residential segregation as persons with more resources and power are able to locate in and advocate for areas with better environmental attributes. In addition, less vehicle-dependence and more walking may also have consequences for changes in land use mix and safety over time.

Like many conceptual models of health inequities, Figure 4.8 highlights some key pathways but cannot represent all possible mechanisms. One important mechanism that is not reflected in the figure is the role of place-based factors in increasing vulnerability to other environmentally patterned exposures. For example, poor neighborhoods may be more vulnerable to the adverse health impacts of climate change.[31] This is because they are often located low lying areas more prone to flooding and can have less green space or tree cover and poorer insulation of homes which makes them more likely to experience high temperatures. Slum areas may also have standing water and other environmental features that can enhance the transmission of vector-borne diseases when temperatures rise. Overcrowding can impact the adverse health consequences of heat. Personal characteristics of the residents of poor neighborhoods can also interact with other exposures. For example, increased airway reactivity related to early childhood infections could magnify the adverse respiratory effects of air pollution exposures.

Although Figure 4.8 emphasizes adverse impacts of segregation, residential sorting is not inevitably linked to adverse environments. A prime example is that of immigrant enclaves which can sometimes (although not always) be linked to improved social support and healthier behaviors (such as healthier diets).[32] Thus, segregation is not inherently bad or good for health, its impact depends on the broader economic and social system in which it is embedded. In the context of structural racism, and as described in Box 4.4, segregation has been a major contributor to health inequities by race in the United States.

Sharrelle Barber

Residential segregation—defined as the systematic separation of individuals into different neighborhoods based on social class and/or race—is considered a "fundamental cause" of racial health inequalities[33] and has received considerable attention in US-based epidemiologic studies (for reviews, see Kershaw and Albrecht[34] Krieger[35] Mehra et al.,[36] Acevedo-Garcia,[37] and Kramer and Hogue[38]). The link between residential segregation and health has been explored for a wide-range of health outcomes including cardio-metabolic risk factors,[34,39-41] cardiovascular disease incidence[42] and mortality,[43,44] and adverse maternal and birth outcomes,[36] among others. The majority of empirical investigations examining links between residential segregation and health have been conducted in the United States. However, other countries that have a history of structural racism and discrimination (e.g., Brazil and South Africa) also experience racialized residential segregation and empirical research in these settings is small but growing.[22]

In the United States, residential segregation represents one manifestation of structural racism[45] with roots that can be traced back to discriminatory federal, state, and local laws and practices such as redlining (i.e., denial or limitation of financing/refinancing to certain neighborhoods based on racial/ethnic composition), restrictive covenants, and racial violence.[46] The Fair Housing Act of 1968 outlawed these discriminatory practices over 50 years ago, yet residential segregation remains one of the most pervasive hallmarks of urban areas across the country[47] and has been most persistent among Blacks. Data from the 2013–2017 American Community Survey shows that among the 51 largest metropolitan areas in the country (metropolitan areas with populations exceeding 1 million), 42 cities have a Black–White dissimilarity index over 50 with the highest Black–White segregation levels found in Milwaukee, Wisconsin (dissimilarity index = 79.8).[48] Related evidence reveals that "the average White person lives in a neighborhood that is 75% White, the average Black person lives in a neighborhood that is 45% Black, and the average Hispanic person lives in a neighborhood that is 46% Hispanic."[49] Residential segregation in its contemporary form is due, in large part, to structural barriers such as discriminatory practices within the housing market[50] and inequalities in accumulated wealth among racial/ethnic minority groups.[51]

However, residential segregation is about far more than the separation of *people*; rather, it is about the separate and unequal residential environments it creates for Blacks and other racial/ethnic minority groups.[52] Decades of disinvestment in segregated neighborhoods has resulted in the clustering of a wide array of adverse exposures in these settings including limited access to economic and educational opportunities,[53-55] limited access to health promoting resources (e.g., access to healthy foods and recreational activities),[56] limited access to high-quality healthcare,[57,58] disproportionate exposure to pollution and environmental toxins,[59-61] and poor housing quality. Moreover, high concentrations of poverty in these neighborhoods coupled with social ills such as higher rates of crime and violence,[62] overpolicing, and racialized trauma that tend to cluster in these settings[33,63] may be sources of chronic stress. This, in turn, may lead to maladaptive coping behaviors (e.g., smoking and high alcohol use) and activate the body's natural "fight or flight" mechanisms, resulting in dysregulation across multiple physiological systems and subsequent disease onset.[64] For Blacks, the impact of residential segregation is experienced across the socioeconomic continuum[65] with Black middle-class neighborhoods experiencing similar levels of economic disinvestment and health-damaging exposures, despite having lower rates of poverty.[66] In short, the deleterious neighborhood environments created by residential segregation predispose Blacks and other racial/ethnic minority populations to behavioral, biological, and psychosocial precursors that become "embodied"[67] and manifest as poor health outcomes for individuals and populations and create striking inequalities within urban settings.

Residential segregation is a complex multidimensional construct that can be defined at various levels and measured in different ways.[24,30] For example, measures for larger areas such as cities, metropolitan areas, or other larger areas such as counties in the United States characterize residential segregation for these larger areas as a whole. They can be used to compare one city to another, one metropolitan area to another, or one county to another. In contrast neighborhood-level measures of residential segregation can be used to compare one neighborhood to another within a given city, metropolitan area, or county. In addition to the geographic level to which they apply, measures of segregation differ in the aspects that they emphasize.[24,30] For example some measures emphasize whether different types of individuals (e.g., different race groups) are evenly distributed in space or clustered in space (sometimes referred to as measures of evenness or clustering). The dissimilarity index reviewed in Box 4.3 is one measure of this type. Other measures emphasize the extent to which different types of individuals are or are not isolated from each other—that is, whether they do or do or do not share the same residential areas (sometimes referred to as measures of exposure or isolation). The isolation index described in Box 4.3 is one measure of this type. Measures can also reflect the segregation of just two groups (e.g. Blacks and whites) or multiple groups (multiple race and ethnic groups). Closely related to the concept of segregation are measures of concentration that capture the composition of areas like racial composition or the index of concentration of the extremes.[68] Box 4.3 summarizes a few commonly used measures of residential segregation and residential concentration.

Much research on urban health inequities has focused on isolating the "independent" impact of neighborhood context on health inequities (after adjusting for individual-level socioeconomic position and race/ethnicity).[69] However, it is important to emphasize that health inequities in urban areas result from the combined effects of social stratification per se (which results in socioeconomic gradients with consequences for health) combined with differences in environmental exposures (broadly defined) resulting from residential segregation. Individual-level differences in social circumstances (by race or socioeconomic position), and health inequities linked to these circumstances, are thus reinforced by neighborhood social and physical environment differences. Breaking this cycle requires acting on social inequality itself as well as on residential segregation, as both approaches are complementary. We will turn to this in the next section where we discuss strategies to reduce urban health inequities.

APPROACHES TO REDUCING URBAN HEALTH INEQUITIES

Reducing health urban inequities is a complex task and requires multipronged approaches. In this section we review three broad approaches to reducing health inequities in cities. They are complementary and all require interdisciplinary teams and engagement of multiple stakeholders.

Making Urban Inequities Visible Through Description and Research

A first step in reducing urban inequities is to make them visible through description and research. The Philadelphia maps shown in Figure 4.5 and the small area life expectancy estimates created by Centers for Disease Control and Prevention[13,70] are excellent examples of how data on health inequities can be provided to community members and other urban health stakeholders so that it can be used for informational and advocacy purposes. Figure

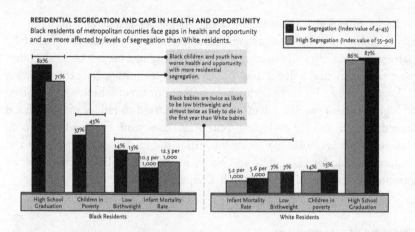

RESIDENTIAL SEGREGATION AND GAPS IN HEALTH AND OPPORTUNITY

Black residents of metropolitan counties face gaps in health and opportunity and are more affected by levels of segregation than White residents.

Legend:
- Low Segregation (Index value of 4–43)
- High Segregation (Index value of 55–90)

Black children and youth have worse health and opportunity with more residential segregation.

Black babies are twice as likely to be low birthweight and almost twice as likely to die in the first year than White babies.

Black Residents:
- High School Graduation: 82%, 71%
- Children in Poverty: 37%, 43%
- Low Birthweight: 14%, 13%
- Infant Mortality Rate: 10.3 per 1,000, 12.3 per 1,000

White Residents:
- Infant Mortality Rate: 5.2 per 1,000, 5.6 per 1,000
- Low Birthweight: 7%, 7%
- Children in poverty: 14%, 15%
- High School Graduation: 86%, 87%

Residential segregation is measured using the index of dissimilarity where higher values indicate greater residential segregation between Black and White country residents. The residential segregation index ranges from 0 (complete integration) to 100 (complete segregation). In this analysis, we measure residential segregation within smaller metro and large urban counties. To learn more about our measure of residential segregation, visit countyhealthrankings.org/segregation. Find your county's residential segregation data, and data by race for children in poverty, low birthweight and infant mortality in your county snapshot.

A CALL TO ACTION

Addressing Neighborhood Opportunity

A range of policies, programs, and systems changes are needed to ensure opportunities for good health exist in all neighborhoods. There is an array of evidence-informed approaches shown to promote inclusive and connected environments, and expand opportunities for health for all. These include:

- Ensure access to safe and affordable housing in mixed-income neighborhoods through inclusionary zoning, taxes to advance affordable housing development, and vouchers for low-income households.

- Support community development and revitalization in ways that avoid displacement of neighborhood residents through policies and incentives to increase economic opportunities, such as jobs that pay a living wage, public transportation systems, and integrated public services.

- Build social connectedness, cultivate empowered communities, and promote civic engagement by addressing barriers to participation in policymaking, information sharing, and collaboration in neighborhoods, schools, and workplaces.

For information on these and other specific strategies that have been proven to work, visit What Works for Health at countyhealthrankings.org/whatworks.

Figure 4.9 Using descriptive data to motivate action to reduce health inequities: An example from the County Health Rankins and Roadmap Initiative.[71]
Source: University of Wisconsin Population Health Institute. 2018 county health rankings key findings report. 2018; https://www.countyhealthrankings.org/resources/2018-county-health-rankings-key-findings-report.

4.9 provides examples of how the County Health Rankings and Roadmaps project,[72] a national initiative that characterizes health and health determinants across US counties, generates descriptive information on the relation between racial segregation and health that can be used by local policymakers and others to stimulate discussion and policy action on urban health inequities.

Research can also make urban health inequities visible and motivate action. For example, studies showing how environmental exposures are spatially patterned and contribute to inequities by race and income can be used to support environmental policies as a tool to reduce inequities. Research showing linkages between lot remediation and violence or mental health can be used to highlight how specific urban policies can be used to reduce neighborhood inequities in health.[73] Developing appropriate communication and dissemination strategies is critical to making inequities and related evidence visible and understandable for the public and policy makers. We return to the topic of communication and dissemination in Chapter 15.

Targeting of Interventions

Some aspects of urban health inequities can be addressed through targeted place-based interventions. Two examples of this approach include slum upgrading in low- and middle-income countries and comprehensive interventions to improve neighborhood conditions in deprived neighborhoods of high-income countries.

Slum upgrading is defined by UN Habitat as

> a process through which informal areas are gradually improved, formalized and incorporated into the city itself, through extending land, services and citizenship to slum dwellers. It involves providing slum dwellers with the economic, social, institutional and community services available to other citizens. These services include legal (land tenure), physical (infrastructure), social (such as crime or education) or economic.[74]

Table 4.2 provides examples of how select components of slum upgrading interventions may impact health.

There is a long tradition of place-based interventions aimed at promoting equity in cities of low- and middle-income countries through upgrading of slums or informal settlements. Examples include the Vila Viva program in Belo Horizonte Brazil,[75] the Neighborhood Recovery Program (Recuperación de Barrios) in Santiago Chile,[76] Kenya's Slum Upgrading Programme,[77] and India's Sum Networking Project.[78] These programs generally include components such as physical improvements of streets and housing, improved access to adequate water and sanitation, social services and job training, and participatory engagement of residents.[79,80] Other examples of place-based interventions with a strong equity component include transportation initiatives like the Metrocable in Medellin[81] or the recent TransMiCable in Bogota[82] aimed at improving public transportation access for disadvantaged neighborhoods located in the periphery of cities.

Table 4.2 EXAMPLES OF HOW SELECT COMPONENTS OF SLUM UPGRADING
INTERVENTIONS MAY IMPACT HEALTH

Slum Upgrading Characteristics (Select)	Health Influences (Examples)
Community empowerment and political recognition via participatory upgrading	Trust, empowerment, control of life decisions
Right to remain (in situ upgrading)	Social connections, collective efficacy, no fear of displacement
Housing improvements and land tenure	Reduced anxiety from fear of displacement, address can result in social services, access to banking, etc.
Safety and security	Reduced gender-based violence, reduced physical violence, improved mental health
Integration of slums into formal city	Transportation and access to employment, education and services, reduced isolation and segregation
Poverty reduction	Income for food, electricity, and other services
Climate change resilience	Reduced health impacts from flooding, heat events, or water scarcity due to drought

Source: Corburn et al.[1]

Initiatives in high-income countries have also focused on comprehensive improvements to deprived neighborhoods. One prominent example is the La Lei de Barrios in Barcelona, Spain.[83] The La Lei de Barrios initiative was focused on the Ciutat Vella region, an inner-city district where poor and minority communities have been increasingly concentrated. Comprehensive interventions were implemented in 117 neighborhoods experiencing high levels of social deprivation from 2004 to 2010.[84] The intervention included (i) improvements to public spaces and green spaces; (ii) physical renovations; (iii) the provision of community facilities; (iv) enhanced communication technologies; (v) implementation and improvement of energy and environmental infrastructure; (vi) the promotion of public spaces; (vii) social, economic, and urban development programs; and (viii) the facilitation of physical accessibility.[84] Another example is the GoWell urban regeneration project in Glasgow Scotland.[85]

An important challenge is the evaluation of the health impact of these interventions. Although some evaluations of slum upgrading programs have been performed, there is still limited empirical evidence of their health effects.[80] An evaluation of the La Lei de Barrios program found that self-rated physical and mental health significantly improved in neighborhoods in which projects were implemented.[83] However, other initiatives have been more difficult to evaluate.[85] Careful planning and partnerships between policymakers, communities, and researchers is critical to generating the evidence base needed to advocate for or modify these policies and interventions so that they can significantly promote health equity in urban areas.

Addressing Fundamental Social Causes of Urban Health Inequities

Eliminating health inequities requires addressing the fundamental drivers of inequities, which are rooted in social inequality. In this sense, urban health inequities are no different than health inequities generally. In urban environments, these fundamental social causes can be addressed through urban policies that impact income and poverty, housing, education, work, and neighborhood conditions, as well as social exclusion, racism, and multiple forms of discrimination. Given their population concentration, urban spaces also provide important opportunities for place-based actions that can reduce health inequities. Place-based approaches can include, for example, neighborhood and community development initiatives (e.g., strengthening of community advocacy groups) and physical improvements to neighborhoods (e.g., urban greening and bike lanes), as well as zoning, regulation, and subsidies (e.g., restricting the density of tobacco outlets and promoting the sale of fresh fruits and vegetables). The urban health in all urban policies approach introduced in Chapter 3 and reviewed in more detail in Chapter 14 is intended to ensure that multisectoral policies are leveraged to reduce urban health often with explicit attention to health inequities.

As we have reviewed earlier in this chapter a key fundamental cause of urban health inequities is residential segregation. The adverse health effects of residential segregation can be addressed by intervening directly on the neighborhood conditions with which segregation is often linked (as reviewed in the section on targeted interventions) or by incentivizing mixed income neighborhoods. One mechanism to promote mixed income neighborhoods is the provision of vouchers that can be used by low-income families to move into neighborhoods that are higher income. The Moving to Opportunity Experiment is one example of this approach.[86] The Moving to Opportunity Experiment found beneficial health effects among women (including reduced risk of diabetes and obesity and improved mental health) and female youth (improved mental health) but some adverse effects among male youth (worse physical health).[87] These results suggest that attention to unintended consequences is important when developing and implementing these types of interventions.

An important unintended consequence of promotion of mixed income housing as well as of interventions in neighborhoods themselves (including those that target the physical conditions of neighborhoods) is gentrification. Gentrification also often occurs as a result of real estate speculation and public policies that promote the real estate development of low-income, often minority neighborhoods. The definitions, causes, and consequences of gentrification have long been debated.[88]

But, in general, gentrification can be thought of as a neighborhood change process that occurs over a period of time, measurable in three predominant ways: (i) compositional demographic shifts in a neighborhood

---

Box 4.5 GENTRIFICATION: EXPLORING THE RELATIONSHIP BETWEEN NEIGHBORHOOD CHANGE, DISPLACEMENT, AND HEALTH

Malo A. Hutson and Carolyn B. Swope

There has recently been increasing concern among policymakers, practitioners, and academics regarding the impact of gentrification on urban residents.[89-91] However, to date, few studies have investigated the impact of gentrification on health.[92] This gap is particularly noteworthy given that the few studies that have been conducted indicate that there indeed appear to be health implications. For example, Gibbons and Barton[93] and Izenberg et al.[94] found that gentrification leads to worse self-rated health for Black residents, but not for residents overall, and Huynh and Maroko[95] found higher risk of preterm birth for Blacks, but not Whites, in gentrified neighborhoods.

There are several mechanisms through which gentrification could impact health. Rents typically rise in gentrifying neighborhoods, which may make it difficult for lower-income original residents to afford their homes. Housing unaffordability experiences are associated with poorer self-rated health, hypertension and arthritis, food insecurity, and forgoing needed medical care.[96] Investigative journalists frequently report landlords disinvesting in maintenance, because they have an incentive for tenants to leave so that they can replace them with higher-paying newcomers.[97] Resulting poor conditions, such as mold or thermal discomfort, are associated with a range of adverse health outcomes.[98]

At a greater extreme, residents could be displaced from their homes and need to move. Quantifying displacement caused by gentrification is controversial: while some researchers find evidence of displacement, others find that displacement is minimal or even lower than in comparable nongentrifying neighborhoods.[99] However, if displacement does occur, it could have health implications. Research on other examples of involuntary displacement has identified a number of ways that it affects health, including stress; move to new housing or neighborhoods that have characteristics associated with poorer health outcomes; disruption of health-protective resources such as social supports; and use of limited resources on resettlement rather than on health-related advantages.[100-102]

Research that examines the effects of gentrification on original residents who remain in the neighborhood suggests that symbolic displacement also often occurs. Such residents experience a loss of place that includes physical, political, social, and cultural components. Beyond the neighborhood's demographic make-up, its amenities, gathering places, and norms of public behavior often change to reflect the preferences of newcomers, who may have disproportionate decision-making power relative to the socially marginalized long-term residents.[103-106]

As new, dissimilar residents move in and other long-term residents move out, long-standing social networks are fractured, removing social support, which has been linked to health. Such social supports may be particularly important for marginalized low-income residents (e.g., by providing otherwise unaffordable child care that is needed to enable caregivers to work outside the home). Community gathering spaces may close,[105] which could erode social cohesion.

Additionally, original residents may face increased exposure to racial discrimination[107] and its adverse health consequences. Members of marginalized racial groups persistently experience and use high-effort and health-compromising coping to manage discrimination and related stressors. These chronic stressors cumulatively disrupt regulation of systems throughout the body and impose a physiological burden that has health consequences.[108] For example, policing has been found to increase in gentrifying neighborhoods.[109] Such increased policing, especially when racially discriminatory, can affect mental or physical health through injury from police brutality or stress due to or in anticipation of a discriminatory policing incident affecting the individual or a loved one.[110]

At the same time that long-standing residents are losing health-protective social and institutional resources, qualitative research indicates that these original residents are excluded from new amenities because of affordability or other alignment with the interests of newcomers.[104,106]

It is important to note that there are also pathways through which gentrification could be hypothesized to benefit the health of original residents who remain, since newer residents' political and cultural capital could bring community improvements to historically marginalized neighborhoods.[104] However, eliminating health-compromising neighborhood characteristics may fuel more rapid gentrification and displacement related to housing conditions and affordability. For example, mitigation of hazardous waste sites has been found to raise housing prices and subsequently lead to increased demographic change and displacement. Anguelovski[111] even argues for reconceptualizing such greening initiatives as new locally unwanted land uses, "green LULUs," because their impact on community stability and resilience is even greater than that of the previous toxic waste sites. Regardless, residents can only accrue such benefits if they are not displaced.

(specifically marked changes in the race or income of residents); (ii) increased property values; and (iii) physical signs of reinvestment, including improved streetscape appearance, beautification, access to healthy food and physical activity resources, and/or signs of housing investment.[112] The key adverse effect of gentrification is the displacement of low-income and non-White residents out of the neighborhoods that are experiencing improvements to their environments. Gentrification can therefore reinforce residential segregation. For this reason, efforts to address residential segregation or neighborhood conditions as a way to reduce health inequities must set in place mechanisms to prevent displacement. The complex ways in which gentrification can affect the health of displaced and nondisplaced original residents is described in more detail in Box 4.5.

URBAN HEALTH INEQUITIES AS A MAJOR CHALLENGE FOR URBAN HEALTH

As discussed in this chapter, urban health inequities are large and pervasive in urban areas all over the world. Their causes are structural and multifactorial, and they manifest themselves across the life course and for many different health outcomes. These inequities are the result of the systems that drive population health in urban areas. The policies and interventions needed to reduce health inequities are necessarily multisectoral and require action on upstream factors outside the purview of the traditional health-care sector or health-care policy. Yet urban health inequities can change and evolve over time, and they are actionable via policy and interventions. Creating continuing awareness of urban health inequities and their causes and motivating, monitoring, and evaluating actions to reduce these inequities remain critical priorities for urban heath researchers and practitioners all over the world.

REFERENCES

1. Whitehead M. *The Concepts and Principles of Equity and Health*. Copenhagen: World Health Organisation; 1990.
2. Braveman P, Arkin E, Orelans T, Plough A. *What Is Health Equity? And What Difference Does a Definition Make?* Princeton, NJ: Robert Wood Johnson Foundation; 2017.
3. Ingram DD, Franco SJ. NCHS urban-rural classification scheme for counties. *Vital and Health Statistics Series 2, Data Evaluation and Methods Research*. 2012(154):1–65.
4. Meit M, Knudson A, Gilbert T, et al. *The 2014 update of the rural–urban chartbook*. Rural Health Research and Policy Centers. October 2014; https://ruralhealth.und.edu/projects/health-reform-policy-research-center/pdf/2014-rural-urban-chartbook-update.pdf.

5. United Nations Department of Economic and Social Affairs Population Division. World urbanization prospects: The 2018 revision, online edition. 2018; https://population.un.org/wup/Download/.

6. UN-Habitat. *World Cities Report* 2016: *Urbanization and Development–Emerging Futures*. Nairobi, Kenya: United Nations Human Settlements Programme; 2016.

7. Harper S, Lynch J. Health inequalities: Measurement and decomposition. *SSRN* 2016; doi:0.2139/ssrn.2887311

8. Galobardes B, Lynch J, Smith GD. Measuring socioeconomic position in health research. *British Medical Bulletin*. 2007;81-82(1):21–37.

9. Krieger N, Williams DR, Moss NE. Measuring social class in US public health research: Concepts, methodologies, and guidelines. *Annual Review of Public Health*. 1997;18(1):341–378.

10. Fleischer NL, Diez Roux AV, Alazraqui M, Spinelli H, De Maio F. Socioeconomic gradients in chronic disease risk factors in middle-income countries: Evidence of effect modification by urbanicity in Argentina. *American Journal of Public Health*. 2011;101(2):294–301.

11. Chetty R, Stepner M, Abraham S, et al. The association between income and life expectancy in the United States, 2001–2014. *JAMA*. 2016;315(16):1750.

12. Stein EM, Gennuso KP, Ugboaja DC, Remington PL. The epidemic of despair among White Americans: Trends in the leading causes of premature death, 1999–2015. *American Journal of Public Health*. 2017;107(10):1541–1547.

13. Arias E, Escobedo LA, Kennedy J, Fu C, Cisewski JA. US small-area life expectancy estimates project: Methodology and results summary. National Center for Health Statistics 2018; https://www.cdc.gov/nchs/data/series/sr_02/sr02_181.pdf

14. Virginia Commonwealth University. Mapping life expectancy: Philadelphia. April 6, 2016; https://societyhealth.vcu.edu/work/the-projects/mapsphiladelphia.html.

15. Philadelphia Department of Public Health, Drexel University Urban Health Collaborative. *Close to home: The health of Philadelphia's neighborhoods*. August 1, 2019; https://www.phila.gov/documents/close-to-home-the-health-of-philadelphias-neighborhoods/.

16. Quick H, Terloyeva D, Wu Y, Moore K, Diez Roux AV. Trends in tract-level prevalence of obesity in Philadelphia by race-ethnicity, space, and time. *Epidemiology*. 2020;31(1):15–21.

17. Pan American Health Organization. *Health in the Americas\+, 2017 edition summary: Regional outlook and country profiles*. Washington, DC: PAHO. 2017.

18. Corburn J, Cohen AK. Why we need urban health equity indicators: Integrating science, policy, and community. *PLoS Medicine*. 2012;9(8):e1001285.

19. Lein A, Slesinski C, Bilal U, Indvik K, Melly S, Diez Roux AV. Mortality and life expectancy in Latin American cities: Data from the SALURBAL project. *Urban Health Network for Latin American and the Caribbean, Data Brief*. 2019;2.

20. Bilal U, Hessel P, Ferrer CP, et al. Variation and predictors of life expectancy across 363 cities in 9 Latin American countries: the SALURBAL study. Unpublished manuscript.

21. Bilal U, Alazraqui M, Caiaffa WT, et al. Inequalities in life expectancy in six large Latin American cities from the SALURBAL study: An ecological analysis. *The Lancet: Planetary Health*. 2019;3(12):e503–e510.

22. Woolf SHB, Paula. Where health disparities begin: The role of social and economic determinants—and why current policies may make matters worse. *Health Affairs*. 2011;30(10):1852–1859.

23. Williams DR, Collins C. Racial residential segregation: A fundamental cause of racial disparities in health. *Public Health Reports*. 2001;116(5):404–416.

24. Louf R, Barthelemy M. Patterns of residential segregation. *PloS ONE*. 2016;11(6):e0157476.

25. Jonathan Spader SR. *Patterns and Trends of Residential Integration in the United States Since 2000*. Cambridge, MA: Joint Center for Housing Studies of Harvard University; 2017.

26. Sabatini F. *The Social Spatial Segregation in the Cities of Latin America*. Washington, DC: Inter-American Development Bank; 2006.

27. López-Morales E, Shin HB, Lees L. Latin American gentrifications. *Urban Geography*. 2016;37(8):1091–1108.

28. Diez Roux AV. Complex systems thinking and current impasses in health disparities research. *American Journal of Public Health*. 2011;101(9):1627–1634.

29. Corburn J. Concepts for studying urban environmental justice. *Current Environmental Health Reports*. 2017;4(1):61–67.

30. Reardon SF, O'Sullivan D. Measures of spatial segregation. *Sociological Methodology*. 2004;34(1):121–162.

31. Voelkel J, Hellman D, Sakuma R, Shandas V. Assessing vulnerability to urban heat: A study of disproportionate heat exposure and access to refuge by sociodemographic status in Portland, Oregon. *International Journal of Environmental Research and Public Health*. 2018;15(4):E640.

32. Osypuk TL, Roux AVD, Hadley C, Kandula NR. Are immigrant enclaves healthy places to live? The multi-ethnic study of atherosclerosis. *Social Science Medicine*. 2009;69(1):110–120.

33. Williams DR, Collins C. Racial residential segregation: A fundamental cause of racial disparities in health. *Public Health Reports*. 2001;116(5):404–416.

34. Kershaw K, Albrecht S. Racial/ethnic residential segregation and cardiovascular disease risk. *Current Cardiovascular Risk Reports*. 2015;9(3):1–12.

35. Krieger N. Discrimination and health inequities. *International Journal of Health Services*. 2014;44(4):643–710.

36. Mehra R, Boyd LM, Ickovics JR. Racial residential segregation and adverse birth outcomes: A systematic review and meta-analysis. *Social Science and Medicine*. 2017;191:237–250.

37. Acevedo-Garcia D, Lochner KA, Osypuk TL, Subramanian SV. Future directions in residential segregation and health research: A multilevel approach. *American Journal of Public Health*. 2003;93(2):215–221.

38. Kramer MR, Hogue CR. Is segregation bad for your health? *Epidemiologic Reviews*. 2009;31:178–194.

39. Kershaw KN, Robinson WR, Gordon-Larsen P, et al. Association of changes in neighborhood-level racial residential segregation with changes in blood pressure among black adults: The cardia study. *JAMA Internal Medicine*. 2017;177(7):996–1002.

40. Do DP, Moore K, Barber S, Diez Roux A. Neighborhood racial/ethnic segregation and BMI: A longitudinal analysis of the Multi-Ethnic Study of Atherosclerosis. *International Journal of Obesity*. 2019;43(8):1601–1610.

41. Barber S, Diez Roux AV, Cardoso L, et al. At the intersection of place, race, and health in Brazil: Residential segregation and cardio-metabolic risk factors in the Brazilian Longitudinal Study of Adult Health (ELSA-Brasil). *Social Science and Medicine*. 2018;199:67–76.

42. Kershaw KN, Osypuk TL, Do DP, De Chavez PJ, Diez Roux AV. Neighborhood-level racial/ethnic residential segregation and incident cardiovascular disease: The Multi-Ethnic Study of Atherosclerosis. *Circulation*. 2015;131(2):141–148.

43. Greer S, Kramer MR, Cook-Smith JN, Casper ML. Metropolitan racial residential segregation and cardiovascular mortality: exploring pathways. *Journal of Urban Health*. 2014;91(3):499–509.

44. Greer S, Casper M, Kramer M, et al. Racial residential segregation and stroke mortality in Atlanta. *Ethnicity and Disease*. 2011;21(4):437–443.

45. Bailey ZD, Krieger N, Agénor M, Graves J, Linos N, Bassett MT. Structural racism and health inequities in the USA: evidence and interventions. *The Lancet*. 2017;389(10077):1453–1463.

46. Rothstein R. *The Color of Law: A Forgotten History of How Our Government Segregated America*. New York: Liveright; 2017.

47. Logan JR. The persistence of segregation in the 21(st) century metropolis. *City & Community*. 2013;12(2). doi:10.1111/cico.12021.

48. Frey WH. *Black–White segregation edges downward since 2000, census shows* The Brookings Institution. December 17, 2018; https://www.brookings.edu/blog/the-avenue/2018/12/17/black-white-segregation-edges-downward-since-2000-census-shows/.

49. Logan JR, Stults B. *The Persistence of Segregation in the Metropolis: New Findings from the 2010 Census*. US2010. March 24, 2011; https://s4.ad.brown.edu/Projects/Diversity/Data/Report/report2.pdf.

50. Turner MA, Santos R, Levy D, Wissoker D, Aranda C, Pitingolo R. *Housing Discrimination Against Racial and Ethnic Minorities 2012*. Washington, DC: U.S. Department of Housing and Urban Development 2013.

51. McKernan S-M, Ratcliffe C, Steuerle E, Zhang S. *Less than Equal: Racial Inequalities in Wealth Accumulation*. Washington, DC: Urban Institute;2013.

52. Osypuk TL, Galea S, McArdle N, Acevedo-Garcia D. Quantifying separate and unequal: Racial-ethnic distributions of neighborhood poverty in metropolitan America. *Urban Affairs Review*. 2009;45(1):25–65.

53. Massey D. Residential segregation and neighborhood conditions in U.S. metropolitan areas. In: Smesler NJ, Wilson WJ, Mitchell F, eds. *America Becoming: Racial Trends and Their Consequences*. Vol 1. Washington, DC: National Academy Press; 2001.

54. Wilson WJ. *When Work Disappears: The World of the New Urban Poor*. New York: Vintage; 1996.

55. Wilson WJ. *The Truly Disadvantage: The Inner City, the Underclass and Social Policy*. Chicago: University of Chicago Press; 1987.

56. Diez Roux AV, Mair C. Neighborhoods and health. *Annals of the New York Academy of Sciences*. 2010;1186:125–145.

57. White K, Haas JS, Williams DR. Elucidating the role of place in health care disparities: The example of racial/ethnic residential segregation. *Health Services Research*. 2012;47(3 Pt 2):1278–1299.

58. Brown EJ, Polsky D, Barbu CM, Seymour JW, Grande D. Racial disparities in geographic access to primary care in Philadelphia. *Health Affairs*. 2016;35(8):1374–1381.

59. Mohai P, Pellow D, Roberts JT. Environmental Justice. *Annual Review of Environment and Resources*. 2009;34(1):405–430.

60. Bravo MA, Anthopolos R, Bell ML, Miranda ML. Racial isolation and exposure to airborne particulate matter and ozone in understudied US populations:

Environmental justice applications of downscaled numerical model output. *Environment International.* 2016;92-93:247–255.

61. Mohai P, Saha R. Which came first, people or pollution? Assessing the disparate siting and post-siting demographic change hypotheses of environmental injustice. *Environmental Research Letters.* 2015;10(11):115008.

62. Sampson RJ, Raudenbush SW, Earls F. Neighborhoods and violent crime: A multilevel study of collective efficacy. *Science.* 1997;277(5328):918–924.

63. White K, Borrell LN. Racial/ethnic residential segregation: Framing the context of health risk and health disparities. *Health and Place.* 2011;17(2):438–448.

64. Juster RP, McEwen BS, Lupien SJ. Allostatic load biomarkers of chronic stress and impact on health and cognition. *Neuroscience and Biobehavioral Reviews.* 2010;35(1):2–16.

65. Alba RD, Logan JR, Stults BJ. How segregated are middle-class African Americans? *Social Problems.* 2000;47(4):543–558.

66. Pattillo M. Black middle-class neighborhoods. *Annual Review of Sociology.* 2005;31:305–329.

67. Krieger N. *Epidemiology and the People's Health: Theory and Context.* New York: Oxford University Press; 2011.

68. Krieger N, Kim R, Feldman J, Waterman PD. Using the index of concentration at the extremes at multiple geographical levels to monitor health inequities in an era of growing spatial social polarization: Massachusetts, USA (2010–14). *International Journal of Epidemiology.* 2018;47(3):788–819.

69. Diez Roux AV, Mair C. Neighborhoods and health. *Annals of the New York Academy of Sciences.* 2010;1186(1):125–145.

70. US Centers for Disease Control and Prevention. Small-Area Life Expectancy Estimates Project (USALEEP). National Center for Health Statistics. 2018; https://www.cdc.gov/nchs/nvss/usaleep/usaleep.html.

71. University of Wisconsin Population Health Institute. *2018 county health rankings key findings report.* 2018; https://www.countyhealthrankings.org/resources/2018-county-health-rankings-key-findings-report.

72. Robert Wood Johnson Foundation, University of Wisconsin Population Health Institute. County Health Rankings and Roadmaps Program. https://www.countyhealthrankings.org/about-us. Accessed October 14, 2019.

73. Branas CC, South E, Kondo MC, et al. Citywide cluster randomized trial to restore blighted vacant land and its effects on violence, crime, and fear. *Proceedings of the National Academy of Sciences.* 2018;115(12):2946–2951.

74. Cities Alliance. Slum Upgrading Fact Sheet. https://www.citiesalliance.org/sites/default/files/CA_Images/SUFactsheet_English_0.pdf. Accessed June 25, 2020.

75. Prefeitura Belo Horizonte. Vila viva. https://prefeitura.pbh.gov.br/urbel/vila-viva. Accessed July 30, 2019.

76. Vio A, ed. *Programa Recuperación de Barrios: Lecciones Aprendidas y Buenas Prácticas.* Santiago, Chile: Gobierno de Chile, Ministerio de Vivienda y Urbanismo; 2009.

77. Meredith T, MacDonald M. Community-supported slum-upgrading: Innovations from Kibera, Nairobi, Kenya. *Habitat International.* 2017;60:1–9.

78. Das AK, Takahashi LM. Evolving institutional arrangements, scaling up, and sustainability. *Journal of Planning Education and Research.* 2009;29(2):213–232.

79. Corburn J, Sverdlik A. Slum upgrading and health equity. *International Journal of Environmental Research and Public Health.* 2017;14(4):342.

80. Turley R, Saith R, Bhan N, Rehfuess E, Carter B. Slum upgrading strategies involving physical environment and infrastructure interventions and their effects on health and socio-economic outcomes. *Cochrane Database of Systematic Reviews*. 2013;1:CD010067.

81. Brand P, Dávila JD. Mobility innovation at the urban margins. *City*. 2011;15(6): 647–661.

82. Alcaldía de Bogotá. TransMiCable le cambiará la cara a Ciudad Bolívar. 2017; https://bogota.gov.co/como-le-cambiara-la-cara-tranmicable-a-ciudad-bolivar.

83. Mehdipanah R, Rodríguez-Sanz M, Malmusi D, et al. The effects of an urban renewal project on health and health inequalities: A quasi-experimental study in Barcelona. *Journal of Epidemiology and Community Health*. 2014;68(9):811–817.

84. Nel·lo O. The challenges of urban renewal: Ten lessons from the Catalan experience. *Análise Social*. 2010;45(197):685–715.

85. Bond L, Egan M, Kearns A, Tannahill C. GoWell: The challenges of evaluating regeneration as a population health intervention. *Preventive Medicine*. 2013;57(6):941–947.

86. Leventhal T, Brooks-Gunn J. Moving to opportunity: An experimental study of neighborhood effects on mental health. *American Journal of Public Health*. 2003;93(9):1576–1582.

87. Ludwig J, Duncan GJ, Gennetian LA, et al. Long-term neighborhood effects on low-income families: Evidence from moving to opportunity. *American Economic Review Papers and Proceedings*. 2013;103(3):226–231.

88. Zuk M, Bierbaum AH, Chapple K, Gorska K, Loukaitou-Sideris A. Gentrification, displacement, and the role of public investment. *Journal of Planning Literature*. 2018;33(1):31–44.

89. O'Brien M. Alameda County: Gentrification could be hurting public health. *The Mercury News*. April 7, 2014.

90. Centers for Disease Control and Prevention. Health effects of gentrification. 2009; https://www.cdc.gov/healthyplaces/healthtopics/gentrification.htm.

91. Atkinson R, Wulff M, Reynolds M, Spinney A. Gentrification and displacement: The household impacts of neighbourhood change. *AHURI Final Report*. 2011;160:1–89.

92. Tulier ME, Reid C, Mujahid MS, Allen AM. "Clear action requires clear thinking": A systematic review of gentrification and health research in the United States. *Health Place*. 2019;59:102173.

93. Gibbons J, Barton MS. The association of minority self-rated health with Black versus White gentrification. *Journal of Urban Health*. 2016;93(6):909–922.

94. Izenberg JM, Mujahid MS, Yen IH. Health in changing neighborhoods: A study of the relationship between gentrification and self-rated health in the state of California. *Health and Place*. 2018;52:188–195.

95. Huynh M, Maroko AR. Gentrification and preterm birth in New York City, 2008–2010. *Journal of Urban Health*. 2013;91(1):211–220.

96. Pollack CE, Griffin BA, Lynch J. Housing affordability and health among homeowners and renters. *American Journal of Preventive Medicine*. 2010;39(6):515–521.

97. Schumaker E. Diagnosing gentrification. *Huffington Post*. February 12, 2018; https://www.huffingtonpost.com/entry/diagnosing-gentrification-health_us_5a7c3af9e4b0c6726e0fd9ec.

98. Krieger J, Higgins DL. Housing and health: Time again for public health action. *American Journal of Public Health*. 2002;92(5):758–768.

99. Brown-Saracino J. Explicating divided approaches to gentrification and growing income inequality. *Annual Review of Sociology.* 2017;43(1):515–539.

100. Fullilove MT. Root shock: The consequences of African American dispossession. *Journal of Urban Health.* 2001;78(1):72–80.

101. Fussell E, Lowe SR. The impact of housing displacement on the mental health of low-income parents after Hurricane Katrina. *Social Science and Medicine.* 2014;113:137–144.

102. Keene DE, Geronimus AT. "Weathering" HOPE VI: The importance of evaluating the population health impact of public housing demolition and displacement. *Journal of Urban Health.* 2011;88(3):417–435.

103. Atkinson R. Losing one's place: Narratives of neighbourhood change, market injustice and symbolic displacement. *Housing, Theory and Society.* 2015;32(4):373–388.

104 Hyra D. The back-to-the-city movement: Neighbourhood redevelopment and processes of political and cultural displacement. *Urban Studies.* 2014;52(10):1753–1773.

105. Parekh T. "They want to live in the Tremé, but they want it for their ways of living": Gentrification and neighborhood practice in Tremé, New Orleans. *Urban Geography.* 2014;36(2):201–220.

106. Shaw KS, Hagemans IW. "Gentrification without displacement" and the consequent loss of place: The effects of class transition on low-income residents of secure housing in gentrifying areas. *International Journal of Urban and Regional Research.* 2015;39(2):323–341.

107. Shmool JLC, Yonas MA, Newman OD, et al. Identifying perceived neighborhood stressors across diverse communities in New York City. *American Journal of Community Psychology.* 2015;56(1-2):145–155.

108. Geronimus AT, Hicken M, Keene D, Bound J. "Weathering" and age patterns of allostatic load scores among Blacks and Whites in the United States. *American Journal of Public Health.* 2006;96(5):826–833.

109. Laniyonu A. Coffee shops and street stops: Policing practices in gentrifying neighborhoods. *Urban Affairs Review.* 2017;54(5):898–930.

110. Alang S, McAlpine D, McCreedy E, Hardeman R. Police brutality and Black health: Setting the agenda for public health scholars. *American Journal of Public Health.* 2017;107(5):662–665.

111. Anguelovski I. From toxic sites to parks as (green) LULUs? New challenges of inequity, privilege, gentrification, and exclusion for urban environmental justice. *Journal of Planning Literature.* 2015;31(1):23–36.

112. Hirsch JA, Schinasi LH. *A Measure of Gentrification for Use in Longitudinal Public Health Studies Based in the United States.* Philadelphia, PA: Drexel University Urban Health Collaborative;2019.

PART II

Identifying and Collecting Data for Urban Health Research

"Science is simply common sense at its best, that is, rigidly accurate in observation, and merciless to fallacy in logic."

—Thomas Henry Huxley

Identifying the most appropriate answers to pressing urban health questions requires data on urban places, how humans react to and utilize such places, and population-based health outcomes. In this section, we emphasize approaches that are relevant to systematically gathering information from multiple sources, which creates the opportunity to subject our assumptions and hypotheses to rigorous real-world testing. Both quantitative and qualitative data play a crucial role in the evidence base to inform strategies to make the urban environment more health supportive. This data allow us to describe reality, generate new knowledge, and evaluate actions. Thus, data can shed light on the pathways linking multilevel urban environment characteristics to multiple health outcomes and on the impact of interventions.

CHAPTER 5

Assessment of the Urban Environment

Measurement Scales, Modes, and Metrics

GINA S. LOVASI

Environmental variation both across and within cities shapes the experience and health of human populations in these settings. Selected examples of what we might measure in the urban environment are shown in Table 5.1. In this chapter, we illustrate the scope and challenges of systematic urban environment assessment and provide guidance on existing resources and emerging tools.

WHY MEASURE THE URBAN ENVIRONMENT

While the specific motivations for assembling data on the urban environment vary widely, we can distinguish these into two broad groupings with implications for our approach to assembling data.

First, some assessments of the environment within a given neighborhood or city reflect an investment in understanding and describing that specific context. Measures of the urban environment can serve to describe variation of health-relevant features of the local area to inform programs and policies, as would often be the case when including urban environmental measures in a community health needs assessment. Likewise, data collection on urban places as a component of an evaluation can help to uncover the setting-specific considerations relevant to understanding consequences of local programs or policies for health. Thus, we can assemble health-relevant data on the urban

Gina S. Lovasi, *Assessment of the Urban Environment* In: *Urban Public Health*. Edited by: Gina S. Lovasi, Ana V. Diez Roux, and Jennifer Kolker, Oxford University Press (2021). © Oxford University Press 2021. DOI: 10.1093/oso/9780190885304.003.0005.

Table 5.1 SELECTED EXAMPLES OF VARIATION IN THE URBAN
ENVIRONMENT THAT MATTERS FOR HEALTH AND CAN BE
SYSTEMATICALLY ASSESSED

Example Measure	Why It Matters for Health	Possible Ways to Assess Variation
Concentrated poverty	A strong socioeconomic gradient is observed for many health outcomes, owing to a combination of material deprivation, social stressors, and processes mediated by individual and collective action	Population census data collected by the government
Availability of healthy food stores	Although food shopping need not necessarily take place locally and cost may be a more important factor than local availability, local availability of supermarkets and other sources of fresh foods may reduce travel time and facilitate intake of nutrient rich foods and a healthy body weight, with consequences for cardiovascular health and other chronic diseases	Obtain via open data portals tools such as the US Department of Agriculture food atlas data; use commercially licensed retail data
Trees, grass, and other green spaces	Availability of green spaces may support physical activity (particularly in the case of large parks available for recreational use) as well as providing psychological benefits such as helping residents recover from stress	Satellite or fly-over imagery to capture land cover, either for green space generally or for more specific measures such as tree canopy coverage
Ambient outdoor levels of particulate air pollution or pollen	Inhaled irritants can exacerbate asthma and other respiratory conditions, and some types of air pollution have strong links to cardiovascular, cancer, and even neurocognitive outcomes	Monitoring using sensors or other devices at fixed locations (see Box 5.1), attached to vehicles, or via personal wear
Neighborhood physical disorder, which captures deterioration or neglect of urban streets and incivilities	Physical disorder may signal a lack of safety and social control, discouraging pedestrian physical activity and reducing health-supportive social interactions among residents	In person or virtual audits (see Box 5.2) of urban streets

environment to address questions such as what is needed here? What happened here and why? For such purposes, getting locally appropriate and detailed data are especially crucial.

Second, beyond or alongside a focus on a given geographic context, we may seek generalizable insights. We might capture variation to further explore the posited connection of area-based change—such as slum upgrading, urban greening, or traffic control—to health, or to identify urban areas at high risk for a given health outcome so as to target program outreach or policy initiatives. Thus, we can address more etiologic questions such as, Does changing urban environments in a certain way lead to more of this health outcome? We can also address descriptive and health equity questions that rely on comparisons across settings, such as, Do disadvantaged populations more often live in harmful contexts, and under what circumstances are such resulting health inequities likely to be attenuated? For such purposes, getting theoretically relevant and consistent data is especially crucial.

As we have reviewed in Chapter 3, the urban environment affects health through multiple pathways including features of urban physical and social environments. Understanding these pathways requires assessment of the health-relevant aspects of the urban environment. Further, making the drivers of health visible can provide an impetus for action.

WHERE AND AT WHAT LEVEL TO MEASURE URBAN FEATURES

The geographic scope and the domains of interest will be driven not only by the goals of the measurement but also by which contrasts are of interest. Planning which urban areas to measure involves addressing questions of geographic extent, level of measurement, and sampling (Table 5.2).

How Widely to Gather Data?

An important guiding consideration is the geographic extent to include. While some efforts to capture environmental variation relevant to health are highly localized, others are national, regional, or even global in scope. Where field work or local partnerships are needed, proximity to the urban health team may limit the range of areas to include. Larger projects that span multiple cities or countries face challenges with comparability of data sources and with communication across a team that may span multiple languages, time zones, and cultures.[1,2] Yet, encompassing a greater area captures more variation and can allow for exploration across multiple levels of geographic organization.

Table 5.2 CONSIDERATIONS FOR WHERE TO ASSESS THE
URBAN ENVIRONMENT

Guiding Question	Perspectives and Priorities to Consider
How big should the study area be? (geographic extent)	Logistical and resource constraints
	Proximity to team and key partners
	Interest in variation across multiple levels
What units of observation should be compared? (level)	Alignment with aims
	Availability of data
	Theoretically appropriate based on pathway of influence on health
	Socially or politically meaningful
	Flexibility to consider multiple levels
Which units in the study area should be assessed? (sampling)	Where cost per unit is low, include all observable units (a census)
	For representativeness, consider random or stratified random sample
	Purposive samples to maximize variation in environmental conditions
	Avoid restricting sample in ways that preclude comparisons of interest
	For efficiency, concentrate observations where population is concentrated

How to Define the Set of Urban Areas to Be Observed?

The urban geographic units of interest can vary in level from entire cities (see discussion of city definitions in Chapter 1) to neighborhoods to specific places such as playgrounds. Central consideration should be given to what set of urban areas is best aligned with the project aims. Since one purpose for measuring the variation across geographic units may be to provide insights into how urban environments contribute to local population health outcomes, alignment with the scale of available health data may guide the choice of units. Often, considerations for data availability favor the use of administrative units such as municipalities, postal codes, or census areas. However, such units may not necessarily capture the most theoretically relevant spatial context when it comes to explaining health effects (e.g., social definitions of neighborhoods may be more relevant to some causal pathways that act through resident perception as discussed in Chapter 6, or in the context of community partnerships as discussed in Chapter 13).

Selecting the level of measurement could also be informed by the perspectives of decision makers in a position to use the resulting information (see Chapter 14). Measuring units that are politically meaningful can help bridge research efforts to subsequent action strategies. As such, city council districts, city planning districts, or municipal boundaries may be especially relevant to some channels of dissemination and advocacy.

Beyond administrative and political boundaries, in studies linking measures of urban environments to individual level data (such as survey or cohort data), geographic units can be personalized based on home address or other locations. Commonly this involves a circular buffer based on distance from the home, though elaborations are possible to account for street networks or for a second location such as school or work.[3] A schematic representation illustrating the range of such personalized neighborhood definitions is shown in Figure 5.1.

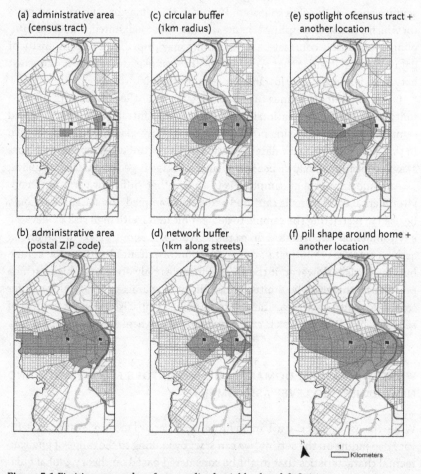

(a) administrative area (census tract)

(b) administrative area (postal ZIP code)

(c) circular buffer (1km radius)

(d) network buffer (1km along streets)

(e) spotlight ofcensus tract + another location

(f) pill shape around home + another location

Figure 5.1 Fictitious examples of personalized neighborhood definitions.
Source: Created by Steve Melly. Adapted from Lovasi GS, Grady S, Rundle A. Steps forward: Review and recommendations for research on walkability, physical activity and cardiovascular health. *Public Health Reviews.* 2012;33(2):484–506.

Measurement of the environment need not be at a single level, and indeed patterns observed across cities or neighborhoods may direct attention to the variation across smaller geographic units.

Observe All Areas or Select a Sample?

Once a geographic extent and level of measurement have been identified, a further consideration is whether all geographic units can be assessed, as may be the case for some secondary data sources such as a population census.

When primary data collection is planned and the cost per area assessed is higher, there may be advantages to focusing attention on a sampled subset of geographic units. Where the units have already been enumerated and characterized, simple random sampling is possible and can help to ensure the representativeness of the data collected. However, there may be strategic contrasts for which a random sampling scheme would not be well-suited. Stratified sampling or purposive contrast-based sampling may prioritize a high intensity of data collection in areas that are of special interest (e.g., to explore the contrast between high income vs. low income neighborhoods).

Other sampling schemes may concentrate data collection efforts in proximity to where the population is concentrated. In contrast, spatially dispersed sampling (such as assessing points along a regularly spaced grid, as discussed in the section on primary data collection across entire urban spaces or across sampled locations) may be used to ensure coverage is geographically inclusive.

An important goal of sampling is to ensure that sufficient variation in environmental conditions is captured across the sampled units. Caution should be used in restricting the sample to geographic units with high risk or elevated environmental exposures. For example, concern about elevated childhood asthma rates may motivate an investigation of potential geographic contributions to risk. However, if the sample includes only areas with high asthma prevalence, there will be limited opportunity to characterize how these differ from areas with low rates. The ability to make comparisons across a range of settings with different risk is crucial to many urban health research questions.

WHAT TO MEASURE: DOMAINS AND INDICATORS FOR CITYWIDE AND NEIGHBORHOOD LEVEL ASSESSMENT

While the aspects of the urban environment that are most relevant to health vary depending on the setting, we can start by looking to the range of environmental characteristics that might be considered based on theory, global guidance, and precedent. From there, a locally tailored plan for what to measure about the environment can be created.

Theory-relevant measures can be selected with an eye to the pathways and frameworks discussed in Chapter 3. Importantly, frameworks may expand our view toward consideration of upstream determinants and downstream consequences of the environmental characteristics of interest, as well as the conditions that may amplify or attenuate a posited health effect.

Globally, measures relevant to health have been identified both at the city-level and for smaller geographic units. The World Health Organization report on environmental health indicators highlights sociodemographic context, shelter, sanitation, access to safe drinking water, food safety, vector control, exposure to air pollution and other hazardous substances, and injury risk environments as key domains.[4] Through the Sustainable Development Goals (introduced in Chapter 2, Box 2.4), the United Nations Development Programme has articulated targets across several domains with clear relevance to the health of current and future urban populations, including indicators for sustainable cities and communities and for good health and well-being.

Looking to prior work in a similar national context can also be useful. For example, a US-based effort to assess neighborhood-level variation may be guided by noting indicators identified by organizations such as the National Neighborhood Indicators Partnership[5] and the Community Indicators Consortium.[6] While measures commonly deployed in neighborhood-level studies in the United States echo many globally relevant domains, particular emphasis has been noted on area-based socioeconomic characteristics, racial or ethnic composition, social environment, and aspects of the built environment relevant to physical activity, food environment, health-care access, and community violence.[7]

Organizations at a local level can also inform domains of interest. An example includes the Bay Area Regional Health Inequities Initiative,[8] which has developed a guide to indicators organized into economic, service, social, and physical domains.

Domains identified globally, nationally, and locally should be viewed with awareness of the need to adapt indicators and measurement approaches to specific population groups. For example, the American Association of Retired Persons Livability Index is particularly designed to capture aspects of the environment relevant to older adults.[9] Indicators or measurement approaches may likewise require adaptation to urban setting types presenting distinct challenges, such as informal settlements, also known as slums,[10-12] helping to identify not only the contrast between formal and informal areas, but also the variation among and within informal settlements.

Finally, the concerns and priorities of the research team, policy and community partner organizations, and residents themselves may guide a shift overtime in the domains included, raising trade-offs between agility to accommodate emerging topics of interest and consistency to allow time trends and

Table 5.3 IDENTIFYING WHICH DOMAINS TO INCLUDE FOR URBAN ENVIRONMENT ASSESSMENT	
Guiding Question	Considerations
Why is urban environment being assessed?	Project-specific goals and research question type
	Theoretical considerations relevant to descriptive, causal, or evaluation question
How can the domains being considered be broadened and aligned with other efforts?	Global or national guidance documents
	Previous research in similar urban settings
	Frameworks or theory of influence on health
How should the domains to be assessed be narrowed or tailored to the local context?	Relevance to identified population groups of interest, such as older adults
	Applicability to setting type, such as informal settlements
	Data availability and variation across the geographic units and time period of interest
	Concerns and priorities raised by research, policy, or community stakeholders

longitudinal analyses. Table 5.3 summarizes factors that may be considered in identifying the domains for measurement.

The Underlying Spatial Pattern for Selected Environmental Indicators Affects Options for Measurement

In planning work with diverse measures of the urban environment, there may be value in considering how the construct of interest varies spatially. A proposed categorization[13] of measures that may be useful distinguishes area-based, event-based, field, and flow types (Table 5.4).

Area-based characteristics are typically assigned to a set of mutually exclusive geographic units with specified boundaries and are further distinguished into integral and derived characteristics.[14] While derived characteristics are based on the aggregated characteristics of area residents, integral characteristics are not reducible to the individual level. For example, the proportion of individuals who smoke cigarettes would be a derived area-based characteristic, whereas a city-wide ban on smoking in bars and restaurants[15] would be an example of an integral area-based characteristic.

Events, for which locations are observable, can be overlaid with and counted within any geographic units, including those that are administratively defined or within personalized neighborhood or activity space areas.[3] Examples taking the form of events include traffic collision locations used to construct a traffic hazard measure[16] and physical activity program sites.[17]

Table 5.4 TYPOLOGY OF URBAN ENVIRONMENT MEASURES BASED
ON SPATIAL DISTRIBUTION

	Notes on Spatial Distribution	Implications for Data Acquisition
Area-based: derived	From the individual level, these have been aggregated to geographic units.	Derived measures are often based on a population census or survey.
Area-based: integral	These are irreducibly area-based, such as policies governing specific jurisdictions.	An understanding of how such characteristics arise may inform the geographic units for measurement.
Event	Events are commonly represented on maps as points, and further have a distinct temporal star.	The pattern of events seen may be geographically stable over time, or may be sensitive to the period of observation selected; often a population census-based denominator is used to create an event rate.
Field	The underlying variation may can be considered as an unseen topographic map, estimated using point-based monitoring and spatial interpolation	Sparse sampling of a field may lead to some spatial variation being overlooked or oversmoothed.
Flow	Directionality from a source to a destination can be represented through arrows, with thickness to show the volume of goods or populations	Documentation should clarify whether the total flow of persons or goods is reflected (which may allow both directions to be represented), as opposed to the net flow.

Fields have underlying variation that is continuous in space, for which observations at specific locations may provide insight into the underlying contours. Without observing every possible point in the urban environment, it may nonetheless be possible to estimate what the observed exposure would have been at unobserved points. Kernel smoothing and kriging can be used for such spatial interpolation, relying on the spatial adjacency to observed points. However, when observations are sparse relative to the underlying spatial variation, the interpolated surface may smooth out and obscure health-relevant variation. Methods such as land use regression allow for the incorporation of other spatially varying characteristics as predictors. Ground-level temperature or the concentration of particulate matter in the air are examples of field-type variation in the physical environment.

Finally, flows have directionality, and can provide insight into movement of substances or individuals, offering a dynamic understanding of the urban environment. Examples include rural-to-urban movement of populations and agricultural products and population displacement due to urban renewal or gentrification.

In the following sections, we discuss how to capture variation in the urban environment using previously assembled secondary data or through systematic collection of primary data.

SECONDARY SPATIAL DATA ON HEALTH DETERMINANTS FROM GOVERNMENTAL, OPEN, AND COMMERCIAL SOURCES

Relative ease of acquisition makes secondary spatial data a common starting point for public health efforts assessing the urban environment. Data sources include governmental agencies, data-sharing portals or nonprofit organizations promoting data access, and data access provided by private entities or using proprietary methods, for which restrictive terms of use or license fees may apply. In the following text, each is discussed with attention to both their potential strengths and relevant cautions.

Governmental Sources for Data: A Spotlight on Population Sociodemographic Characteristics

Population census data are perhaps the most used source of geographic context data. Sociodemographic characteristics of area residents commonly collected include age, poverty, and household composition. Sociodemographic characteristics can include measures that signal social disadvantage and corresponding stressors in a given setting. As discussed in Chapter 4, area-based population composition in terms of class, race, employment type may be linked to access to resources and health-supportive environments, although availability of such data varies considerably by national context.[18]

The aggregated data made available by governments for census districts or larger urban geographic units such as municipalities will often take the form of counts or proportions, such as the number of households stratified by poverty status or the proportion of households with plumbing connected to the formal sanitation infrastructure. Other manipulations of interest when working with population census data at a neighborhood level include measures of central tendency (e.g., median household income) or of isolation (e.g., distance to affluent area[19]). Population census data may also be of interest as indicators of an underlying construct such as deprivation which brings together information from several variables.[20] In addition, measures of inequality[21] or segregation[22] can be constructed within multilevel data structures.

The frequency with which governments collect population census data varies, although decennial data collection is common and has been recommended.[23] In the United States, economic and demographic data previously sourced from decennial census data have since 2006 been available from the American Communities Survey on a rolling basis.[24] Longitudinal census data, if consistently collected or longitudinally harmonized over time,[25] can be used to construct metrics of change. An increasing population density may be used to operationalize urbanization, while socioeconomic status and housing cost increases in a formerly low-income area may be labeled as gentrification.[26]

In addition to the role in characterizing the environment, population counts within demographic strata may be used as denominators when analyzing event counts; the importance of such denominators for health outcomes is discussed further in Chapter 7. While, by nature, a population census attempts to enumerate the entire population across all geographic units, undercounting or misclassification may remain important. Marginalized urban groups—including racial and ethnic minorities, impoverished households and those in transient or informal living situations—are particularly likely to be underrepresented.[27-29]

Other public sector data beyond population characteristics include data on the availability of goods and services from economic or city planning agencies. Publicly provided infrastructure such as transportation systems may be captured through publicly available data on how both access to and use of these systems varies spatially. Licensing and inspection data available public health agencies may provide insights into the spatial distribution of tobacco or alcohol sources and the condition of parks and restaurants.

The requirements for establishing data sharing agreements and access arrangements vary among governmental data sources, ranging from freely available data to download to those accessible only within a secured facility.

A key caution to keep in mind when working with governmentally sourced data, as with all secondary data sources, is that there may be limited alignment with the domains of interest. Further, consistency in the quality of data across political boundaries is challenging to assure or assess. These cautions make triangulating across alternative data sources a useful strategy.

Open Data Portals

Open data portals provide access to a range of available data, including crowdsourced data or data assembled at global, national, and local levels. Working through an authorized application programing interface is the safest way to ensure data acquisition is done in accordance with the terms of use and appropriate permissions obtained. Web-scraping from sites not designed or authorized as portals requires attention to legal requirements.

Globally, portals of city-level data may be assembled by global intergovernmental organizations such as UN Habitat. The data assembled through national efforts may allow for comparison across an entire nation (e.g., the US Department of Agriculture food atlas[30]). Of emerging importance are spatial data contributed by users such as OpenStreetMap[31] and other crowd sourced or sensor-based data,[32] which have developed data infrastructure that may be relevant to supporting participatory data collection efforts discussed in Chapter 13.

When working with open data portals, caution is warranted as data have not necessarily been validated or harmonized for comparisons across cities and countries, although standards and opportunities to improve data quality continue to be identified.[33] In some instances (e.g., the New York City Community Air Survey [NYCCAS][34]) the resolution of the data provided through open data portals is limited, and contact with the source organization can be pursued to explore further detail.

Paid Data Access Through Commercial Licensing or Contracting With Private Organizations

Commercial entities license or distribute data relevant to characterizing the urban environment, often for a fee.

Data for which there is a cost for bulk data acquisition include Web interfaces such as WalkScore[35]—a tool used to assign a number to how pedestrian supportive the surrounding environment is, expressed in values from zero to 100. Likewise, Google maintains a broad range of data, but their terms of service restrict long-term storage that would typically be required to fully leverage such data for urban health research projects. Notably, however, some noncommercial uses of data, such as for academic research, may fall under copyright allowances such as Fair Use[36] in the United States or analogous legal frameworks in other countries. Also, the geographic information system (GIS) software company Esri provides access to data elements, along with documentation that helps the user to understand the data.

Another business model is to package data access on a fee-for-service basis. For health-care organizations, such companies may provide georeferencing and linkage of patient records to a range of data sources, some of which are governmental or open source. This is an expeditious but potentially expensive alternative to contracting to academic partner organizations or developing in house GIS capacity.

Data cleaning and coding efforts can add value to such a commercially sourced urban environment data. Contextual data that are longitudinal offer extra challenges in the data cleaning and processing phase, as illustrated by work with the National Establishment Time Series data on retail across the United States.[37]

Cautions to note when working with commercially sourced data are that terms of use may impose restrictions on data sharing or integration of multiple data sources. Importantly, measures constructed by commercial entities the methods may also be proprietary and incompletely disclosed.

PRIMARY DATA COLLECTION ACROSS ENTIRE URBAN SPACES OR ACROSS SAMPLED LOCATIONS

While secondary data are useful in urban health research, several cautions and limitations have already been noted. When secondary data do not offer the needed spatial or temporal coverage, or the specific domains and indicators of interest, primary data collection may be preferred. However, given the potential for greater costs per observation, logistical considerations and trade-offs may constrain the geographic extent or number of spatial locations to observe.

To optimize the investment of time and resources for assessing the environment, complementary data may be needed on resident perspectives, and health outcomes, which are discussed in Chapters 6 and 7, respectively. However, primary data collection that focuses on the environment alone, as described in this chapter, may be a useful starting point.

For primary data collection on the urban environment, the level of measurement and sampling of urban spaces can be closely aligned with goals and priorities. A well-described plan for which areas get observed, and how each observation is conducted, is crucial to transparency and rigor of systematic observation. To illustrate how such observations take place, we highlight data collection based on remote sensing, through deployment of monitoring devices, by auditing streets or establishments, and using survey-based derived measures.

A View From the Sky: Using Satellite Imagery and Aerial Photos for Remote Sensing of Green Space and Other Physical Environment Measurement

In their raw form, stored imagery from satellites or fly-over campaigns may take the form of geographically referenced pixels with varying value across a two-dimensional representation of the ground, or occasionally throughout a three-dimensional representation of space. As an example of the latter, reflectance at different heights can be used to characterize land cover.[38] In addition, thermal spectral or multispectral imagery allows for quantification of aspects beyond the visible range, such as measurement of urban heat island effects using infrared imagery.

Remote sensing of ground conditions can be used to quantify urban green spaces, or conversely to quantify the coverage of impermeable surfaces. Metrics such as Normalized Difference Vegetation Index can be obtained or more tailored measures relevant to physical activity or psychosocial pathways to health can be created. Work to construct variables of interest such as tree canopy coverage from remote-sensing data benefit from algorithmic approaches, through processes such as object detection,[38] which may be deployed in combination with the value added through human checking and inspection. Triangulation with ground-level data can further help to quantify and understand sources of error. In addition to working with stored imagery, urban health research teams may consider deploying drones to obtain desired imagery properties and frequency. Regulations and the potential for property damage or theft should be considered in planning drone-based data collection in urban settings.[39]

Work with satellite and aerial imagery to estimate conditions experienced on the ground is included here with our discussion of primary data collection with attention to the substantial data manipulation and value added in the process of some research applications. However, we also note that data derived from such imagery may be also at times be accessible as secondary data, such as through open data portals. In addition, the use of satellite imagery in identifying boundaries of built-up urban areas was discussed in Part I (Box 1.3 and Box 2.1).

Device-Based Environmental Monitoring of Ambient Physical Conditions

Despite the potential for satellite imagery and fly-over data to inform estimation of a range of physical environment conditions including air pollution,[40] monitoring ground conditions remains an important strategy. Sensors and related technologies continue to evolve, making monitoring more efficient.[41]

While relevant global, regional and national data have been compiled to monitor conditions and compliance with standards, cities have led the way in creating outdoor air quality data resources useful for studying within city differences, as illustrated by the NYCCAS.[42] Beyond size fractions, the composition of particulate air pollution matters for urban health. Some components may be notably connected to a source type, allowing sensitivity to emissions reduction efforts. For example, the NYCCAS data on nitric oxide exposure were selected for an investigation of taxi emissions reductions, as nitric oxide varies spatially and responds to traffic conditions in the immediate environment.[43] Other ambient measures may be of great interest because their respiratory or other health impact is pronounced compared to other particles of a similar size. This is the case for trace metals, as well as for allergenic particles such as tree pollen (see Box 5.1).

Box 5.1 MONITORING SPATIAL PATTERNS IN POLLEN EXPOSURE TO BETTER UNDERSTAND THE LINK BETWEEN URBAN TREES AND ALLERGIC DISEASE

Kate Weinberger, Faizan Shaikh, Guy Robinson, and Gina S. Lovasi

In recent years, cities around the world have undertaken massive urban tree planting campaigns (e.g., Million Trees NYC, Million Trees LA). The rationale for such campaigns draws on the broad range of ecological, social, and public health benefits provided by trees.[44] Indeed, a large body of literature links urban greenspace—including trees lining streets and in parks—to improved health.

At the same time, some tree species commonly planted in urban areas produce allergenic pollen, a key trigger of symptoms of allergic rhinitis (commonly referred to as "hay fever").[45,46] In the United States, approximately 8.2% of adults and 8.4% children had been diagnosed with allergic rhinitis in 2015, making it the sixth leading cause of chronic disease.[47] In 2005, health services and prescription medication sales for allergic rhinitis in the United States totaled $11.2 billion.[48] Exposure to certain types of pollen is also associated with the exacerbation of allergic asthma.[46,49] Thus, urban trees may lead to more frequent or severe allergic disease symptoms.

Little is known about the spatial distribution of allergenic pollen and its relationship to urban trees. Many studies assessing the health impacts of tree pollen rely on data from only a single pollen monitoring station located within a city.[50] To better understand intra-urban variation in pollen levels across New York City, our team conducted a sampling campaign encompassing 45 sites distributed across the city's five boroughs in 2013. These sites were chosen from among those included in the NYCCAS, a study of the spatial distribution of air pollutants.[42] We installed modified Tauber traps (Figure 5.2) on utility poles at a uniform height in late February and removed them in November of the same year to capture a single, integrated sample for the entire pollen season at each site.

Results from this sampling campaign suggest that exposure to tree pollen varies substantially across the city. Specifically, we found that the total amount of tree pollen ranged from 2,942 to 17,463 grains per square centimeter across monitoring sites and that levels of some types of tree pollen varied to an even greater degree. In addition, we found that the urban tree canopy coverage within circular buffers around pollen sites was positively correlated with tree pollen levels. For example, we found that percentage tree canopy cover within a half kilometer radial buffer around each monitoring site explained approximately 39% of spatial variance in tree pollen.[51] In subsequent work,[52] we have explored the robustness of

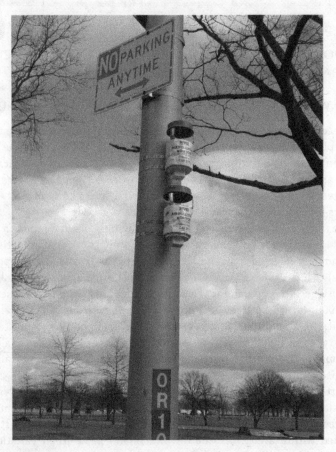

Figure 5.2 Two Tauber traps mounted for urban pollen monitoring.

this spatial pattern in a second year of monitoring, as well as the sensitivity of our measurements to the height and direction at which monitors are mounted. These results suggest that urban trees may be a key driver of exposure to tree pollen and highlight the importance of considering allergenicity when selecting species for inclusion in future tree planting campaigns.

As illustrated by the case of pollen monitoring, controlled monitoring conditions and comparison to other place-based characteristics help to ensure that variation of interest is captured while avoiding variation that is not of interest (e.g., distinguishing spatial patterning from variation based on monitoring height).

Beyond device-based monitoring of ambient conditions, devices have been deployed to capture indoor air quality, physical conditions such as temperature and humidity, or activity contributing to emissions such as traffic counts. Further, personal monitoring or use of biomarkers of exposure can more directly characterize the conditions experienced by an individual as they move through their environment. Such approaches can be coupled with information about human perception of and responses to the context, providing insight into ways that stressors and behaviors may exacerbate or mitigate time-varying exposures.

In Person or Virtual Audits of the Environment: Food Sources and Pedestrian Supportive Environments

Beyond the exposures to harmful substances within the urban context, we may plan primary data collection to characterize availability of health-supportive amenities. Systematic audits have been designed to capture aspects of physical spaces that influence health behaviors, and we illustrate this with audits of establishments selling food and of streets that may encourage residents to walk.

While secondary sources such as retail data were mentioned earlier in this chapter, questions may remain as to the specific foods available for sale and the marketing messages on display. Food establishments can themselves be sampled to capture variation across urban spaces using tools such as the Nutrition Environment Measures Survey.[53,54] Versions are available for both restaurants and food stores, though in some cases this distinction may be blurred.[55] Other measures are available that differ in emphasis or in the intensity of training needed before deployment. In many global cities, integration of both formal and informal[56] sources of food is relevant to health, with in person audits having potential to capture mobile or unregistered food distribution sites and vendors and hygienic conditions.[11] Other actions such as food purchases can be monitored via bag checks or collection of receipts.

On the other side of the energy balance equation, we turn to how urban environments affect physical activity. Streets are the most common site for urban residents to get daily physical activity, often while walking and biking for transportation or leisure.[57] Streets themselves can be audited to understand characteristics relevant to walkability and pedestrian supports.[58] Aesthetic amenities, road safety infrastructure, and physical disorder[59] are relatively unlikely to be well-captured by secondary data sources and thus have been commonly included in physical activity focused street audits.

Traditional strategies for audits include field teams carrying out structured assessments on clipboards. Increasingly, smartphones or tablets are used to allow data entry while in the field.[10] The use of smartphones allows for photos to be captured, allowing flexibility for additional coding after field data collection has concluded. However, since issues arise due to battery life, Internet access, and other technical issues, back-up paper forms are advised.

Unfortunately, travel time adds to the costs of many street environment audits, resulting in a limited geographical extent or reduction in the fraction of streets sampled. An alternative strategy for auditing streets has emerged through virtual street audits that leverage available images.[60] While research teams at one time needed to gather images of streets themselves,[61] online sources such as Google Street View have emerged, allowing virtual audits to become an efficient option. Globally, several teams have deployed such an approach, and more information about one such team and their user interface tool[62] is illustrated in Box 5.2. This virtual audit method has been used on a spatially dispersed sample of streets, with a higher density of sampling near addresses from a multicity cohort study.[63] In contrast, other virtual audit efforts have prioritized observing all streets within selected contiguous areas, as exemplified by a study in Madrid;[64] after selecting target neighborhoods with distinct contextual character, the contiguous sampling approach included all observable streets within selected neighborhoods. As automated methods to scale up virtual audit approaches[65,66] become more widespread, the cost per observation may be reduced to the point where sampling is no longer required to contain costs.

Box 5.2 GOOGLE STREET VIEW AUDITS USING CANVAS

Stephen J. Mooney, Michael Bader, Andrew Rundle, and Gina S. Lovasi

Assessing the impact of neighborhood conditions on health outcomes requires valid and reliable measurement. Systematic social observation offers a technique to collect these data. Researchers design standard protocols to measure features of the neighborhood and then train auditors to reliably measure those features. Trained auditors traditionally travel to systematically sampled locations (e.g., intersections or street segments) and then assess each location using the protocol. Existing protocols measure physical disorder (e.g., presence of litter and graffiti), pedestrian infrastructure (e.g., presence of traffic lights, medians, condition of sidewalk), and urban design features (e.g., variation in facades, setbacks). The method provides reliable and valid data but is expensive due to the time and travel costs of transporting the auditors to the streets. Moreover, auditors may face physical danger when collecting data on streets in some neighborhoods.[67]

Google Street View, a feature of Google Maps that provides street-level imagery throughout much of the world, has made virtual audits an efficient alternative to sending auditors to each sample location. Virtual audits collect data analogous to those collected in-person without the time and travel costs of physically visiting a location.[67-69] Street View imagery now covers most urban streets and is updated as often as several times a year. Google makes the historical imagery available through their user interface. Virtual audits allow researchers to collect neighborhood data on a very large scale, including entire cities or regions.[70,71]

Supporting software has the potential to improve virtual audit efficiency and reliability. The Computer Assisted Neighborhood Visual Assessment System (CANVAS) is a Web-based tool to deploy virtual audits. CANVAS provides interfaces (i) for study managers to develop the systematic protocol, including developing samples of locations, assigning locations to auditors, and monitoring study progress and reliability, and (ii) for auditors to enter data into standardized street audit forms ensuring the correct location using the Street View application programing interface. Many commonly used audit tools have been programmed into CANVAS.[72] Researchers have used CANVAS to collect neighborhood environment data across entire cities, including New York, NY; Detroit, MI; San Jose, CA; Washington, DC; and Philadelphia, PA, as well as six counties in New Jersey.[70-73]

Existing tools use automated image-analysis techniques to measure selected built environment features (e.g., greenspace,[74,75] utility poles,[76] on-premises advertising,[77] cars[78]) as well as overall streetscape complexity.[79-86] Google's Terms of Use and its copyright notification, however, expressly prohibit downloading and automated image processing at this writing.[87,88] Accordingly, virtual neighborhood audit studies conducted by human auditors provide an appealing method to measure neighborhood features.[67,69,70,72,73,89,90]

Sampling for virtual audits presents ethical concerns. Some audit studies seek to measure specific locations, such as study subject addresses. Transmitting these addresses to Google could represent the release of personally identifiable information and should not be used.[67,91] Spatial inference based on a sample of locations provides an alternative strategy that avoids releasing personally identifiable information.

Survey and Surveillance: Aggregated Reports From Residents and Public Space Observations

In some assessments, questionnaire-based derived measures or place-based observations provide a window into the characteristics of urban spaces.

While perceptions of the urban environment are complex, as discussed in the next chapter, surveyed residents can be considered as informants about characteristics of the areas where they live. An ecometric approach has been developed that integrates the perceptions of multiple area residents.[92,93] Agreement among area residents can be quantified to provide insights into uncertainty. This ecometric approach is particularly suitable for social dynamics or other aspects of the environment that are more credibly reported by residents than by trained outside observers.

Place-based observations by trained observers can be used to systematically assess public space use. For example, the System for Observing Play and Recreation in Communities (SOPARC) has been developed to take a rapid inventory of park use and levels of physical activity across playgrounds, ball fields, or other predefined areas. A range of physical activity studies have used the SOPARC protocol to identify where within-park physical activity is taking place,[94] including some with an explicit focus on equity.[95,96] More broadly, inclusiveness of public life may also be of interest, and potentially relevant to safety.[97] An important consideration in understanding how urban spaces are used is the possibility of behavioral reactivity; since study participants or the users of public spaces change their behavior patterns in response to being observed,[98] resultant patterns may reflect dynamics beyond the intended characterization of the urban environment. Moreover, public space observations are particularly challenging in urban environments where safety considerations or other complexities may require working in pairs, modification to existing training materials, or other adjustments to data collection.

CLOSING THOUGHTS ON MEASURING HEALTH-RELEVANT ASPECTS OF THE URBAN ENVIRONMENT

Considerations and methods for classifying urban health measures presented in this chapter (Figure 5.3) provide an entry point to understanding the complexity of characterizing variation across urban environments. Teams spanning disciplines from environmental health sciences to engineering have technical expertise to offer for those interested to learn more, as do local, national, and international organizations that draw our attention to priority aspects of the environment.

The complexity is further increased when a retrospective or prospective longitudinal sequence of measurements is of interest, allowing for longitudinal analysis strategies discussed in Chapter 9.

While improved environmental measures have been recommended as key to advancing our understanding of how local contexts can support health,[99] complementary assessment of how people view and understand their environment is also needed, and we turn to this important topic in our next chapter.

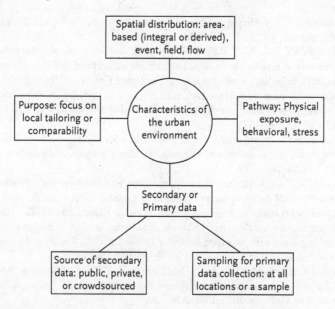

Figure 5.3 Ways to categorize measures of the urban environment.

REFERENCES

1. Diez Roux AV, Slesinski SC, Alazraqui M, et al. A novel international partnership for actionable evidence on urban health in Latin America: LAC-urban health and SALURBAL. *Global Challenges*. 2019;3(4):1800013.
2. Quistberg DA, Diez Roux AV, Bilal U, et al. Building a data platform for cross-country urban health studies: The SALURBAL study. *Journal of Urban Health*. 2019;96(2):311–337.
3. Lovasi GS, Grady S, Rundle A. Steps forward: Review and recommendations for research on walkability, physical activity and cardiovascular health. *Public Health Reviews*. 2012;33(2):484–506.
4. Briggs DJ. *Environmental Health Indicators: Framework and Methodologies*. Geneva: World Health Organization, 1999.
5. Kahn C, Kingsley GT, Taylor G. *National Neighborhood Indicators Partnership (NNIP) Shared Indicators Initiative: Framework*. Washington, DC: Urban Institute; 2012.
6. Farnam J, Holden M. Community indicators consortium. In: Michalos AC, ed. *Encyclopedia of Quality of Life and Well-Being Research*. New York: Springer; 2014: 1062–1066.
7. Arcaya MC, Tucker-Seeley RD, Kim R, Schnake-Mahl A, So M, Subramanian S. Research on neighborhood effects on health in the United States: A systematic review of study characteristics. *Social Science & Medicine*. 2016;168:16–29.
8. Prentice B, Thomas N. Exploring the intersection of public health and social justice: The bay area regional health inequities initiative. In: Hofrichter R, Rajiv B, eds. *Tackling Health Inequities Through Public Health Practice: Theory to Action*. New York: Oxford University Press; 2010: 283–295.

9.   Scharlach A. Creating aging-friendly communities in the United States. *Ageing International*. 2012;37(1):25–38.

10.   Remigio RV, Zulaika G, Rabello RS, et al. A local view of informal urban environments: A mobile phone-based neighborhood audit of street-level factors in a Brazilian informal community. *Journal of Urban Health*. 2019:96(4):537–548.

11.   Nizame FA, Alam MU, Masud AA, et al. Hygiene in restaurants and among street food vendors in Bangladesh. *American Journal of Tropical Medicine and Hygiene*. 2019;101(3):566–575.

12.   Hachmann S, Arsanjani JJ, Vaz E. Spatial data for slum upgrading: Volunteered geographic information and the role of citizen science. *Habitat International*. 2018;72:18–26.

13.   Bailey TC, Gatrell AC. *Interactive Spatial Data Analysis*. New York: Wiley; 1995.

14.   Diez-Roux AV. Bringing context back into epidemiology: Variables and fallacies in multilevel analysis. *American Journal of Public Health*. 1998;88(2):216–222.

15.   Mayne SL, Auchincloss AH, Tabb LP, et al. Associations of bar and restaurant smoking bans with smoking behavior in the CARDIA Study: A 25-year study. *American Journal of Epidemiology*. 2018;187(6):1250–1258.

16.   Lovasi GS, Bader MD, Quinn J, Neckerman K, Weiss C, Rundle A. Body mass index, safety hazards, and neighborhood attractiveness. *American Journal of Preventive Medicine*. 2012;43(4):378–384.

17.   Fernandes AP, Andrade ACdS, Costa DAdS, Dias MAdS, Malta DC, Caiaffa WT. Health Academies Program and the promotion of physical activity in the city: The experience of Belo Horizonte, Minas Gerais State, Brazil. *Ciencia & Saude Coletiva*. 2017;22(12):3903–3914.

18.   Simon P, Piché V, Gagnon Amélie A. *Social Statistics and Ethnic Diversity: Cross-National Perspectives in Classifications and Identity Politics*. Cham, Switzerland: Springer; 2015.

19.   Auchincloss AH, Diez Roux AV, Brown DG, O'Meara ES, Raghunathan TE. Association of insulin resistance with distance to wealthy areas: The multi-ethnic study of atherosclerosis. *American Journal of Epidemiology*. 2007;165(4):389–397.

20.   Diez-Roux AV, Kiefe CI, Jacobs DR, Jr., et al. Area characteristics and individual-level socioeconomic position indicators in three population-based epidemiologic studies. *Annals of Epidemiology*. 2001;11(6):395–405.

21.   Wilkinson RG, Pickett KE. Income inequality and population health: A review and explanation of the evidence. *Social Science & Medicine*. 2006;62(7):1768–1784.

22.   Williams DR, Collins C. Racial residential segregation: A fundamental cause of racial disparities in health. *Public Health Reports*. 2001;116(5):404–416.

23.   United Nations Department of Economic and Social Affairs. Principles and Recommendations for Population and Housing Censuses. Revision 2. 2008; https://unstats.un.org/unsd/demographic-social/Standards-and-Methods/files/Principles_and_Recommendations/Population-and-Housing-Censuses/Series_M67Rev2-E.pdf.

24.   MacDonald H. The American Community Survey: Warmer (more current), but fuzzier (less precise) than the decennial census. *Journal of the American Planning Association*. 2006;72(4):491–503.

25.   Logan JR, Stults BJ, Xu Z. Validating population estimates for harmonized census tract data, 2000–2010. *Annals of the American Association of Geographers*. 2016;106(5):1013–1029.

26. Hirsch JA, Schinasi LH. *A Measure of Gentrification for Use in Longitudinal Public Health Studies Based in the United States.* Philadelphia, PA: Drexel University Urban Health Collaborative; 2019.

27. Maantay J, Maroko A. Mapping urban risk: Flood hazards, race, & environmental justice in New York. *Applied Geography.* 2009;29(1):111–124.

28. Ebenstein A, Zhao Y. Tracking rural-to-urban migration in China: Lessons from the 2005 inter-census population survey. *Population Studies.* 2015;69(3): 337–353.

29. Rotondi MA, O'Campo P, O'Brien K, et al. Our Health Counts Toronto: Using respondent-driven sampling to unmask census undercounts of an urban indigenous population in Toronto, Canada. *BMJ Open.* 2017;7(12):e018936.

30. Chi S-H, Grigsby-Toussaint DS, Bradford N, Choi J. Can geographically weighted regression improve our contextual understanding of obesity in the us? Findings from the USDA Food Atlas. *Applied Geography.* 2013;44:134–142.

31. Haklay M, Weber P. OpenStreetMap: User-generated street maps. *IEEE Pervasive Computing.* 2008;7(4):12–18.

32. Boulos MNK, Resch B, Crowley DN, et al. Crowdsourcing, citizen sensing and sensor web technologies for public and environmental health surveillance and crisis management: trends, OGC standards and application examples. *International Journal of Health Geographics.* 2011;10(1):67.

33. Martin EG, Law J, Ran W, Helbig N, Birkhead GS. Evaluating the quality and usability of open data for public health research: A systematic review of data offerings on 3 open data platforms. *Journal of Public Health Management and Practice.* 2017;23(4):e5–e13.

34. Clougherty JE, Kheirbek I, Eisl HM, et al. Intra-urban spatial variability in wintertime street-level concentrations of multiple combustion-related air pollutants: The New York City Community Air Survey (NYCCAS). *Journal of Exposure Science and Environmental Epidemiology.* 2013;23(3):232–240.

35. Manaugh K, El-Geneidy A. Validating walkability indices: How do different households respond to the walkability of their neighborhood? *Transportation Research Part D: Transport and Environment.* 2011;16(4):309–315.

36. Samuelson P. Copyright's fair use doctrine and digital data. *Communications of the ACM.* 1994;37(1):21–28.

37. Kaufman TK, Sheehan DM, Rundle A, et al. Measuring health-relevant businesses over 21 years: Refining the National Establishment Time-Series (NETS), a dynamic longitudinal data set. *BMC Research Notes.* 2015;8:507.

38. MacFaden SW, O'Neil-Dunne JPM, Royar AR, Lu JWT, Rundle A. High-resolution tree canopy mapping for New York City using LiDAR and object-based image analysis. *Journal of Applied Remote Sensing.* 2012;6(1):063567.

39. Gallagher K, Lawrence P. Unmanned Systems and managing from above: The practical implications of UAVs for research applications addressing urban sustainability. In: Gatrell JD, Jensen RR, Patterson MW, Hoalst-Pullen N, eds. *Urban Sustainability: Policy and Praxis.* New York: Springer; 2016: 217–232.

40. Van Donkelaar A, Martin RV, Brauer M, et al. Global estimates of ambient fine particulate matter concentrations from satellite-based aerosol optical depth: Development and application. *Environmental Health Perspectives.* 2010;118(6): 847–855.

41. Cavaliere A, Carotenuto F, Di Gennaro F, et al. Development of low-cost air quality stations for next generation monitoring networks: Calibration and validation of PM2. 5 and PM10 sensors. *Sensors.* 2018;18(9):2843.

42. Matte T, Ross Z, Kheirbek I, et al. Monitoring intraurban spatial patterns of multiple combustion air pollutants in New York City: Design and implementation. *Journal of Exposure Science and Environmental Epidemiology*. 2013;23:223–231.

43. Fry D, Kioumourtzoglou M-A, Treat CA, et al. Development and validation of a method to quantify benefits of clean-air taxi legislation. *Journal of Exposure Science & Environmental Epidemiology*. 2019. doi:10.1038/s41370-019-0141-6.

44. City of New York. PlaNYC: A greener, greater New York. 2007; http://www.nyc.gov/html/planyc/downloads/pdf/publications/planyc_2011_planyc_full_report.pdf

45. Cakmak S, Dales RE, Burnett RT, Judek S, Coates F, Brook JR. Effect of airborne allergens on emergency visits by children for conjunctivitis and rhinitis. *The Lancet*. 2002;359(9310):947–948.

46. Ito K, Weinberger KR, Robinson GS, et al. The associations between daily spring pollen counts, over-the-counter allergy medication sales, and asthma syndrome emergency department visits in New York City, 2002–2012. *Environmental Health*. 2015;14:71.

47. Asthma and Allergy Foundation of America. Allergy Facts and Figures. https://www.aafa.org/allergy-facts/. Accessed June 25, 2020.

48. Soni A. *Allergic Rhinitis: Trends In Use And Expenditures, 2000 and 2005: Medical Expenditure Panel Survey*. Washington, DC: Agency for Healthcare Research and Quality; 2008.

49. Darrow LA, Hess J, Rogers CA, Tolbert PE, Klein M, Sarnat SE. Ambient pollen concentrations and emergency department visits for asthma and wheeze. *Journal of Allergy and Clinical Immunology*. 2012;130(3):630–638.e4.

50. Weinberger KR, Kinney PL, Lovasi GS. A review of spatial variation of allergenic tree pollen within cities. *Arboriculture & Urban Forestry*. 2015;41(2):57–68.

51. Weinberger KR, Kinney PL, Robinson GS, et al. Levels and determinants of tree pollen in New York City. *Journal of Exposure Science & Environmental Epidemiology*. 2018;28(2):119–124.

52. Weinberger K, Shaikh F, Robinson G, Kinney P, Lovasi G. Intra-urban pollen data to inform buffer selection for greenspace research. *Environmental Epidemiology*. 2019;3:433.

53. Neckerman KM, Lovasi L, Yousefzadeh P, et al. Comparing nutrition environments in bodegas and fast-food restaurants. *Journal of the Academy of Nutrition and Dietetics*. 2013;114(4):595–602.

54. Saelens BE, Glanz K, Sallis JF, Frank LD. Nutrition Environment Measures Study in restaurants (NEMS-R): Development and evaluation. *American Journal of Preventative Medicine*. 2007;32(4):273–281.

55. Neckerman KM, Lovasi L, Yousefzadeh P, et al. Comparing nutrition environments in bodegas and fast-food restaurants. *Journal of the Academy of Nutrition and Dietetics*. 2014;114(4):595–602.

56. Crush J, Frayne B. Supermarket expansion and the informal food economy in Southern African cities: Implications for urban food security. *Journal of Southern African Studies*. 2011;37(4):781–807.

57. Eyler AA, Brownson RC, Bacak SJ, Housemann RA. The epidemiology of walking for physical activity in the United States. *Medicine and Science in Sports and Exercise*. 2003;35(9):1529–1536.

58. Neckerman KM, Lovasi GS, Davies S, et al. Disparities in urban neighborhood conditions: Evidence from GIS measures and field observation in New York City. *Journal of Public Health and Policy*. 2009;30(Suppl 1):S264–S285.

59. Ndjila S, Lovasi GS, Fry D, Friche AA. Measuring neighborhood order and disorder: A rapid literature review. *Current Environmental Health Reports*. 2019;6(4):316–326.

60. Rzotkiewicz A, Pearson AL, Dougherty BV, Shortridge A, Wilson N. Systematic review of the use of Google Street View in health research: Major themes, strengths, weaknesses and possibilities for future research. *Health & Place* 2018;52:240–246.

61. Sampson RJ. The making of the Chicago Project. In: Maltz MD, Rice SK, eds. *Envisioning Criminology*: Cham, Switzerland: Springer; 2015: 99–107.

62. Bader MD, Mooney SJ, Lee YJ, et al. Development and deployment of the Computer Assisted Neighborhood Visual Assessment System (CANVAS) to measure health-related neighborhood conditions. *Health & Place*. 2015;31: 163–172.

63. Mooney SJ, Bader MDM, Lovasi GS, Neckerman KM, Teitler JO, Rundle AG. Validity of an ecometric neighborhood physical disorder measure constructed by virtual street audit. *American Journal of Epidemiology*. 2014;180(6):626–635.

64. Gullón P, Badland HM, Alfayate S, et al. Assessing walking and cycling environments in the streets of Madrid: Comparing on-field and virtual audits. *Journal of Urban Health*. 2015;92(5):923–939.

65. Naik N, Kominers SD, Raskar R, Glaeser EL, Hidalgo CA. Computer vision uncovers predictors of physical urban change. *Proceedings of the National Academy of Sciences* 2017;114(29):7571–7576.

66. Olafenwa M. Object detection with 10 lines of code. 2018; https://towardsdata-science.com/object-detection-with-10-lines-of-code-d6cb4d86f606.

67. Bader M, Mooney S, Bennet B, Rundle A. The promise, practicalities, and perils of virtually auditing neighborhoods using Google Street View. *The annals of the American Academy of Political and Social Sciences*. 2016;669(1):18–40.

68. Mooney SJ, Bader MDM, Lovasi GS, et al. Street audits to measure neighborhood disorder: Virtual or in-person? *American Journal of Epidemiology*. 2017;186(3):265–273.

69. Rundle AG, Bader MD, Richards CA, Neckerman KM, Teitler JO. Using Google Street View to audit neighborhood environments. *American Journal of Preventive Medicine*. 2011;40(1):94–100.

70. Mooney SJ, Bader MDM, Lovasi GS, Neckerman KM, Teitler JO, Rundle AG. Validity of an ecometric neighborhood physical disorder measure constructed by Virtual Street Audit. *American Journal of Epidemiology* 2014;180(6):626–635.

71. Plascak JJ, Llanos AAM, Chavali LB, et al. Sidewalk conditions in northern New Jersey: Using Google Street View imagery and ordinary kriging to assess infrastructure for walking. *Preventing Chronic Disease*. 2019;16:E60.

72. Bader MDM, Mooney SJ, Lee Y, et al. Development and Deployment of the Computer Assisted Neighborhood Visual Audit System (CANVAS) to measure health-related neighborhood conditions. *Health & Place*. 2015;31:163–172.

73. Quinn J, Mooney SJ, Sheehan D, et al. Neighborhood physical disorder in New York City. *Journal of Maps*. 2016;12(1):53–60.

74. Larkin A, Hystad P. Evaluating street view exposure measures of visible green space for health research. *Journal of Exposure Science and Environmental Epidemiology*. 2019;29(4):447–456.

75. Helbich M, Yao Y, Liu Y, Zhang J, Liu P, Wang R. Using deep learning to examine street view green and blue spaces and their associations with geriatric depression in Beijing, China. *Environmental International*. 2019;126:107–117.

76. Zhang W, Witharana C, Li W, Zhang C, Li X, Parent J. Using deep learning to identify utility poles with crossarms and estimate their locations from Google Street View images. *Sensors (Basel)*. 2018;18(8):E2484.

77. Tsai TH, Cheng WH, You CW, Hu MC, Tsui AW, Chi HY. Learning and recognition of on-premise signs from weakly labeled street view images. *IEEE Transactions on Image Processing*. 2014;23(3):1047–1059.

78. Gebru T, Krause J, Wang Y, et al. Using deep learning and Google Street View to estimate the demographic makeup of neighborhoods across the United States. *Proceedings of the National Academy of Sciences of the United States of America*. 2017;114(50):13108–13113.

79. Cavalcante A, Mansouri A, Kacha L, et al. Measuring streetscape complexity based on the statistics of local contrast and spatial frequency. *PLoS One*. 2014;9(2):e87097.

80. Elsheshtawy Y. Urban complexity: Toward the measurements of the physical complexity of street-scapes. *Journal of Architectural and Planning Research*. 1997;14:301–316.

81. Cooper J. Fractal assessment of street-level skylines: A possible means of assessing and comparing character. *Urban Morphology*. 2003;7:73–82.

82. Kacha L, Mansouri L, Matsumoto N, Cavalcante A, Mansouri A. Study on visual complexity and RMS image contrast statistics in streetscapes in Algeria and Japan. *Journal of Architectural and Planning*. 2013;78:625–633.

83. Forsythe A, Nadal M, Sheehy N, Cela-Conde CJ, Sawey M. Predicting beauty: Fractal dimension and visual complexity in art. *British Journal of Psychology*. 2011;102(1):49–70.

84. Forsythe A, Sheehy N, Sawey M. Measuring icon complexity: An automated analysis. *Behavior Research Methods, Instruments, & Computers*. 2003;35(2):334–342.

85. Rosenholtz R, Li Y, Nakano L. Measuring visual clutter. *Journal of Vision*. 2007;7(2):1–22.

86. Nasanen R, Kukkonen H, Rovamo J. Spatial integration of band-pass filtered patterns in noise. *Vision Research*. 1993;33(7):903–911.

87. Goggle Inc. Using Street View imagery—prohibited uses. https://www.google.com/permissions/geoguidelines/. Accessed October 10, 2018.

88. Google Inc. Google Maps/Google Earth additional terms of service. https://www.google.com/intl/ALL/help/terms_maps.html. Accessed October 22, 2018.

89. Mooney SJ, DiMaggio CJ, Lovasi GS, et al. Use of Google Street View to assess environmental contributions to pedestrian injury. *American Journal of Public Health* 2016;106(3):462–469.

90. Mooney SJ, Rundle A. *Using CANVAS with Built Environment Natural Experiments*. Clearwater FL: Active Living Research; 2016.

91. Bader MD, Mooney SJ, Rundle AG. Protecting personally identifiable information when using online geographic tools for public health research. *American Journal of Public Health* 2016;106(2):206–208.

92. Mujahid MS, Diez Roux AV, Morenoff JD, Raghunathan T. Assessing the measurement properties of neighborhood scales: From psychometrics to ecometrics. *American Journal of Epidemiology*. 2007;165(8):858–867.

93. Raudenbush SW, Sampson RJ. Ecometrics: Toward a science of assessing ecological settings, with application to the systematic social observation of neighborhoods. *Sociological Methodology*. 1999;29(1):1–41.

94. Evenson KR, Jones SA, Holliday KM, Cohen DA, McKenzie TL. Park characteristics, use, and physical activity: A review of studies using SOPARC (System

for Observing Play and Recreation in Communities). *Preventive Medicine.* 2016;86:153–166.

95. Marquet O, Aaron Hipp J, Alberico C, et al. Park use preferences and physical activity among ethnic minority children in low-income neighborhoods in New York City. *Urban Forestry & Urban Greening.* 2019;38:346–353.

96. Marquet O, Hipp JA, Alberico C, et al. Use of SOPARC to assess physical activity in parks: Do race/ethnicity, contextual conditions, and settings of the target area, affect reliability? *BMC Public Health.* 2019;19(1):1730.

97. Begault L. Crime prevention through environmental design: A public life approach. Gehl Institute. 2017; https://gehlinstitute.org/wp-content/uploads/2017/02/CPTED-Public-Life-Approach.pdf

98. Wray TB, Merrill JE, Monti PM. Using ecological momentary assessment (EMA) to assess situation-level predictors of alcohol use and alcohol-related consequences. *Alcohol Research: Current Reviews.* 2014;36(1):19–27.

99. Story M, Giles-Corti B, Yaroch AL, et al. Work group IV: Future directions for measures of the food and physical activity environments. *American Journal of Preventative Medicine.* 2009;36(4 Suppl):S182–S188.

CHAPTER 6

Human Perceptions and Reflections on the Urban Context

GINA S. LOVASI AND STEPHEN E. LANKENAU

While the previous chapter focused on characterizing cities and the smaller spaces that make up urban environments, we now turn to the roles of human perception and reflections on the environment, which are crucial to several causal pathways connecting urban environments to health as discussed in Chapter 3. Efforts to understand and elevate resident perceptions and reflections benefit from a range of data collection strategies and place-based quantitative and qualitative approaches.

OVERVIEW OF DATA ON HUMAN PERCEPTIONS AND REFLECTIONS ABOUT THE ENVIRONMENT

Pathways linking environments to health may act through individual behavioral or stress pathways, in which case the health consequences will depend on how people perceive and respond to their environment. Where environments have been modified to become more health supportive, realization of health benefits may require that residents are aware of, feel positively about, and are empowered to act on the environmental change.

What residents know about the environment, such as awareness of services and resources is a requisite for taking full advantage of available health supportive opportunities and avoiding harm. This cognitive aspect of perception may be assessed through structured questionnaires or more open-ended attempts to elicit information. The field of environmental cognition reflects a

Gina S. Lovasi and Stephen E. Lankenau, *Human Perceptions and Reflections on the Urban Context* In: *Urban Public Health*. Edited by: Gina S. Lovasi, Ana V. Diez Roux, and Jennifer Kolker, Oxford University Press (2021).
© Oxford University Press 2021. DOI: 10.1093/oso/9780190885304.003.0006.

long-standing interest in understanding how and under what circumstances what people "know" about their environment diverges from what is independently observable.[1] Communication and marketing strategies may be needed to overcome lack of awareness and resultant underutilization of urban features.

Beyond knowing what is available in the environment, resident responses will be importantly shaped by their sense of emotional attachment or distance.[2] Thus, how residents feel about local amenities and disamenities may importantly shape their behavioral and health response. This aspect of how people react to their environments may be particularly important when planning to address health inequities, as past injustices or traumas may affect the understanding of and emotional reaction to environmental characteristics and neighborhood change.

In addition to knowledge and feelings about the environment, residents can be engaged to reflect on what should be. Whether residents are empowered to feel ownership of a space or program may, in fact, be crucial to whether utilization is sufficient to result in health benefits. Participatory research, which can play a key role in addressing health inequities,[3] is highlighted in the examples in Boxes 6.1 to 6.3, and may be instrumental in shifting what people know, feel, and are empowered to envision for their environment.

As we consider approaches to gathering data on perceptions and reflections, an important consideration is whether the data collection will take place while residents are in the urban spaces being studied. Beyond inviting reporting or reflections on past experiences of the urban environment, there are complementary quantitative and qualitative approaches that may be more sensitive to situational factors by collecting data while participants are experiencing urban contexts. Figure 6.1 schematically represents this and several other key aspects of data collection on perception of the urban environment.

QUANTITATIVE DATA TO CAPTURE PERCEPTIONS OF THE ENVIRONMENT

We begin with a discussion of traditional questionnaires and then highlight opportunities to embed questions about perception into device-based data collection to capture reactions in context. Quantitative approaches often have larger sample sizes as compared with qualitative data and, as such, may be especially well suited to investigating patterns between multiple previously identified variables or testing for systematic variation in perception across population groups.

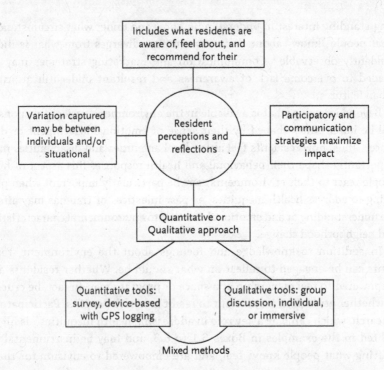

Figure 6.1 Summary of information on perceptions and reflections on the environment.

Questionnaire-Based Data Collection on Perceptions of and Use of the Environment: Considerations for Survey Sampling

A population-based survey is a common way to capture structured answers to questions about what features people report awareness of, as well as more evaluative questions about, neighborhood satisfaction or neighborhood problems. In designing such surveys, a number of logistical and scientific considerations come into play.

Some recruitment strategies may depend on available information such as an inventory of households and require adaptation depending on the setting. For example, in informal urban communities, sampling by address from a list may not be feasible, requiring instead an on-the-ground strategy to ensure the sample will be systematic, with known sampling probabilities. Recruitment strategies may be nested within selected urban areas. Key issues to consider in the selection of such areas were discussed in Chapter 5.

While random digit dial or household surveys continue to play an important role in health research, response rates have been falling.[4] Thus, intercept surveys, which have recruited people based on where they are in the moment rather than where they live, and other emerging approaches should be considered as complementary to traditional household surveys.[5,6]

Box 6.1 UTILIZING THE *OUR VOICE* CITIZEN SCIENCE
MODEL TO SUPPORT AND PROMOTE ACTIVE URBAN
ENVIRONMENTS: THE CASE OF THE CICLOVÍA OF BOGOTÁ

Olga L. Sarmiento, Silvia A. González, Diana Rocio Higuera-Mendieta,
and Abby C. King

The *Our Voice* "by the people" citizen science model is a community-based participatory research approach that uses information and communications technology.[7] Through this model, "citizen scientists" have a channel for providing feedback on existing programs, and the model also empowers community members to actively promote data-driven changes in the local built and social environments.[7,8] Citizen scientists use the Stanford Healthy Neighborhood Discovery Tool, which is a mobile data-gathering application that allows residents to document neighborhood characteristics and perceptions through geocoded photographs, audio narratives, and GPS-tracked walking routes.[7] The tool was designed to ensure ease of use regardless of age, education, culture, language, or technology literacy.[7,8]

CASE STUDY

Our Voice in the Ciclovía is part of the *Our Voice* Global Citizen Science for Health Equity Initiative.[8,9] The Ciclovías comprise worldwide programs in which streets are temporary closed to motor vehicles and open to individuals for leisure activities.[10] As of 2018, there are about 490 programs in 24 countries from all continents.[9] The Ciclovía of Bogotá is the largest in the world, with about 1 million participants per event in 121 km city streets during a 7-hour period (Sundays and holidays).[10]

Our Voice in the Ciclovía assessed residents' perceptions of the barriers and facilitators of the program for engaging in active living in the city. Following a training, Ciclovía users documented their perceptions of the Ciclovía environment with geocoded photos and narrative recordings, taken while walking, biking, or skating along their usual routes during the Ciclovía and also during a weekday with normal traffic on the roads. The study sample comprised 32 users of the Ciclovía program, including 5 homeless adults who reported that the Ciclovía was a program that they used for recreation. Participants held eight meetings at the community level to discuss their findings and establish priorities for the improvement of the program and one meeting with policymakers. With the legal guidance, the citizen scientists were involved subsequently in an advocacy process with policymakers of the Ciclovía program.

The main topics that emerged from the Discovery Tool data and surveys were safety, services/activities, signaling, street features, and friendliness of the environment. Policymakers were pleased with the information provided, including the positive features of the Ciclovía that were noted and expressed their willingness to act on the suggestions made by the citizen scientists. The reports of barriers by the citizen scientists were considered valuable inputs for future and current improvement of the program. An extension of 3.6 km to the program circuit coincided with the advocacy-based recommendations made by the citizen scientists, as did the installation of some new portable toilets along the Ciclovía route. *Our Voice* in the Ciclovía provides evidence that a participatory approach that involves resident's voices creates community-engaged citizen scientists that can contribute to the improvement of programs and policies to promote active living.

A fact sheet and information regarding Our Voice Global Network can be found at http://med.stanford.edu/ourvoice/the-global-network-right.html.

Box 6.2 PARTICIPATORY ACTION RESEARCH IN USING PHOTOVOICE IN MADRID

Pedro Gullón, Julia Díez, and Manuel Franco

Photovoice is a participatory visual research method, emanating from the community-based participatory research and participatory action research paradigms. Within these paradigms, participants act as equal partners throughout the research and action processes.[11,12] Photovoice is defined as "a process by which people can identify, represent, and enhance their community through a specific photographic technique."[13]

We have developed two different photovoice projects in the city of Madrid between 2015 and 2017, aimed to identify environmental factors (both facilitators and barriers) related to residents' physical activity[14] and diet[15,16] in two neighborhoods of contrasting socioeconomic status. Following Wang's[13] methodology, we organized the photovoice process in five group discussion sessions. The initial session introduced the project aims and discussed the planned schedule with participants. Participants received a digital camera and training on photographic techniques and ethical issues. Then, we asked participants to photograph all the features they felt related to the food/physical activity environment in their neighborhood.

Participants could take as many photographs as they wanted, but we asked them to bring five of the most meaningful photos to the next sessions. In the following sessions, participants reviewed and discussed the content and meaning of their photographs with other group members. Finally, we conducted participatory data analysis, where participants code the data and identify themes emerging from photographs and group discussions. Figure 6.2. shows two example photos relevant to themes that emerged from photovoice groups.

Once the group discussion sessions were completed, participants translated their results into concrete policy recommendations to improve their food and physical activity environment.[17] For this purpose, we used an adapted logical framework approach for intervention planning.[18] Recommendations were categorized as relevant to the physical environment (e.g., redesigning the current bus network), the sociocultural environment (e.g., supporting local small retailers), or the policy/economic environment (e.g., adjust sport facilities fees based on the socioeconomic status of the area). Within each category, recommendations were arrayed from the macro level (e.g., improving the design of nutritional labels) to the micro level (e.g., putting out benches in the streets for the older people).

Importantly, photovoice is itself a potential force for change, as at different stages, citizens, policymakers, health professionals, and researchers come together to create policy-relevant neighborhood and health research[17,19] and to contribute to community empowerment.[16] Indeed, such community partnership could lead to a "spillover effect" where new collaborations may become even more influential than the original design.

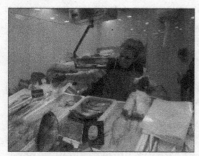

Photograph title: 'My fish shop'

Category: 'social relationships and social trust'; theme: 'social local influences'

(Photographer: Encarnación, resident of Villaverde)

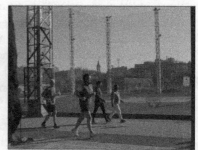

Photograph title: '4 persons, 4 towers: David vs Goliath'

Category: 'physical activity at Canal Park'; theme: 'sport in the city'

(Photographer: Carlos, resident of Chamberí)

Figure 6.2 Example photos related to diet (left) and physical activity (right) from photovoice project in Madrid.

To foster these community and policy changes, it is also key to develop an effective communication and dissemination strategy engaging participants.[12] In our projects, participants chose the final photographs to be included in the photobook and in the photographic exhibition of the projects.[14,15] Other dissemination activities can include videos, policy briefs, and public meetings, where participants, researchers, and decision makers come together and discuss participants' results and policy recommendations. The developed dissemination materials are available on our website: https://hhhproject.eu/hhh-sub-studies/photovoice/project/.

Box 6.3 A CASE STUDY ON USING MIXED METHODS TO BETTER UNDERSTAND HEALTH DISPARITIES

Bridgette M. Brawner

Immersed in Philadelphia's HIV prevention landscape for more than a decade, colleagues and I sought to develop a better understanding of the ways in which individual, social, and structural factors shaped the local HIV epidemic. We recognized the role of place in disparate HIV outcomes among the city's Black residents (i.e., higher incidence, greater morbidity and mortality) and selected a community-engaged approach to understand perception and behavior patterns with relevance to potential solutions. This resulted in a multiphase, mixed methods study with focus groups, ethnographic observation, community mapping, GIS mapping, and secondary analysis of health department data. Through integration of these data sources, the researchers and community partners were able to provide a contextualized picture of experiences contributing to or buffering risk.

To begin, the team conducted a focused discussion with 10 key stakeholders—community residents, direct service providers, and administrators—in January 2012. This provided an opportunity to hear directly from community members what beliefs they held about causes of the local epidemic. Despite the small sample size, this provided an important foundation for the subsequent research phases, and in response to interest from others in the field, we published our methodology and findings in 2017.[20] Gender equity, social capital, and cultural mores such as monogamy were perceived to be the main protective factors. The long-term effects of racial residential segregation, poverty, and incarceration were the leading perceived contributors to risk.

The research team was able to validate the investigator-developed conceptual model, confirming that those affected by the local epidemic agreed with the hypothesized concepts, relationships, and directionality. Through years of extensive community-engaged work, Brawner also coined the term *geobehavioral vulnerability to HIV*. According to Brawner,[21p634]

> it is not just what you do, but also where you do it, and with whom, that increases your risk of HIV infection. Geosocial spaces, geographic areas where people interact, such as housing developments, census tracts, or cities, with high HIV prevalence produce a greater probability of being exposed to HIV. . . . Therefore, individual risk behavior is only one part of the equation when a person's geography and network/community associations influence HIV risk. . . . Although individual risk-related behaviors do increase transmission risk, the probability of exposure is increased at the outset for those who have geobehavioral vulnerability to HIV

The aforementioned endeavors guided a formative comparative community-based case study to further investigate individual, social, and structural factors that contributed to the HIV/AIDS epidemic among Black Philadelphians. The team selected four Philadelphia census tracts across quadrants defined by predominant race and HIV/AIDS disease burden. Within selected census tracts, the research team engaged in ethnographic and GIS mapping based on observations of individual behaviors and their interaction with environmental features, informal conversations with residents and business owners, and secondary analyses of census tract-level data.[22] A key finding was that HIV/AIDS burden appeared to reflect social and structural inequities beyond the area's racial composition. Specifically, areas with less favorable social and structural conditions (i.e., more vacant parcels) had higher HIV/AIDS burden even after restricting to predominately White tracts, and those with more favorable social and structural conditions (i.e., fewer narcotics violations) had lower HIV/AIDS burden, even after restricting to predominantly Black tracts.

This led to a more in-depth secondary analysis of health department data on HIV-positive cases to examine racial/ethnic and geographic disparities in HIV transmission and disease burden.[23] We discovered differences in mode of HIV transmission by race/ethnicity and census tract, with greater transmission due to heterosexual contact and injection drug use in predominantly Black census tracts, whereas in other contexts male-to-male sexual contact had a greater role in transmission. The findings underscore the need to continue to address multiple HIV risk behaviors, including those most relevant to specific populations and geographic settings.

We have since has extended this approach to other topics. In the Black Hearts Matter protocol, we are combining biobehavioral strategies with location logging to explore neighborhood-level influences on cardiovascular disease risk factors among Black emerging adult men. Coordinates for locations where participants worked, purchased food, and were exposed to tobacco retailers and advertisements were used to conduct an audit to examine ways in which the environment (e.g., unhealthy food retailers) affect individuals' potential to live heart-healthy lifestyles.

Altogether, the findings from this mixed methods research program in urban health illustrates how the search for community-level insights and interventions to address health disparities unfold across multiple phases of data collection, crucially including and elevating the voices of those affected in the planning process.

Perceptions of area characteristics collected through structured questionnaires have been central to research on how urban neighborhoods affect health-relevant stress and behavioral outcomes. Often, when perceived measures are compared to objectively assessed versions of the same characteristics, the perceptions more strongly predict behavioral outcomes such as physical activity.[24] This suggests perceptions themselves may play a key mediating role. However, doubts have been raised as to whether this reflects biased patterns of self-report, such as being more likely to report environment–behavior combinations that are seen as socially desirable: having reported their neighborhood as unsafe, a participant may be nudged toward underreporting their child's time playing outdoors; conversely, having reported a low level of fruit and vegetable consumption, a respondent may overemphasize barriers to access within their food environment.

An alternative, which leverages residents' perceptions, is to use an ecometric approach that integrates the perceptions of multiple area residents.[25,26] Residents of an area are considered as informants, and responses are combined to create an area-based derived measure (see discussion in Chapter 5). Although derived from perceptions, the aggregation of multiple resident responses (which can average across subjectivities and errors) can sometimes result in more valid measures of objective features.

While resident perceptions are influenced the objectively measurable characteristics of the environment, perception may also vary across population groups.[24] For example, the ecometric Health in Beaga Study[27] notes that older age and higher levels of educational attainment predicted perceiving lower levels of physical disorder that other residents. Ecometric techniques can be used to create measures that account for systematic differences in perceptions across characteristics like age and sex when creating survey derived area-based measures.[28]

Use of mobile phones can allow the integration of survey-style inquiries in multiple settings, commonly taking the form of ecological momentary assessment. At a prespecified schedule, participants are prompted to respond to brief assessments that may include aspects of their social and physical context, as well as their mood (e.g., levels of happiness or anxiety). When the geographic location is salient to such data collection, the label geographically explicit ecological momentary assessment (GEMA) is used,[29] and new possibilities and challenges emerge.[30]

Approaches such as GEMA and other device-based data collection result in intensive longitudinal data, with many observations on the same individual over a short period of time. A key advantage is to be able to study situational triggers of thoughts, feelings, or choices relevant to health while holding stable personal traits constant. However, in anticipation of threats to validity that emerge in longitudinal analyses (see Chapter 9), measurement of potential time-varying confounders (such as intentions or the presence and behavior of other people) should be included during data collection.

Passive device-based data collection from the individuals whose health is in question may offer additional detail without the high level of participant burden imposed by asking questions throughout the day. Common approaches include global positioning system (GPS) logging to measure location during daily travel. Location information from GPS logger devices requires additional processing to estimate where participants spend time while accounting for the potential for differential error depending on the urban environment[31] and may benefit from strategies to address locational error in animal ecology studies.[32] Other wearables can include heart rate monitors or cameras (from which the resulting abundance of images may be efficiently handled by emerging image-processing algorithms[33,34]). Several relevant challenges to managing and linking such data are discussed in Chapter 8.

Device-based data collection approaches require training and communication to ensure the ethical treatment of participants and the quality of data returned.[35] Prior efforts have identified privacy infringement through real-time tracking and device loss as salient participant concerns.[36] In addition, integrity of the data and participant burden can be affected by device battery life. Minimizing or eliminating the need for participants to charge the device may require using a device with longer battery life or deploying team members to retrieve depleted devices and replace them with charged devices. As the hardware available continues to improve with regard to transmission and integration of sensing data with other data sources, additional sensing studies including those with multiple sensors used simultaneously will be more widespread.[33] Other strategies that may be considered depending on the data collection goals include variation of wear instructions (e.g., wrist instead of hip, allowing placement in a bag vs. on the body) and integration of multiple capabilities into a single device (e.g., a study-provided smartphone or the participant's own communication device).[37]

Participatory methods offer a way to build communications and capacity, as illustrated by the example in Box 6.1 on how dedicated recreational use of city streets can result in maximal health benefits. For both quantitative and qualitative data collection efforts, we note participatory approaches (discussed further in Chapter 13) can face particular challenges, such as providing appropriate training in human subjects research to a team with variable prior experience with research methods.[38]

QUALITATIVE AND MIXED METHODS RESEARCH TO UNDERSTAND HOW RESIDENTS VIEW AND REFLECT ON URBAN ENVIRONMENTS

Qualitative approaches can inform our understanding of how urban environments affect health in several ways.

Qualitative approaches are uniquely suited to tap into the life experiences and local expertise possessed by community residents and may be a crucial component of participatory research efforts as discussed in Chapter 13. Such approaches provide an enriched theoretical understanding of health-relevant processes occurring in urban spaces. Qualitative data can help identify the features of an urban environments most important to the health of residents. In addition, qualitative research is critical to understanding how residents relate, use, and react to their environments and can, therefore, be of major utility in understanding the processes through which environment characteristics affect health.

Qualitative investigations can additionally inform the design of quantitative studies. For example, qualitative data gathered through interviews with Hispanic mothers in New York City, which emphasized the value placed on foods direct from farmers markets and slaughterhouses, was later used to develop quantitative measures of the urban food retail environment as part of a mixed methods food environment study.[39]

Distinguishing Characteristics of Qualitative Research

Understanding how residents see and make sense of their environment benefits from the complementary strengths of qualitative and quantitative data.[40] Whereas quantitative and qualitative data and analyses differ in multiple ways,[41] here we highlight just two.

First, whereas quantitative data are typically summarized and compared numerically, qualitative data are characterized by quotes, themes, and insights captured in narrative form.

A second difference pertains to assumptions about reality: while training in quantitative methods is typically positivist, assuming a reality that exists independent of human perception, qualitative training emphasizes a constructivist view that allows for discordant but equally valid understandings of reality to be held by different observers.[42]

The distinct role of qualitative data for understanding perception in urban environments relates to both the narrative form and constructivist understanding of reality. The kinds of insights that can be gained from qualitative approaches in place-based research range from developing theories and explaining pathways to providing holistic and community-driven input to inform action.[43]

The qualitative and quantitative approaches reviewed in this chapter, as well as the measures of the environment discussed in the previous chapter, can be integrated.[44] Notably when using a mixed methods framework,[45,46] the broader team engaged may not all have qualitative research expertise. The framework method, with origins in policy research,[47] may be useful to such teams, by offering a highly systematic approach to categorizing and organizing documentation of qualitative data in a way that may be more readily understood by quantitatively trained members of a team.

Integration of Place into Qualitative Data Collection Using Focus Groups, In-Depth Interviews, and Ethnography

Gathering information on the explicitly stated and inferred preferences of urban residents may occur through commonly deployed qualitative data collection strategies, such as focus groups, in-depth interviews, or ethnographic observation. These data collection techniques, and the corresponding data analysis and reporting guidelines, are described elsewhere in detail.[48,49] While not exhaustive, we highlight here select strategies for anchoring these qualitative data collection approaches to the nearby urban environment.

Focus groups are a commonly deployed mode of qualitative data collection, which may engage area residents in conversation about concerns about the environment or proposed changes to an area. An option to anchor these conversations—or other community meetings—in physical spaces include using large-form maps to elicit spatially-referenced information on perceived hazards and assets.[50] An example of this approach emerged in a collaboration led by the New York Restoration Project in New York City's South Bronx.[51] Community members were convened to discuss neighborhood change and to annotate maps of their neighborhood. The event, convened in anticipation of a new pedestrian walkway connected to a large park, was intended to gather data for a design team on barriers and safety hazards that could impede park use. The resulting data were used to inform design strategies to complement and activate use of a new pedestrian bridge from the South Bronx to Randall's Island. A crucial component that emerged was the identification of community points of pride that could be highlighted by the new design, both for the for the enjoyment of area residents and for others who discovered the neighborhood by way of the pedestrian connector. Such spatially explicit group processes have been integrated into a broader approach originating outside of public health called public participation geographic information systems (GIS).[52-54]

In contrast to a group-based approach, one-on-one qualitative data collection strategies, such as in-depth interviews, can be particularly appropriate when specialized knowledge or sensitive topics are discussed. When such data collection efforts focus on experts or leaders, the approach is referred to as key informant interviews,[55] although in recognition of the first-hand expertise that residents have, residents may themselves be considered as key informants. Perceptions reported during in-depth interviews may depend on the characteristics of individuals included and whether representation extends to groups such as youth who may have distinct insights to offer.[56] Interviews can be augmented with visual representations or immersive experiences in the urban environment. Photovoice[57,58] and walk-along[59] interviews can uniquely reveal how individuals understand their surroundings, including aspects that are perceived as health supportive or harming. In urban health photovoice projects such as the one described in Box 6.2, residents may photograph their environment and then retrospectively narrate health-supportive and harmful aspects; in contrast, walk-along interviews elicit narrative descriptions in real time while within the urban contexts of interest.

Beyond the planned information gathered from focus groups and individuals, ethnographic observation has an important history within place-based health research.[43] While this observation approach is by definition intensely specific and local, the utility of ethnographies to generate generalizable knowledge is increasingly recognized.[60] Ethnography that is focused on comparison across urban settings can further be anchored to variation within the urban context through integration with GIS data.[22] Ethnographic accounts from areas with different population characteristics and health burdens may provide insight into the social perceptions and processes. The integration of mixed methods and multiple measurement approaches can provide insights into how urban contexts affects health, and expanding such investigations across multiple areas offers insights that would likely be missed by investigations using GIS data alone or ethnography in a single area, as illustrated in Box 6.3.

Each of these qualitative data collection strategies (see overview in Table 6.1), deployed within a broader framework of qualitative investigation, has the potential to guide our understanding of how people react to and feel about their environment.

Table 6.1 INNOVATIONS FOR ADAPTING SELECTED QUALITATIVE DATA
COLLECTION METHODS TO PLACE-BASED URBAN RESEARCH

Traditional Qualitative Method	Place-Based Adaptation
Focus group	Integration of mapping through PPGIS
In-depth interviews (including key informant interviews)	Photo-voice or walk-along interviews
Ethnography	Selection for observation using GIS-derived characteristics

Abbreviation: PPGIS, public participation geographic information systems.

Recruitment for Qualitative Data Collection: Criteria for Inclusion and for Ending Data Collection

Qualitative approaches have the benefit of allowing urban health teams to engage directly with and hear from a wide range of residents and other stakeholders. Sampling strategies vary across qualitative studies, with research teams and their community partners weighing the importance of ease of recruitment (often by using a convenience sample or snowball sampling) and ensuring the widest range of perspectives is included (through purposive sampling). The goals of sampling, sampling options, and the implications for validity, are viewed differently in quantitative and qualitative data collection efforts.[61] Specifically, qualitative research places less emphasis on obtaining a representative sample (e.g., through random sampling), with more emphasis being placed on informativeness and inclusion.

Once a plan to initiate recruitment has been outlined, teams also need a guideline for when data collection should end. Resource or time limitations may dictate a prespecified sample size or end date. However, particularly for thematic analyses (see brief discussion of qualitative analysis methods in Box 6.4), a saturation criterion is often used to determine when to stop collecting qualitative data.[62] Generally, a sample is thought to reach saturation when themes raised become repetitive, with evidently diminishing returns. However, the operationalization of such a criterion has been challenging and remains controversial.[62,63]

CLOSING THOUGHTS ON IMPROVING OUR UNDERSTANDING OF PERCEPTION AND REFLECTION IN URBAN CONTEXTS

In addition to strategic and systematic measurement, further development or refinement of theory has been strongly recommended for urban health research.[64] The mix of retrospective and situational data collection methods

Box 6.4 QUALITATIVE DATA ANALYSES: REVEALING RECURRENT THEMES AND ELEVATING THE VOICE OF RESIDENTS

Stephen Lankenau

A primary goal of qualitative research methods and data analysis is to convey the perspectives and experiences of research participants in a meaningful and organized manner. A single quote or set of quotes carefully identified from a sea of qualitative data is sometimes the most impactful result from a qualitative analysis. A primary challenge for a qualitative analyst is to convey both depth and breadth of participant experiences so that a full picture of the individuals under study emerge. Much like descriptive quantitative data, qualitative data may be deployed to convey a range of viewpoints on a particular topic as well the most typical sentiment among research participants.

The immediate outcome of qualitative research methods, such as face-to-face interviews, focus groups, and field observations, is raw qualitative data, such as interview transcripts or field notes ready for subsequent analysis. However, transcripts that result from audio recordings of face-to-face interviews or focus groups, while often perceived as objective verbatim recreations of an interview, often involve subjective decision-making by a transcriber (i.e., deciding how to represent an ambiguous section of the interview). Similarly, notes of observations or conversations jotted down in the field must later be converted to organized accounts in the form of written field notes. Hence, these textual data files are created through an initial kind of analytical process. Once developed, textual files can be efficiently organized for more formalized analysis using qualitative software programs (e.g., NVivo, Atlas.ti). These software programs by no means replace the critical thinking required to conduct qualitative data analysis. Rather, these programs are tools to manage, sort through, and code enormous amounts of qualitative data.

To begin the data coding process, a recommended first step is reading through an entire interview transcript or field note to gain an understanding of the person or dynamic among persons captured as a whole during data collection. This is a particularly important step if the data analyst did not conduct the interview or field research themselves, as a way to begin to immerse themselves in the data. Next, blocks of text are tagged with codes within and across multiple transcripts or field notes. Codes can be created through an emergent process as an understanding of the qualitative data unfolds or developed prior to coding and based upon existing theories or research questions. During this coding process, maintaining a broader understanding of the research participants, such as knowing relevant demographic characteristics such as age, gender, race/ethnicity, is important so that individuals are not reduced to decontextualized text or quotes.

Once the coding process is completed, one or more codes may point to a particular theme or themes across multiple participants. Ultimately, themes become the primary set of results emerging from a qualitative analysis. Illustrative participant quotes are often used to highlight particular themes or salient participant sentiments. In this way, presenting the voices of individual participants is a unique and powerful characteristic of qualitive analysis. The validity of qualitative results can be checked by involving multiple coders or analysts from a single research team as well as presenting results to research participants (i.e., "member checking") for their feedback and input. Ultimately, research participants should see themselves clearly and accurately represented in the themes and quotes comprising a finalized qualitative data analysis.

described in this chapter provide fertile ground for theory development and refinement.

Collaboration with a range of qualitative and quantitative experts is important to the data collection strategies described in this chapter, as is collaboration with substantively relevant fields such as environmental psychology.[65] In addition, community and participant relationships and trust are crucial to obtaining data that reflect candid perceptions, concerns, and ideas. Without these, we may misunderstand the causes of the geographically patterned health outcomes described in the following chapter.

REFERENCES

1. Moore GT. Knowing about environmental knowing: The current state of theory and research on environmental cognition. *Environment and Behavior.* 1979;11(1):33–70.
2. Mesch GS, Manor O. Social ties, environmental perception, and local attachment. *Environment and Behavior.* 1998;30(4):504–519.
3. Travers KD. Reducing inequities through participatory research and community empowerment. *Health Education & Behavior.* 1997;24(3):344–356.
4. Beullens K, Loosveldt G, Vandenplas C. Interviewer effects among older respondents in the European social survey. *International Journal of Public Opinion Research.* 2019;31(4):609–625.
5. Couper MP. New developments in survey data collection. *Annual Review of Sociology.* 2017;43:121–145.

6. Rosenbaum DP, Lurigio AJ, Lavrakas PJ. Crime stoppers: A national evaluation of program operations and effects, 1984. Inter-university Consortium for Political and Social Research. Updated January 12, 2006; https://doi.org/10.3886/ICPSR09349.v1.

7. King AC, Winter SJ, Sheats JL, et al. Leveraging citizen science and information technology for population physical activity promotion. *Translational Journal of the American College of Sports Medicine.* 2016;1(4):30.

8. King AC, Winter SJ, Chrisinger BW, Hua J, Banchoff AW. Maximizing the promise of citizen science to advance health and prevent disease. *Preventive Medicine.* 2019;119:44.

9. Zieff SG, Musselman EA, Sarmiento OL, et al. Talking the walk: Perceptions of neighborhood characteristics from users of Open Streets Programs in Latin America and the USA. *Journal of Urban Health.* 2018;95(6):899–912.

10. Sarmiento OL, del Castillo AD, Triana CA, Acevedo MJ, Gonzalez SA, Pratt M. Reclaiming the streets for people: Insights from Ciclovías Recreativas in Latin America. *Preventive Medicine.* 2017;103:S34–S40.

11. Caldwell WB, Reyes AG, Rowe Z, Weinert J, Israel BA. Community partner perspectives on benefits, challenges, facilitating factors, and lessons learned from community-based participatory research partnerships in Detroit. *Progress in Community Health Partnerships.* 2015;9(2):299–311.

12. Ronzi S, Pope D, Orton L, Bruce N. Using photovoice methods to explore older people's perceptions of respect and social inclusion in cities: Opportunities, challenges and solutions. *SSM—Population Health.* 2016;2:732–745.

13. Wang C, Burris MA. Photovoice: Concept, methodology, and use for participatory needs assessment. *Health Education & Behavior.* 1997;24(3):369–387.

14. Gullón P, Díez J, Conde P, et al. Using photovoice to examine physical activity in the urban context and generate policy recommendations: The Heart Healthy Hoods study. *International Journal of Environmental Research and Public Health.* 2019;16(5):749.

15. Díez J, Conde P, Sandin M, et al. Understanding the local food environment: A participatory photovoice project in a low-income area in Madrid, Spain. *Health & Place.* 2017;43:95–103.

16. Budig K, Diez J, Conde P, Sastre M, Hernán M, Franco M. Photovoice and empowerment: Evaluating the transformative potential of a participatory action research project. *BMC Public Health.* 2018;18(1):432.

17. Díez J, Gullón P, Sandín Vázquez M, et al. A community-driven approach to generate urban policy recommendations for obesity prevention. *International Journal of Environmental Research and Public Health.* 2018;15(4):E635.

18. Norwegian Agency for Development Cooperation. *The Logical Framework Approach (LFA): Handbook For Objectives-Oriented Planning.* Oslo, Norway: NORAD; 1996.

19. Franco M, Díez J, Gullón P, et al. Towards a policy relevant neighborhoods and health agenda: Engaging citizens, researchers, policy makers and public health professionals. SESPAS Report 2018. *Gaceta Sanitaria.* 2018;32:69–73.

20. Brawner BM, Reason JL, Hanlon K, Guthrie B, Schensul JJ. Stakeholder conceptualisation of multi-level HIV and AIDS determinants in a Black epicentre. *Culture, Health & Sexuality.* 2017;19(9):948–963.

21. Brawner BM. A multilevel understanding of HIV/AIDS disease burden among African American women. *Journal of Obstetric, Gynecologic, and Neonatal Nursing.* 2014;43(5):E633–E650.

22. Brawner BM, Reason JL, Goodman BA, Schensul JJ, Guthrie B. Multilevel drivers of human immunodeficiency virus/acquired immune deficiency syndrome among Black Philadelphians: Exploration using community ethnography and geographic information systems. *Nursing Research*. 2015;64(2):100–110.

23. Brawner BM, Guthrie B, Stevens R, Taylor L, Eberhart M, Schensul JJ. Place still matters: Racial/ethnic and geographic disparities in HIV transmission and disease burden. *Journal of Urban Health*. 2017;94(5):716–729.

24. Blacksher E, Lovasi GS. Place-focused physical activity research, human agency, and social justice in public health: Taking agency seriously in studies of the built environment. *Health & Place*. 2012;18(2):172–179.

25. Mujahid MS, Diez Roux AV, Morenoff JD, Raghunathan T. Assessing the measurement properties of neighborhood scales: From psychometrics to ecometrics. *American Journal of Epidemiology*. 2007;165(8):858–867.

26. Raudenbush SW, Sampson RJ. Ecometrics: Toward a science of assessing ecological settings, with application to the systematic social observation of neighborhoods. *Sociological Methodology*. 1999;29(1):1–41.

27. Friche AAdL, Diez-Roux AV, César CC, Xavier CC, Proietti FA, Caiaffa WT. Assessing the psychometric and ecometric properties of neighborhood scales in developing countries: Saúde em Beagá Study, Belo Horizonte, Brazil, 2008–2009. *Journal of Urban Health*. 2012;90(2):246–261.

28. Sánchez BN, Raghunathan TE, Diez Roux AV, Zhu Y, Lee O. Combining data from primary and ancillary surveys to assess the association between neighborhood-level characteristics and health outcomes: The Multi-Ethnic Study of Artherosclerosis. *Statistics in Medicine*. 2008;27(27):5745–5763.

29. McQuoid J, Thrul J, Ling P. A geographically explicit ecological momentary assessment (GEMA) mixed method for understanding substance use. *Social Science & Medicine*. 2018;202:89–98.

30. Mennis J, Mason M, Ambrus A, Way T, Henry K. The spatial accuracy of geographic ecological momentary assessment (GEMA): Error and bias due to subject and environmental characteristics. *Drug and Alcohol Dependence*. 2017;178:188–193.

31. Mooney SJ, Sheehan DM, Zulaika G, et al. Quantifying distance overestimation from global positioning system in urban spaces. *American Journal of Public Health*. 2016;106(4):651–653.

32. Jonsen I. Joint estimation over multiple individuals improves behavioural state inference from animal movement data. *Scientific Reports*. 2016;6:20625.

33. Chaix B. Mobile sensing in environmental health and neighborhood research. *Annual Review of Public Health*. 2018;39(1):367–384.

34. Mehra M, Bagri A, Jiang X, Ortiz J. Image Analysis for Identifying Mosquito Breeding Grounds. Paper presented at: 2016 IEEE International Conference on Sensing, Communication and Networking (SECON Workshops); June 27, 2016, London.

35. Oliver M, Badland H, Mavoa S, Duncan MJ, Duncan S. Combining GPS, GIS, and accelerometry: Methodological issues in the assessment of location and intensity of travel behaviors. *Journal of Physical Activity and Health*. 2010;7(1):102–108.

36. Paz-Soldan VA, Stoddard ST, Vazquez-Prokopec G, et al. Assessing and maximizing the acceptability of global positioning system device use for studying the role of human movement in dengue virus transmission in Iquitos, Peru. *American Journal of Tropical Medicine and Hygiene*. 2010;82(4):723–730.

37. Ben-Zeev D, Schueller SM, Begale M, Duffecy J, Kane JM, Mohr DC. Strategies for mHealth Research: Lessons from 3 mobile intervention studies. *Administration and Policy in Mental Health and Mental Health Services Research.* 2014;42(2):157–167.

38. Makosky Daley C, James AS, Ulrey E, et al. Using focus groups in community-based participatory research: Challenges and resolutions. *Qualitative Health Research.* 2010;20(5):697–706.

39. Park Y, Quinn J, Florez K, Neckerman K, Jacobson J, Rundle A. Understanding how the retail food environment supports dietary goals among Hispanics in New York City. *Epidemiology.* 2011;22(1):S261.

40. Diez Roux AV. Investigating neighborhood and area effects on health. *American Journal of Public Health.* 2001;91(11):1783–1789.

41. Creswell JW, Creswell JD. *Research Design: Qualitative, Quantitative, and Mixed Methods Approaches.* Thousand Oaks, CA: SAGE; 2017.

42. Sale JEM, Lohfeld LH, Brazil K. Revisiting the quantitative-qualitative debate: Implications for mixed-methods research. *Quality and Quantity.* 2002;36(1):43–53.

43. Keene DE. Qualitative methods and neighborhood health research. In: Duncan DT, Kawachi I, eds. *Neighborhoods and Health.* 2nd ed. New York: Oxford University Press; 2018:193–218.

44. Thompson S, Paine G, Judd B, Randolph B. Towards a nuanced understanding of health-supportive place using composite research methods. *Geographical Research.* 2019;57(1):24–39.

45. Creswell JW, Clark VLP. *Designing and Conducting Mixed Methods Research.* 3rd ed. Los Angeles, CA: SAGE; 2017.

46. Creswell JW, Klassen AC, Plano Clark VL, Smith KC. *Best practices for mixed methods research in the health sciences.* Washington, DC:Office of Behavioral and Social Sciences Research, National Institutes of Health; 2011.

47. Gale NK, Heath G, Cameron E, Rashid S, Redwood S. Using the framework method for the analysis of qualitative data in multi-disciplinary health research. *BMC Medical Research Methodology.* 2013;13:117.

48. Ulin PR, Robinson ET, Tolley E. *Qualitative Methods in Public Health: A Field Guide for Applied Research.* New York: Wiley; 2005.

49. Tong A, Sainsbury P, Craig J. Consolidated criteria for reporting qualitative research (COREQ): A 32-item checklist for interviews and focus groups. *International Journal for Quality in Health Care.* 2007;19(6):349–357.

50. Kahila-Tani M, Broberg A, Kyttä M, Tyger T. Let the citizens map: Public participation GIS as a planning support system in the Helsinki Master Plan process. *Planning Practice & Research.* 2016;31(2):195–214.

51. Charlotte T, Unite SB, Design H. The Haven Project of the New York Restoration Project. *Landscape Architecture Frontiers.* 2016;4(4):82–93.

52. Brown G, Kyttä M. Key issues and research priorities for public participation GIS (PPGIS): A synthesis based on empirical research. *Applied Geography.* 2014;46:122–136.

53. Cinderby S, Forrester J. Facilitating the local governance of air pollution using GIS for participation. *Applied Geography.* 2005;25(2):143–158.

54. Lowery DR, Morse WC. A qualitative method for collecting spatial data on important places for recreation, livelihoods, and ecological meanings: Integrating focus groups with public participation geographic information systems. *Society & Natural Resources.* 2013;26(12):1422–1437.

55. Ong BN, Humphris G, Annett H, Rifkin S. Rapid appraisal in an urban setting, an example from the developed world. *Social Science & Medicine.* 1991;32(8): 909–915.

56. Morrow V. Using qualitative methods to elicit young people's perspectives on their environments: Some ideas for community health initiatives. *Health Education Research.* 2001;16(3):255–268.

57. Lewinson T, Robinson-Dooley V, Grant KW. Exploring "home" through residents' lenses: Assisted living facility residents identify homelike characteristics using photovoice. *Journal of Gerontological Social Work.* 2012;55(8):745–756.

58. Hergenrather K. Photovoice as community-based participatory research: A qualitative review. *American Journal of Health Behavior.* 2009;33(6).

59. Van Cauwenberg J, Van Holle V, Simons D, et al. Environmental factors influencing older adults' walking for transportation: A study using walk-along interviews. *International Journal of Behavioral Nutrition and Physical Activity.* 2012;9(1):85.

60. Merry SE. Crossing Boundaries: Ethnography in the Twenty-First Century. In: Darian-Smith E, ed. *Ethnography and Law.* London: Routledge; 2017:115–121.

61. Winter G. A comparative discussion of the notion of "validity" in qualitative and quantitative research. *The Qualitative Report.* 2000;4(3):1–14.

62. Saunders B, Sim J, Kingstone T, et al. Saturation in qualitative research: Exploring its conceptualization and operationalization. *Quality & Quantity.* 2018;52(4):1893–1907.

63. Nelson J. Using conceptual depth criteria: Addressing the challenge of reaching saturation in qualitative research. *Qualitative Research.* 2017;17(5):554–570.

64. Story M, Giles-Corti B, Yaroch AL, et al. Work group IV: Future directions for measures of the food and physical activity environments. *American Journal of Preventative Medicine.* 2009;36(4 Suppl):S182–S188.

65. Steg L. *Environmental Psychology: An Introduction.* New York: Wiley-Blackwell; 2018.

CHAPTER 7

Characterizing and Mapping Health in Urban Areas

GINA S. LOVASI AND STEVE MELLY

A key element of urban health introduced in Chapter 1 is the attention to multiple outcomes. Injury and mental health are considered alongside infectious and noncommunicable diseases. Urban health research considers a range of health-related outcomes from risks factors to subclinical disease to clinical disease to functional and quality of life outcomes. The selection of the most appropriate outcome is often driven by hypotheses regarding how multilevel factors in the urban environment affect health related processes.

Several health outcomes of interest, while not comprehensive, are displayed in Table 7.1 to spark thinking about the breadth of potential health outcomes, corresponding data sources, and the goals these data can help to address. Another traditional way to organize health outcomes is based on the organ system most affected. The heart, lung, bones, muscles, brain, digestive system, kidneys, immune system, and many others have corresponding indicators of normal functioning, and indicators of vulnerability to, or progression toward, disfunction and disease states. However, such a focus should not be allowed to obscure the interdependence between them or the importance of more integrative measures such as healthy child development or frailty among the elderly.

In this chapter, we first focus on the goals that shape which health outcomes are of interest. We then turn to common sources of health data and related cautions for their use in an urban context. Because of the place-based focus of urban health, we present information about working with geographically referenced health data as a way to describe spatial variability.

Gina S. Lovasi and Steve Melly, *Characterizing and Mapping Health in Urban Areas* In: *Urban Public Health*. Edited by: Gina S. Lovasi, Ana V. Diez Roux, and Jennifer Kolker, Oxford University Press (2021). © Oxford University Press 2021. DOI: 10.1093/oso/9780190885304.003.0007.

Table 7.1 SELECTED EXAMPLES OF HEALTH OUTCOMES AND MEASUREMENT TYPES FOR CONSIDERATION IN URBAN HEALTH RESEARCH

	Notes Relevant to Urban Health Goals	Common Sources and Cautions for Their Use in Urban Contexts	Noncommunicable Disease	Infectious Disease	Injury	Mental Health
Risk factors	Could be influenced by the urban environment or modify the influence of the urban environment	Sources commonly include surveys and cohort studies; caution is warranted if error masks signal or is different by place or population	Life's Simple 7 for cardiovascular risk; cotinine as a biomarker of tobacco exposure	Sexual risk behaviors, intravenous substance use, medical care settings	Medications that impair balance, intoxication and related behaviors	Family history of mental health conditions, adverse childhood experiences
Early manifestation (subclinical)	Could reflect cumulative exposures in the urban environment or be used to target place-based programs and interventions to slow disease progression	Sources commonly include cohort studies or electronic health records	Atherosclerosis, subclinical emphysema assessed using computed tomography, infections or growths associated with subsequent cancer development	Seropositive without symptoms (latent phase or asymptomatic carrier), colonization of the skin (e.g., with methicillin-resistant *Staphylococcus aureus*)	For older adults, this could include impaired balance or osteoporosis as early manifestations of frailty, which will later result in falls	Subclinical symptoms that indicate potential for progression toward diagnosed mental illness

(continued)

Table 7.1 CONTINUED

	Notes Relevant to Urban Health Goals	Common Sources and Cautions for Their Use in Urban Contexts	Noncommunicable Disease	Infectious Disease	Injury	Mental Health
Diagnosed illness (incidence or prevalence)	Central to community needs assessments and surveillance of health within and across cities	Sources commonly include disease registries, electronic health records; denominators are needed to convert these to rates, and undercounting in both the numerator and denominator may differ by city	Events such as stroke or screening (blood or biopsy) findings resulting in diagnosis	Infection symptoms triggering diagnostic testing with positive results confirming infectious organism, may be reportable to public health agencies	Injury occurrence and severity, may be documented via reports to public authorities (e.g., police report) or hospitalization	Meeting DSM diagnostic criteria, may be detectable through assistance program eligibility or mental health care service utilization
Downstream consequences (harms due to illness)	Economic and patient-oriented outcomes may be of particular interest in community needs assessment and evaluation, and for research or surveillance integrating information across multiple outcomes	Common sources include vital statistics, electronic health records, cohorts; urban neighborhood influence may be obscured if living situation is shifted in response to health challenges	Community susceptibility to further illness / Health-related quality of life and related losses of resilience and productivity / Mortality and years of life lost / Costs for admissions, procedures, and medications to individuals and payor systems / Unequal distribution of health-related burdens may reinforce inequities and block social mobility			

Abbreviation: DSM, *Diagnostic and Statistical Manual of Mental Disorders*.

As an orientation to the multiple health outcomes that may be included in urban health research, we consider goals of description via community needs assessment and surveillance of within and across city differences, as well as etiologic research and evaluation.

Community Health Needs (and Assets) Assessment and the Inclusion of Locally Valued Health Outcomes

Descriptive analyses are often used in an assessment of community needs and assets, which may be labeled a community needs assessment, community diagnosis, or community profile. The term *community* in this context refers to geographic areas; usually these communities are smaller than an entire city, although city-level profiles[1] share many of the features with community needs assessments. A key data requirement is that the health outcome data be geographically aligned with community boundaries or other characteristics defining the population of interest.

Community needs assessments vary in the level of community engagement (discussed in Chapter 13) and in the resources and time allotted to their completion.[2] Because of the local focus of such assessments, selection of health outcomes reflects the priorities of local stakeholders and populations.

Health needs assessments can include medical needs but are broader as well. Indeed, such assessments often point to opportunities to engage with the transportation, social services, educational, or other sectors to address fundamental or "upstream" causes of ill health that are difficult to treat within the doctor's office.

In discussing community diagnoses or community health needs assessments, which can be a basis for population health improvement,[3] we deliberately balance attention to deficits and to assets. Communities understandably are wary of research investigations that may stigmatize or negatively stereotype area residents. A balanced focus may point to opportunities to invest in infrastructure to alleviate disease burden, as well as ways to leverage strengths and sources of health resilience in the existing community.

Urban Health Surveillance Requires Comprehensive or Representative Data and Consistent Methods

Like community health needs assessment, health surveillance can be used to guide action to protect the health of populations.[4] However, health surveillance typically have less engagement with community stakeholders and are often more narrowly focused on selected types of outcomes. Surveillance of specific health outcomes may be particularly helpful in spatial optimization of where relevant facilities or programs should be located.

In contrast to community health needs assessments, which typically take a snapshot of recent community health needs, surveillance is an ongoing and continuous process. Thus, a key data requirement is consistency over time and the availability to incorporate regular updates. Consistency of measurement across different geographic areas is also needed. Thus, the geographic extent and data availability for surveillance will potentially affect which measures can be included. The need for harmonization across location often dictates that a more limited set of data is available for surveillance efforts as they extend to include multiple cities, as the dashboard featuring cities across the United States described in Box 7.1.

Etiologic Research With a Focus on Unbiased Health Outcome Data, Independent of Environment Measurement Error

Research on the urban environment features that influence health outcomes requires special attention to potential biases and measurement error in assessment of health outcomes. As with surveillance, there is an emphasis on measurement of health outcomes that is systematic and comparable across space and time.

Attention to potential bias makes the need for appropriate denominators when estimating rates crucial to etiologic research. For comparisons at a national or state level, rates can reasonably be estimated using the number of diagnoses or deaths in the numerator and the number of residents in the denominator. However, defining such denominators within urban environments can be complex because of population mobility. Individuals can be at risk for experiencing health crises such as injury or cardiac arrest[5] in a location other than their home neighborhood. Places where people spend time, such as parks and streets, are expected to experience a correspondingly high count of health outcomes. As such, in traffic-related injury studies the appropriate denominator may be some measure of pedestrian or vehicular activity, rather than the more commonly used count of residents in that location. While the concentration of individuals walking and engaged in other active transportation activity may lead to a high count of injuries in spaces that attract such activity; we should be cautious to interpret that as indicating high risk, and, in fact, the concentration of active transportation activity may itself improve safety.[6]

Marc N. Gourevitch, Shoshanna Levine, Benjamin Spoer, Becky Ofrane, Neil Kleiman, and Lorna Thorpe

Box 7.1 CITY HEALTH DASHBOARD

Over 80% of the US population lives in urban areas, yet for mayors, city managers, and local health officials seeking to drive health improvements, there are no standardized tools for understanding and benchmarking a city's performance and relative standing on actionable and widely accepted indicators of health and health risk. In an era in which information and data are essential in shaping policies and programs, this lack of common guideposts is one of the most significant challenges to urban health improvement in the United States.

Although data on many key indicators of health and its determinants (e.g., income, housing, education, access to healthy food, air quality) exist for larger geographies (county, state, or national), a core challenge is that these data are not systematically extracted, synthesized, or organized into a useful, standardized set of measures at the city level. Municipal decision makers and community stakeholders thus lack a common framework for focusing on and prioritizing efforts to improve city- or community-level population health and health equity.

To address this gap, with Robert Wood Johnson Foundation support, we developed the City Health Dashboard (www.cityhealthdashboard.com) as a resource for the largest 500 US cities (those with a population of at least 66,000 residents), comprising 33% of the US population. City selection matched that of the 500 Cities Project of the Centers for Disease Control and Prevention. This national resource includes data on 37 measures of health, drivers of health, and health equity that can guide actionable recommendations for urban population health by galvanizing municipal action for health. Responding to stakeholder input during the development process, the site is organized from a city user's perspective: upon selecting one's city, data on the 37 measures are shown for that city's boundaries (and in many cases to its census tracts). Data are fully comparable across cities. Reliance on national data sets rather than primary data collection from cities facilitated feasibility, comparability and scalability.

Inclusion criteria for metrics were defined with city partners, and specified metrics were

1. derived from national-level data sets with rigorous methodological underpinnings, sufficiently granular to permit city-level calculation, and accessible to our team;

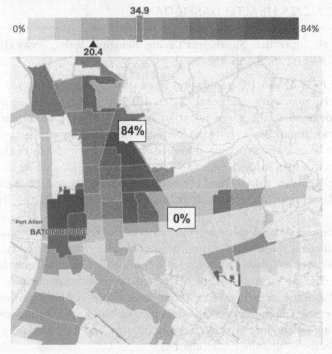

City Value for Children in Poverty in Baton Rouge, LA

Figure 7.1 City value for children in poverty in Baton Rouge, Louisiana.

2. addressed one of five prespecified domains of health and determinants (social and economic factors, physical environment, health behaviors, health outcomes, and clinical care; see examples in Figure 7.1 and 7.2);
3. were important to and could be actionable by city- and community-level stakeholders; and
4. were updated regularly, preferably annually.

Evidence of the Dashboard's adoption and application is increasing rapidly since its launch in mid-2018. In Waco, Texas, the Dashboard is being used to guide community health workers and engage businesses in neighborhood improvement. In Providence, Rhode Island, the Dashboard was used to refocus an effort to improve physical activity. In Grand Rapids, Michigan, the Dashboard was used to spur a specific health focus in the city's strategic plan. In its first year, the website had more than 50,000 unique visitors.

The Dashboard initiative is led by the NYU School of Medicine's Department of Population Health and New York University's Robert F. Wagner School of Public Service, in partnership with the National

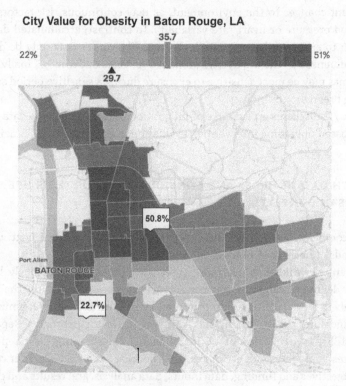

Figure 7.2 City value for obesity in Baton Rouge, Louisiana.[7]

Resource Network, the National League of Cities, and International City/ County Management Association.

Policy Evaluation Requires Health Outcomes Sensitive to Change Over the Study Period

Consistency of measurement quality and low risk of bias, noted previously as priorities for surveillance and etiologic research, are likewise crucial to selection of health outcomes evaluation efforts. Without these, interpretation of evaluation results will be complicated by having multiple plausible explanations.

In the context of an evaluation, health outcomes are selected based on being potentially responsive to the change being evaluated within the timeframe of the study. Conditions with rapid onset or exacerbations may respond to recent changes to the environment, as may continuous risk factors such as blood pressure or heart rate variability. In contrast, accumulated damage leading to susceptibility or chronic diseases like cancer may only be detectably influenced by the urban environment over years or decades. Finally, some outcomes may be most sensitive to exposure during a sensitive period such as during pregnancy or infancy.

Box 7.2 discusses an example of integration of health outcome data into a place-based upgrading intervention evaluation in Belo Horizonte, Brazil.

HEALTH DATA SOURCES AND CONSIDERATION FOR THEIR USE IN URBAN CONTEXTS

With complementary strengths, health data sources discussed next vary in the kinds of health outcomes they include (Table 7.1).

Potential weaknesses warrant attention, although as previously hinted at the degree of emphasis on consistency and bias depend on the goals. Assembled by a working group convened by the World Health Organization, the Guidelines for Accurate and Transparent Health Estimates Reporting (GATHER), is a checklist of 18 items, aimed at promoting best reporting practices of global health estimates. The checklist is divided into four categories: objectives and funding, data inputs, data analysis, and results and discussion. The goal of the checklist is to provide the minimum essential items that should be reported to best serve researchers and decision makers.[8]

Vital Statistics

Birth and death certificate data are among commonly referred to as vital statistics or vital records data. Reports to the national government may be required for births and deaths. Availability of maternal and paternal characteristics relevant to perinatal risk varies by location based on national or state-level systems for data collection. Access to comprehensive data on vital statistics is an ideal that many nations strive toward.

However, this ideal is achieved to varying degrees, with potential for undercounting and misclassification of cause of death. Data from population census records and demographic methods can be used for statistical tuning to compensate for spatial variation in the completeness of death vital statistics data.[9,10]

Box 7.2 BH-VIVA PROJECT: USING SECONDARY DATA TO UNDERSTAND URBAN INTERVENTIONS IN BELO HORIZONTE, BRAZIL

Amélia Augusta de Lima Friche and Waleska Teixeira Caiaffa

A BRIEF DESCRIPTION OF VILA VIVA PROGRAM AND OF BH-VIVA RESEARCH PROJECT

In Belo Horizonte, since 2005, City Hall has been carrying out actions of urban upgrading in slum areas within the scope of Vila Viva Program (VVP), funded by national and international agencies, and investments of the Program of Acceleration of Growth, a policy of the Brazilian Federal Government.[11]

The VVP comprises planning, intervention, and participatory evaluation, based on community participation. For each area, the intervention is designed based on a document called the Global Specific Plan, which is the main planning tool.[11,12] The interventions comprise improvement of the housing, road/street system, sanitation (water, sewage), slope stabilization, land tenure regularization, and promotion of the communities' socioeconomic development to improve the quality of life of residents.[12]

To evaluate the Vila Viva interventions, the Observatory on Urban Health in Belo Horizonte (OSUBH) has been carrying out the BH-Viva Research Project, since 2013. This multiphase, multimethod, and multifunded study includes both qualitative and quantitative components, using secondary and primary data.

The main objective of this research is to evaluate the impact of VVP interventions on health and quality of life of the residents of vulnerable areas and their surroundings compared to the results of the formal city. The conceptual model of the BH-Viva is presented in Figure 7.3. In the next sections, we will focus on collecting, georeferencing and ethical issues regarding secondary health data.[13]

SELECTING STUDY AREAS AND SECONDARY HEALTH DATA SOURCES

A sample of areas was selected based on comparability of their historical characteristics, demographics, occupations, and location in the municipality. Presence or absence of any intervention, location, and timing of interventions was assessed, drawing on

Conceptual framework BH Viva Project

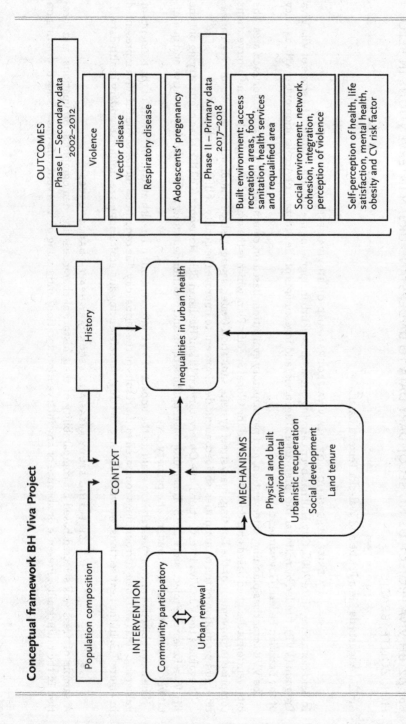

Figure 7.3 Conceptual model of community slum interventions and their effects on health outcomes.
Source: Adapted Mehdipanah R, Manzano A, Borrell C, et al. Exploring complex causal pathways between urban renewal, health and health inequality using a theory-driven realist approach. *Social Science & Medicine.* 2015;124:266–274.

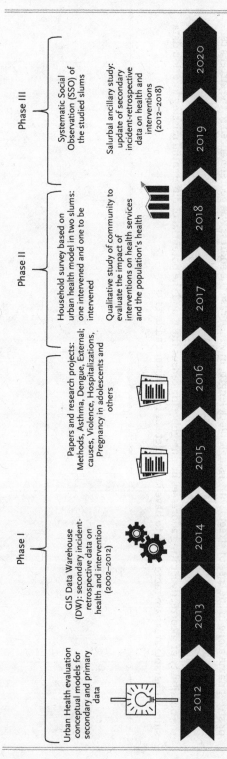

Figure 7.4 Phases and timeline of the BH-Viva Project.

official documents and information gathered in meetings with staff at the central, regional, and local levels of Belo Horizonte Urban Development Company (URBEL). Five slums with and five without intervention were selected to be compared to each other and to the entire formal city (defined as the remainder of Belo Horizonte excluding the slums). The selected areas with and without intervention showed baseline similarities in terms of their health indicators and organization of health services.[13]

Secondary data on mortality and morbidity were obtained through the Health Secretariat of Belo Horizonte, which compiles the health information for the Information Technology Department of the Unified Health System (DATASUS) of the Ministry of Health.[14] A historical series of 11-years (2002–2012), containing the residence addresses of individuals, were initially compiled in a data warehouse. Subsequently, the data warehouse has been expanded with all information from 2013 to 2018 (Figure 7.4).

Based on their importance as health markers for the urban population and their potential sensitivity to the urban intervention, the following events, and respective data sources were selected: (i) mortality due to external causes and cardiovascular diseases from the Mortality Information System (SIM); (ii) hospitalization due to asthma, external causes, and cardiovascular diseases from the Hospital Information System (SIH); and (iii) dengue and tuberculosis occurrence from the Compulsory Notification Disease Information System.[13,14]

Georeferencing of health information was done based on residential addresses of individuals into census tracts, including those that made up selected slum areas. Georeferencing was conducted using the municipal GIS, a local tool managed by the Belo Horizonte Data Processing Company (PRODABEL) through the Intersect Operator Mapinfo software version 8.5. The BH-VIVA Project was approved by the Ethics Research Committees of Federal University of Minas Gerais and SMSA-BH (CAAE 11548913.3.0000.5149).

About 90% of the addresses were georeferenced to the street address level using automatic georeferencing; 5% were based on the closest address on the same street with a street number, of ±100, when the given address was not found in the geographic database or street name alone in the case of streets with a single block length, in which case the address was georeferenced to the street's centroid. The last 5% of the addresses were considered as missing location data.

Challenges noted in this process include the identification of changes of census tracts boundaries and demographics over time,[13,15] the possibility of incorrectly locating addresses in a neighboring census tract, and the potential of differential missing location data since vulnerable areas are more likely to have incomplete or nonexistent addresses.

In the United States, a range of data portals to access such data exist for accessing vital statistics data, including the Center for Disease Control and Prevention's tool, CDC WONDER.[16] The SALURBAL team (introduced in Chapter 1) has assembled vital statistics data available for cities and subcity units in Latin America.[17]

Disease Registries and Notifiable Illness

In addition to collecting vital statistics data, government agencies may require registration of new cases for key conditions as part of ongoing health surveillance. Often, this includes communicable or foodborne illness, although there are also registries for cancers and other chronic diseases. Globally, cases of yellow fever, plague, and cholera are required to be reported to the World Health Organization, although other conditions are notifiable for cases within particular countries.

The individuals whose health is represented in disease registries and records of notifiable illness have not typically provided informed consent for the sharing of their data, as would be typical of human subjects research. Thus, government agencies may treat as sensitive and highly confidential the individual-level records, releasing publicly or for-research-use-only data that has been aggregated across larger geographies such as municipalities or states/provinces. Nonetheless, such aggregated data are useful in estimation of incidence or prevalence rates, life expectancy, and corresponding metrics of inequity.

Cross-Sectional Telephone-Based and In-Person Data Collection

Cross-sectional studies may include telephone-based data collection such as Behavioral Risk Factor Surveillance System or in-person data collection such as National Health and Nutrition Examination Survey. Either approach can provide a snapshot of how risk factors and conditions vary geographically and may be repeated in subsequent years to inform how observed patterns are changing.

An in-person approach may limit reporting bias and provide additional options for assessing subclinical disease burden through direct measurement (i.e., anthropometrics such as height and weight, and other biometrics such as blood pressure), observation during structured tasks (such as a timed-walk or cognitive assessment), and biological samples collected for later analysis (often blood spots, blood serum or plasma, or urine).

The limitations of gathering such data cross-sectionally are important to acknowledge. Often the observed patterns are compatible with more than one plausible explanation and do not provide a clear picture as to whether a purported cause was present prior to disease onset.

Cohort Studies

Cohort studies, which enroll and follow the health of a set of individuals over time, are uniquely suited to focus on the emergence of health outcomes over time. Using approaches like those previously mentioned for in-person cross-sectional data collection, cohort studies can combine multiple time points on the same individual to detect changes in health. Such changes may represent early stages of disease that arise even before symptoms trigger the affected individuals to seek medical care, making cohort studies especially important for our understanding of primary prevention.

Loss to follow-up, however, is a threat to the validity of cohort studies. Not all individuals may stay engaged and available for health measurements over the period of follow-up, and in urban contexts, individuals from socially disadvantaged groups or with unstable living situations are among the most likely to have incomplete follow-up data.

Further, health challenges may themselves precipitate loss to follow-up or relocation,[18] making attention to not only health but also location over time important.

Electronic Health Records

Illness resulting in care from a medical professional may be captured by records kept for patient care and billing purposes—as well as for ongoing quality improvement. Such data may be maintained by governmental, private for-profit, or nonprofit entities. Such data have also been repurposed for exploratory or hypothesis testing investigations.

There is variation in the systems used to record patient information and associated diagnostic and cost data. Further, there may be multiple health systems capturing some data on a given individual, making the data within one health record an incomplete picture of diagnoses and services received. In addition, overlapping catchment areas across multiple hospitals or other organizations in urban areas makes it challenging to identify the population at risk, which is commonly needed for use in denominators when creating rates.

Novel Data Collection Including Sensors and Social Media

Beyond the previously mentioned sources, the increasing abundance of online data has led to innovation in capturing health outcome data using sensor-based data,[19] search terms,[20] and social media text.[21] Such novel data are often accompanied by geographic location, making it potentially useful for the promotion of healthy cities.[22]

While some geographic location information may accompany health data from the various previously discussed sources, the form varies, including address-level, census or postal area, or city-level location information. With the availability of geographic information system (GIS) technology, mapping health data often involves creating spatial data sets that incorporate location information as well as related attribute data including health outcomes. GIS software can be used to query and analyze spatial data sets and link them to other spatial data such as data on environmental exposures. Next, we focus on common processes for creating spatial data sets from tabular health outcome data and visualizing health outcomes using different mapping approaches.

Georeferencing

Data containing addresses for individuals (or for establishments relevant to urban health, such as medical facilities or food stores) can be converted using GIS software to a spatial data set, a process called georeferencing. Longitude, latitude, and attributes based on location can be used along with health outcome data both to create maps to visualize health outcomes and in statistical analyses.

To georeference a health record address, a reference file is used. This reference file can take one of two main forms:

1. a list of street addresses and associated locations (which may include multiple variations of street addresses to accommodate potential ambiguities such as renaming of streets over time), or
2. a street network with included address ranges for each segment between a pair of intersections, allowing for addresses to be assigned a location based on prespecified rules (e.g., assuming that addresses occur throughout the address range with equal spacing along the street, that buildings are a fixed "offset" distance from the center of the street).

Consideration should be given to the software and settings, and depending on the expertise of the team and the scope of the project, it may be appropriate to incorporate multiple reference files in sequence.[23] The address fields themselves may include substantial error that will prevent them from being matched to records in the reference file, which may either result in an incorrect match or missing location data, depending on whether settings allow matching that is less geographically precise, such as based only on postal code.[24]

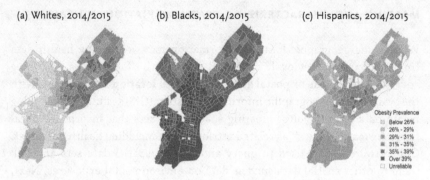

(a) Whites, 2014/2015 **(b) Blacks, 2014/2015** **(c) Hispanics, 2014/2015**

Obesity Prevalence
- Below 26%
- 26% - 29%
- 29% - 31%
- 31% - 35%
- 35% - 39%
- Over 39%
- Unreliable

Figure 7.5 Age/sex-adjusted obesity prevalence in Philadelphia County by race in 2014/2015
Source: Quick H, Terloyeva D, Wu Y, Moore K, Diez Roux AV. Trends in tract- level prevalence of obesity in Philadelphia by race- ethnicity, space, and time. *Epidemiology.* 2020;1(1):15– 21.

The previous discussion uses the more general term *georeferencing* versus *geocoding,*[24,25] as some reserve the term *geocoding* for the process of assigning a numeric code (such as a census tract ID) based on location; georeferencing more generally describes making data mappable, as by assigning longitude and latitude. Nonetheless, a common use of the term *geocoding* is to describe the use of addresses, in combination with a reference street file, to assign longitude and latitude or *xy* coordinates.[26,27]

Mapping Observations and Health Outcomes

Geographic visualizations of health conditions and death have long had a role to play in public health surveillance. Such maps may support both exploratory investigations and hypothesis testing. While cartographic practices cannot be completely covered here, we offer an orientation as a starting point to learning more.

In GIS, data can be thought of as taking the form of either vectors or a raster surface.

Vector data take the form of

- Polygons—geographic areas contained by identified boundaries, such as neighborhoods or parks;
- Lines—defined by connecting an ordered sequence of locations, as to represent streets or transit paths; or
- Points—defined by a single location, often used for homes of other buildings and for intersections.

These labels do not fully capture the complexity with which each can appear on a map. Polygons need not be regular polygons such as squares but can have intricate boundaries, including concave shapes where part of the boundary curves into or intrudes into the main shape, as though a bite or a slice has been removed; shapes simplified to not allow concave parts (minimizing the length of the boundary as though it were a rubber band trying to stretch around the whole shape) are referred to as convex polygons. Likewise, lines on a map need not be unbending and can include paths that appear to curve or change direction. Finally, points need not be represented by a dot, but can instead be shown by a marker such as a star, photo, or even a small chart. Often, a point is used to represent the approximate center or "centroid" of a building or even a neighborhood, which could instead be shown as a polygon in a map zoomed in to show more detail.

Polygons, lines, and points can all be represented in different colors or other aspects of their appearance, which are commonly used to convey differences in the underlying data values. Health outcomes may be shown in an unadjusted fashion or differences in demographic characteristics such as age and sex may be accounted for through methods such as standardization.

In contrast to vector data, raster data are made up of uniform pixels, giving raster maps a grid-like appearance (see Figure 7.5). Once again, color or shade can be used to display values in the underlying data. Some continuous health determinants and risk factors are suitable to being represented in this fashion.

A common strategy to visually compare levels of health (or other attributes) across different pixels or polygons with varied color or shade in accordance a categorized metric of interest, termed choropleth maps. In a cloropleth map, variation in an outcome (e.g., prevalence of violent crime[28]) over space can be easily visualized. Choropleth maps work best when the geographic areas shown are approximately the same size. If the size of the geographic areas varies greatly, the geographically largest areas (which do not necessarily correspond to where data are most reliable) will stand out, and variation in risk among smaller areas may not be noticeable. Cross-hatching or a given color may be identified in the map legend as indicating geographic areas where estimates have a high level of uncertainty or are missing due to insufficient data.

Describing Spatial Variation: Quantifying Autocorrelation

Whether health outcomes are more clustered than would be expected by chance can be described using approaches such as an intraclass correlation.[29] However, other approaches account not only for the multilevel structure of the data, but also for spatial adjacency.

Procedures to detect whether adjacent areas are more similar than expected have been developed, such as Moran's I.[30] Also, spatial scan statistics use arbitrary aggregations (e.g., many concentric circles of different scales centered on the point of each event) to look for higher than expected rates, while accounting for multiple comparisons. Example applications include use of such scans in detection of cancer clusters.[31]

Small-Area Estimation With Attention to Sparse Data

One limitation that may arise when working with aggregated data is having sparse data. Rates or other health outcomes estimated based on a small number of observations are more likely to result in extreme but unreliable values. Fortunately, emerging quantitative methods allow for improved estimates of rates for a specific location, borrowing strength from similar or geographically proximate areas (see Box 7.3).

Box 7.3 SMALL AREA ESTIMATES

Harrison Quick

The growing recognition of often substantial neighborhood variation in health within cities has motivated greater demand for reliable data on small-scale variations in health outcomes. This interest in spatial variation over small geographic areas leads to the challenge of small area estimation (i.e., making inference at a level of geography where the observations within that area do not by themselves provide reliable estimates). To put this in context, a minimum of 16 to 20 events per area for an estimated rate have been recommended to be deemed "reliable."[32]

Obtaining reliable small area-specific estimates for a given subpopulation can be challenging using census, vital statistics, or registry data and perhaps even more so using survey data. To illustrate this, we use our study of census tract-level trends in obesity in Philadelphia[33] based on data with an average of approximately 10 survey respondents per census tract per survey year. Assuming an average obesity prevalence of 30%, this implies that the survey data will fail to provide reliable tract-level estimates not just for subsets of the population (e.g., strata defined by gender and race/ethnicity), but even for the entire population of a given tract.

To overcome this challenge, we considered the use of spatiotemporal Bayesian statistical models.[33] Specifically, using a Bayesian framework facilitates the ability of statistical models to leverage complex correlation structures to obtain more precise estimates of the tract-specific prevalence of obesity for non-Hispanic Whites, non-Hispanic Blacks, and Hispanics.

In addition to leveraging spatial (i.e., between neighboring census tracts) and temporal sources of dependence, our model also accounts for correlation across gender and race/ethnicity. In our Philadelphia-based data, this additional model structure is particularly useful for estimating the prevalence among Hispanics, whose sample sizes are much lower than those for non-Hispanic Whites and Blacks and thus whose small area estimates stand to be most informed by leveraging additional sources of information.

While the primary strength of using a Bayesian approach is its seamless ability to incorporate complex model structures, an often overlooked benefit of Bayesian methods is the flexible nature of the output from Bayesian analyses. For instance, while our model was designed to produce tract-level estimates by race/ethnicity, gender, age, poverty status, and survey year, it is simple to implement population-weighting such that these estimates are recombined to estimate quantities such as the city-level prevalence of obesity by race/ethnicity and gender, complete with point and uncertainty interval estimates. Furthermore, while maps of obesity prevalence like those in (Figure 7.5) may be of chief interest, we can also make formal inference on comparisons between rates, such as the probability of an increase in prevalence or the probability of racial disparities in prevalence.[33]

CLOSING NOTE ON ALIGNMENT ACROSS GOALS, DATA SOURCES, AND VISUALIZATION STRATEGIES

As we close this chapter on mapping health, we note the important role of visuals for reaching the range of community and policy audiences is discussed further in Part III. Excellence in mapping can make the objective and key messages of map easy for a viewer to understand and navigate. Maps of health outcomes, from the time of John Snow to the more recent obesity epidemic, have played an important role in public health priority setting, even though sources of error and representation choices can distort or distract from the spatial patterns observed.[34]

REFERENCES

1. Webster P, Lipp A. The evolution of the WHO city health profiles: A content review. *Health Promotion International*. 2009;24(Suppl 1):i56–i63.
2. de Leeuw E. Evidence for healthy cities: Reflections on practice, method and theory. *Health Promotion International*. 2009;24(Suppl 1):i19–i36.

3. Pennel CL, McLeroy KR, Burdine JN, Matarrita-Cascante D, Wang J. Community health needs assessment: Potential for population health improvement. *Population Health Management*. 2016;19(3):178–186.

4. Thorpe LE. Surveillance as our sextant. *American Journal of Public Health*. 2017;107(6):847–848.

5. Goh CE, Mooney SJ, Siscovick DS, et al. Medical facilities in the neighborhood and incidence of sudden cardiac arrest. *Resuscitation*. 2018;130:118–123.

6. Jacobsen PL. Safety in numbers: More walkers and bicyclists, safer walking and bicycling. *Injury Prevention*. 2015;21(4):271–275.

7. Mehdipanah R, Manzano A, Borrell C, et al. Exploring complex causal pathways between urban renewal, health and health inequality using a theory-driven realist approach. *Social Science & Medicine*. 2015;124:266–274.

8. Stevens GA, Alkema L, Black RE, et al. Guidelines for accurate and transparent health estimates reporting: The GATHER statement. *The Lancet*. 2016;388(10062): e19–e23.

9. Hill K. Estimating census and death registration completeness. *Asian and Pacific Population Forum/East-West Population Institute, East-West Center*. 1987;1(3): 8–13, 23.

10. Bennett NG, Horiuchi S. Mortality estimation from registered deaths in less developed countries. *Demography*. 1984;21(2):217–233.

11. Afonso AS, Magalhães MCF. Programa Vila Viva: Intervenção estrutural em assentamentos precários. In. Revista Urbanização e Habitação. Vol 1. Belo Horizonte: Cia. Urbanizadora e de Habitação de Belo Horizonte - Urbel; 2014.

12. Silveira DC, Carmo RF, Luz ZMPd. O planejamento de quatro áreas do Programa Vila Viva na cidade de Belo Horizonte, Brasil: Uma análise documental. *Ciência & Saúde Coletiva*. 2019;24:1165–1174.

13. Friche AAdL, Dias MAdS, Reis PBd, Dias CS, Caiaffa WT. Urban upgrading and its impact on health: a "quasi-experimental" mixed-methods study protocol for the BH-Viva Project. *Cadernos de saúde pública*. 2015;31:51–64.

14. de Araujo Lima CR, Leal CD, Dias EP, et al. Departamento de Informática do SUS–DATASUS: A experiência de disseminação de informações em Saúde. In: Ministério da Saúde, ed. *A experiência brasileira em sistemas de informação em saúde: Vol. 1. Produção e disseminação de informações sobre saúde no Brasil*. Brasilia, Brazil: Ministério da Saúde, 2009;109–128.

15. Duchesne L. Proyecciones de población, por sexo y edad, para áreas intermedias y menores: Método relación de cohortes. In: del Pilar Granados M, ed. *Métodos para Proyecciones Subnacionales de Población*. Bogotá, Columbia: DANE, 1989: 71–126.

16. Friede A, Reid JA, Ory HW. CDC WONDER: A comprehensive on-line public health information system of the Centers for Disease Control and Prevention. *American Journal of Public Health*. 1993;83(9):1289–1294.

17. Quistberg DA, Diez Roux AV, Bilal U, et al. Building a data platform for cross-country urban health studies: The SALURBAL Study. *Journal of Urban Health*. 2018;96(2) 311–337.

18. Lovasi GS, Richardson JM, Rodriguez CJ, et al. Residential relocation by older adults in response to incident cardiovascular health events: A case-crossover analysis. *Journal of Environmental and Public Health*. 2014;2014:951971.

19. Swan M. Sensor mania! The Internet of things, wearable computing, objective metrics, and the quantified self 2.0. *Journal of Sensor and Actuator Networks*. 2012;1(3):217–253.

20. Green HK, Edeghere O, Elliot AJ, et al. Google search patterns monitoring the daily health impact of heatwaves in England: How do the findings compare to established syndromic surveillance systems from 2013 to 2017? *Environmental Research*. 2018;166:707–712.

21. Curtis B, Giorgi S, Buffone AE, et al. Can Twitter be used to predict county excessive alcohol consumption rates? *PloS ONE*. 2018;13(4):e0194290.

22. Boulos MNK, Al-Shorbaji NM. On the Internet of Things, Smart Cities and the WHO Healthy Cities. *International Journal of Health Geographics*. 2014;13:10.

23. Lovasi GS, Weiss JC, Hoskins R, et al. Comparing a single-stage geocoding method to a multi-stage geocoding method: How much and where do they disagree? *International Journal of Health Geographics*. 2007;6:12.

24. Ribeiro AI, Olhero A, Teixeira H, Magalhães A, Pina MF. Tools for address georeferencing: Limitations and opportunities every public health professional should be aware of. *PLoS ONE*. 2014;9(12):e114130.

25. Reibel M. Geographic information systems and spatial data processing in demography: A review. *Population Research and Policy Review*. 2007;26(5–6):601–618.

26. Krieger N, Waterman P, Lemieux K, Zierler S, Hogan JW. On the wrong side of the tracts? Evaluating the accuracy of geocoding in public health research. *American Journal of Public Health*. 2001;91(7):1114–1116.

27. Rushton G, Armstrong MP, Gittler J, et al. Geocoding in cancer research: A review. *American Journal of Preventive Medicine*. 2006;30(2):S16–S24.

28. Joseph S, Gibson B, Nadji A, Sestito S, Carroll-Scott A. *Community Violence Profile: Eastern North Philadelphia*. Philadelphia, PA: Drexel University Urban Health Collaborative; 2018.

29. Merlo J. A brief conceptual tutorial of multilevel analysis in social epidemiology: Using measures of clustering in multilevel logistic regression to investigate contextual phenomena. *Journal of Epidemiology & Community Health*. 2006;60(4):290–297.

30. Arcaya M, Brewster M, Zigler CM, Subramanian S. Area variations in health: A spatial multilevel modeling approach. *Health & Place*. 2012;18(4):824–831.

31. Sheehan TJ, DeChello LM, Kulldorff M, Gregorio DI, Gershman S, Mroszczyk M. The geographic distribution of breast cancer incidence in Massachusetts 1988 to 1997, adjusted for covariates. *International Journal of Health Geographics*. 2004;3(1):17.

32. US Cancer Statistics Working Group. *United States Cancer Statistics, 1999–2012: Incidence and Mortality Web-Based Report*. Atlanta: US Department of Health and Human Services, Centers for Disease Control and Prevention and National Cancer Institute; 2015.

33. Quick H, Terloyeva D, Wu Y, Moore K, Diez Roux AV. Trends in tract-level prevalence of obesity in Philadelphia by race-ethnicity, space, and time. *Epidemiology*. 2020;31(1):15–21.

34. Monmonier M. *How to Lie With Maps*. 2nd ed. Chicago: University of Chicago Press; 1996.

PART III

Tools for Working With Urban Health Data

"The trick to being a scientist is to be open to using a wide variety of tools."
— Leo Breiman,[1p214]

Bringing together diverse urban health data and using these data to obtain insights and answers to pressing urban health questions requires a flexible repertoire of research tools. We discuss data management and linkage, analysis strategies for investigations that consider the health effects of urban places, the synthesis of results across multiple investigations, and system-oriented approaches to explore the consequences of planned actions. All these strategies serve the ultimate goals of understanding the pathways connecting urban environments to health and guiding action toward improved population health and health equity. While different types of tools are discussed in different chapters, they are all complementary.

REFERENCE

1. Breiman L. Statistical modeling: The two cultures (with comments and a rejoinder by the author). *Statistical Science*. 2001;16(3):199–231.

CHAPTER 8

Managing and Integrating Diverse Sources of Urban Data

GINA S. LOVASI AND STEVE MELLY

In Part II, we have discussed obtaining data on the environment, perceptions of and reflections on that environment, and geographically referenced
health outcomes. In this chapter, we turn to the ways that multiple types of
data can be managed and aligned.

We start with discussion of unique identifiers and other variables. We then
expand our attention to consider naming and linkage of multiple data files,
and documentation of metadata (data about data). Finally, we look at data
linkage, with special attention to linkage of electronic health record (EHR)
data to area-based characteristics. Note that the terms *observations*, *variables*,
and *data sets* will be used but that geographic information systems (GIS) specialists use somewhat parallel terms: *features, attributes*, and *geographic data
sets* (represented visually as layers; see Box 8.1).

VARIABLE CREATION AND MANIPULATION TO FACILITATE LINKAGE

Within a data set to be used for analyses in urban health, key variables include the identifiers of unique observations, along with relevant dates and
distances.

Gina S. Lovasi and Steve Melly, *Managing and Integrating Diverse Sources of Urban Data* In: *Urban Public Health*.
Edited by: Gina S. Lovasi, Ana V. Diez Roux, and Jennifer Kolker, Oxford University Press (2021). © Oxford University
Press 2021. DOI: 10.1093/oso/9780190885304.003.0008.

Box 8.1 DECODING TERMS USED BY GEOGRAPHIC
INFORMATION SYSTEM SPECIALISTS

GIS computer applications have become commonly used in population research.[1] Specialists in their use commonly use terms that have analogues in non-spatial data management. We highlight a few such terms here, and many more have been compiled elsewhere for reference.[2]

A *feature* is a single record or observation that can be mapped, such as the geocoded home address of a study subject.

An *attribute* is a characteristic (analogous to a variable) associated with a feature, for example a person's age or the air pollution level of a census tract.

A *layer* is a visual representation of a geographic data set. In ESRI software layers define how the data should be symbolized and could restrict the visible features to a subset of the features in the data set.

A *spatial overlay* is a technique used to create attributes from one layer based on another layer; for example, a layer of patient home addresses might be used together with a layer of air pollution estimates to create new attributes for the home address layer based on the pollution levels within 1 km.

A *geographic projection* is a method for showing the three-dimensional Earth's surface on a flat screen or other two-dimensional surface; trade-offs are made among preserving distance, area, and shape.

Variable Naming Conventions

Inconsistent variable naming and value formats across data sets can contribute to confusion or even to overwriting data unintentionally if variables with the same name are stored across different data sets.

Naming conventions can be guided by rules established by the team at the outset, with attention to potential trade-offs. For example, there may be a tension between naming that is descriptive of the content and recognizable to most users and naming that links clearly to data collection instruments (e.g., "baselineage" vs. "CATI_Q3" to indicate the third question on a computer-assisted telephone interview, which asks the participant's age).

Variable naming with a fixed placement and length for components such as neighborhood definition or data source may help analysts seeking to identify sets of related variables or conduct sensitivity analyses.

Unique Identification of Observations

While variables are represented as columns within the data, each row represents an observation. Observations may represent individuals, geographic areas, or other instances of data collection (e.g., street observations or environmental samples). A unique identifier variable can be used to refer specifically to each observation in the data set and also to link together multiple data sets pertaining to the same set of observations.

When working with individual data on the health of individuals, confidentiality considerations usually dictate that personal identifiers such as name or medical record number should not be used as the unique identifier for research purposes, nor should we use geographically identifying characteristics such as address (see Box 8.2 for alternative approaches).

Box 8.2 OPTIONS FOR CREATING UNIQUE IDENTIFIERS IN URBAN HEALTH RESEARCH AND EXAMPLE FROM SALURBAL

There are several options for creating unique identifiers, ranging from sequential numbers to more complex structures.

Despite being simple and easy to implement, several problems arise when using sequential numbers to uniquely identify observations. First, the sequence may reveal something (such as recruitment order) that should not be known to the analyst or other research personnel who are meant to be blinded. Second, transpositions or other data entry errors can easily occur that result in an in range but incorrect identifier. For example, "142" may be miswritten or mistyped as "124," which could also be a valid identifier. Training and ongoing checks are key to limiting errors. Finally, if data are simultaneously being collected across multiple sites, sequentially assigned numbers may not, in fact, be unique once multiple data sets are combined.

Another potential strategy to creating unique identifiers is to use globally unique identifiers (GUIDs), which have previously been used for health data.[3,4] The resulting identifier consists of 32 letters and numbers (called hexadecimal digits, since only the 10 numeric digits and the first 6 letters of the alphabet are used). An example of a randomly generated GUID (from www.guidgenerator.com) is "d84e43f6-ba45-4a0a-ad56-09075687773f"—note that there are 8, 4, 4, 4, and 12 digits grouped together, separated by dashes. Rather than directly sharing and using personally identifying information, the GUID system can incorporate such information using a one-way encryption algorithm. Such identifiers

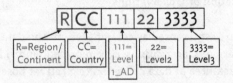

R	CC	111	22	3333
R=Region/ Continent	CC= Country	111= Level 1_AD	22= Level2	3333= Level3

Figure 8.1 Example structure for an identifier in multilevel data from the SALURBAL study. R is a placeholder for a single-digit indicator of region, to potentially be used in future collaborations beyond the Latin American region; the parts of the identifier representing country and city (CC111) are used together as an identifier for city (a variable named "SALID1"); correspondingly, the country, city, and subcity (CC11122) make up an identifier for subcity (a variable named "SALID2"); finally, the smallest geographic units have country, city, and subcity information as well as neighborhood (CC111223333; "SALID3").

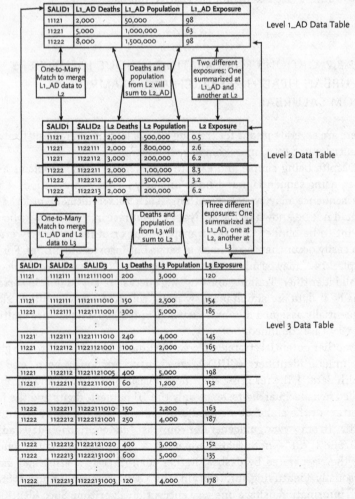

Figure 8.2 Schematic representation of multi-level linkage from city to sub-city to neighborhood units in SALURBAL.

have sufficient complexity to prevent analysts from re-identifying the data, even though using identical values in the original fields would result in the same GUID—this allows for observations representing the same individual to be recognized. Coded data sets do not contain but can be linked to personally identifying variables, in which case linkage files should be kept separate and secure.

Given the multilevel nature of data used for urban health research, an option is to structure the ID numbers in a way that reflects the structure of the data, such as with a prefix that indicates the broader geographic area from which a sample was obtained. For example, from the SALURBAL data structure protocol, the identifying variable for small spatial units are shown in Figure 8.1. The global region (R), two-letter country code (CC), a numeric code for the administratively defined urban area (111) and large subcity units (22), are each embedded within the identifying variable of smaller level 3 units (with an ending of 3333). Here the number of digits for each part is fixed, such that there will always be the same structure, allowing the parts to be parsed to facilitate linkage of data at multiple levels.

When studying environmental characteristics assessed at multiple levels as predictors of health outcomes (such as cause-specific mortality rates) at the smallest geographic unit, linkage across levels would be use the information in common between the identifying variables for larger and smaller geographic units (Figure 8.2).

Dates and Distance

Date and distance variables notably require attention to the format and units used to facilitate ease of use and interpretation.

For variable names incorporating dates or variables whose values represent dates, a format of four-digit year, two-digit month, and two-digit day (yyyymmdd) has the advantage of sorting chronologically. We also note that treatment of dates may vary across software.

For variables related to distance, units of observation can be incorporated into variable names (e.g., adding "_ft" or "_m" for the names of distance variables to indicate feet or meters, respectively). Given the aspirations of urban health research to connect local and global efforts, the international system of units (SI units, also known as metric units) should be preferred,[5] except when there are overriding considerations such as preference of a key stakeholder audience.

FILE NAMING AND METADATA TO EASE NAVIGATION AND LINKAGE

As with the identification of unique observations and the naming of variables, file naming and archiving of metadata can be planned to facilitate navigation and reduce errors in use of the data.

Naming Files to Reflect the Content of Files and Their Relationship to Each Other

For complex projects with many files, file naming can signal not only the type of data in a given file, but also where the file fits within a hierarchy in the data structure. Often, if files are to be organized by the geographic area they represent, using the beginning of the file name to signal the broadest level of this hierarchy eases sorting and identification of geographically similar files (e.g., by country or city). Additional elements of the file naming may signal the sequence within data collection or which release of the data is represented (while some projects update data on a rolling basis, it is common to provide periodic releases or "freezes" of the data, reflecting data collection and cleaning through a certain date).

In naming files that are specific to individual study participants, such as documents containing interview transcripts or data sets of an individual's recorded GPS points, considerations of confidentiality in file naming are similar to those that exist in creating a unique identifier. When necessary, use of a coded study identifier in the file name is preferable to personally identifying information such as name or medical record number.

Considerations Related to Temporal Scale: From Days to Decades

Urban health is shaped by processes that unfold over time, yet the relevant time scale varies. Exposures such as extreme temperatures[6,7] or elevated pollen counts[8-10] appear to affect health outcomes in a matter of days. Other short-term effects of urban places on health have been shown such as for community violence and test performance in the following week.[11] On the other hand, place-based exposures that affect fundamental causes of health, such as educational attainment, may require decades or generations to take full effect.

For relatively uncommon occurrences, such as homicides, pooling of multiple years may be desirable to obtain stable spatial patterns. Multiple years of data may also be used together to obtain stable estimates for small geographic areas are of interest in a given year.

Thus, as choices are made to combine data across dates or maintain temporal detail, there may be temporal structure that should be reflected in the file naming. This may require not only distinguishing which date the data represents, but also which files contain original data with detailed variation over time or versions that reflect combinations across time, such as to approximate stable annual or five-year pooled estimates.

Data About the Data Set: Maintaining Metadata

Although thoughtful approaches to the naming of data files and the variables within them can signal their contents to data users, it is rare for file and variable names to include all necessary information about the data sets. Each data set will have idiosyncrasies that should be considered during its use that need to be captured in separate documentation about the data, or metadata.

Standards for metadata have been proposed across several fields and catalogued. Of particular note is the International Organization for Standardization (ISO) technical committee on geographic information/geomatics,[12] which provides updated guidance every five years. Metadata documents can vary widely in length. Even longer data dictionaries or codebooks designed to provide variable-specific information to analysts (e.g., on missing data or labels for response options).

Metadata including details on the sources of secondary data or the protocols used to collect primary data collection help to ensure this information is available at the analysis stage. This can include the construction of analytic or complex survey weights,[13] to be used for better approximation of what would be seen in the population from which the data were sampled. Later modification of these weights may be needed, including for analyses at a finer geographic unit than was originally planned.[14,15]

Restrictions on use or redistribution of the data can also be noted, such as those reflecting terms specified by governmental or commercial providers of secondary data. Metadata documents can also to draw attention to important cautions and caveats that become salient through early experience cleaning and using the data. For spatially referenced data in particular, information should include the geographic projection used (see definition in Box 8.1) and any known locational error in each data set.

BRINGING IT ALL TOGETHER: LINKING AND SHARING DATA SETS AND ASSOCIATED DOCUMENTATION

Other important considerations in preparing for analysis pertain to how data are structured and combined and how data and associated documentation are shared.

Longer or Wider: Options for Combining Data Sets

Data sets with the same variables (or that can be manipulated to have the same variables) can be combined by stacking or "appending" observations. This may be possible, for example, when data are collected across multiple urban settings using the same protocol and data entry system. Resources have been developed on working with data in a tidy form,[16] as well as responsible work with spreadsheets,[17] which can ease the process of bringing observations from multiple data sets together.

When data of different types need to be combined, such as environmental characteristics to be merged with individual-level health data, we need to envision the structure we want the resulting data to have. A format with many observations (e.g., with repeated measurements of the same park represented across multiple rows) can be described as being in a "long" format. This is contrasted with a "wide" representation of the same data with many variables (e.g., with one row containing all information on a given park, with multiple variables to represent the multiple rounds of observation). Projects with a large volume of data may also consider alternatives such as normalized relational databases, designed to limit redundancy.[18]

Spatial data can be viewed and modified using GIS software. Metrics can be constructed for the areas around home address or for other personalized neighborhood definitions.[19] Spatial information across different layers may be used to bring them together. This is usually through either a table join (e.g., using a census district identifier that is common to all data elements) or using spatial operations (e.g., spatial overlay to create new attributes for features in one layer based on spatially adjacent or overlapping features in another).

Making Files Available With Attention to Accessibility and Data Security

While on the one hand a shared mission to assemble timely evidence on urban health may motivate open data sharing, countervailing considerations include any required confidentiality protections or restrictions due to licensed data or terms of use.[20] For project management and to avoid duplicated effort and conflict, many projects document proposed use of data resources, allowing the group to come to preliminary agreement on the scope and approach, as well as to evaluate the level of sensitivity of the required data and how such data should be shared. Tracking data access can be helpful to ensure that users are alerted to updated versions that become available or errors that have been identified.

For metadata, data collection protocols, and other elements with low sensitivity, sharing can often be done at minimal cost via cloud storage systems such as Google Drive or Dropbox or via institutional intranet and server systems. A front end can be developed (e.g., Google sites, internal study website) to help users navigate documentation. Clear guidance should also be provided to ensure that any such storage systems are used only as intended by the team and that protected human subjects' information such as location of residence or health characteristics are never shared without adequate protections and ethical committee oversight.

For personally or geographically identifying information and individual-level health data, protection from potential breach of confidentiality often requires that all individuals using the data be named on a corresponding human subjects research protocol, having previously completed appropriate certification in the responsible handling of human subjects data. Such protocols may specify acceptable secure methods of file transfer and whether data may need to be stored and accessed exclusively through encrypted server space or encrypted endpoint devices (using tools such as bitlocker or filevault). For extremely sensitive individual-level data, there may be a requirement to access data in a secure on-site data center.[20,21]

SPOTLIGHT ON STRATEGIES FOR INTEGRATING GEOGRAPHIC DATA WITH CLINICAL RECORDS

While the increasingly widespread adoption of EHRs[22] was introduced in the previous chapter, here we emphasize the scope of research questions that can be addressed when information about geographic context is integrated with individual health data (see Box 8.3 for a summary of prior work and Box 8.4 for an example).

Both clinical and place-based researchers increasingly recognize the ways in which neighborhood- and community-level factors affect both the health of individuals and persistent social, economic, and racial/ethnic health disparities,[23,24] motivating linkage of geographic data with clinical records. Linked data can then be used to

1. Understand the geographic scope and pattern of health threats or opportunities to improve health,[25-28] as would be incorporated into a community health needs assessment;
2. Provide geographically specific information to residents or local organizations[29];
3. Conduct etiologic research relevant to how where patients live, work, or play affects their health risks, either directly or by modifying the effects of clinical care decisions[30-34]; and/or
4. Deploy locally descriptive data in combination with generalizable research findings to inform local action on modifiable aspects of the environment,[35-37] including future policies and programs.[38]

EHRs are a vast source of patient information, often recorded with a high level of precision and containing a variety of indicators from which to extract indicators of health status. A recent systematic literature review summarized the characteristics of studies linking EHRs to geospatial data.[39]

Of note, only a limited number of health outcomes have been the focus of population health research studies. Of these, the most common outcomes studied were health care utilization, cardiometabolic health, and obesity.

Area-based socioeconomic measures, including area-level median household income or percentage of area residents living below the poverty line, were the most common type of environmental measure that was linked with EHR data. Studies have also examined whether proximity to medical facilities affects utilization rate of health-care services, such as receiving colonoscopy screenings or psychiatric services. Built environment characteristics were used, especially in studies that focused on cardiometabolic health outcomes. For example, living in closer proximity to fast-food restaurants and convenience stores was associated with a higher body mass index.[40] Some studies also explored the relationship between environmental contaminants or outdoor air pollutants with a range of health outcomes, including birth outcomes and respiratory outcomes such as asthma.

The review noted that EHRs contain accurate location information for patients, which can be used to conduct highly efficient environmental research studies. The spatial units used to assign environmental exposures to patient records varied across studies, commonly including census tracts, postal codes, or municipalities. A minority of studies used geocoded patient addresses to assign environmental exposures within a buffer defined by distance from the home address. Finally, beyond ongoing exposures in the vicinity of the home address, some studies focused on temporal variation (e.g., in area-level pollutant or meteorological variables) or on characteristics of the area surrounding the clinical care location.

The existing research illustrates the potential that EHR data offer for conducting efficient, low-cost, and urban health research. Future research innovation may expand the use of narrative information stored in EHRs, opening new avenues to assess health inequities and environmental-health associations across a variety of clinical health outcomes.

Source: Adapted by Vaishnavi Vaidya from a review by Schinasi et al.[39]

Box 8.4 LINKING GEOGRAPHIC AND PEDIATRIC HEALTH RECORDS IN PHILADELPHIA

The Urban Health Collaborative (UHC) at Dornsife School of Public Health Drexel University is working in close collaboration with Children's Hospital of Philadelphia (CHOP) to link a broad suite of place-based measures to EHR to investigate predictors of pediatric health concerns, including avoidable hospitalizations, obesity, and asthma.[41] This project titled "Pediatric Big Data" (PBD) leverages robust environmental data capabilities including big data, machine learning and traditional epidemiology methods.

Patients' home addresses from CHOP EHR were linked to Census tracts and blocks, as well as to 30 m and 250 m grids created throughout the metropolitan Philadelphia area (Figure 8.3). Examples of geospatial measures created include

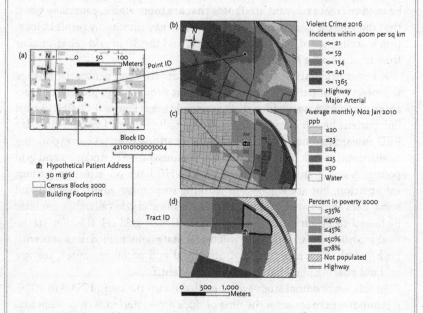

Figure 8.3 Linking addresses to data at different spatial scales.[42]

Sources: Panel A: 30 m grid, Urban Health Collaborative; Census Blocks 2000, US Census; Building Footprints, OpenDataPhilly.org; City of Philadelphia Department of Licenses and Inspections & Office of Innovation and Technology, 2015. Panel B: Crime Incidents, OpenDataPhilly.org; Philadelphia Police Department, 2016; Street Center Lines, OpenDataPhilly.org; City of Philadelphia Streets Department, 2016. Panel C: Average monthly NO$_2$ from Bechle MJ, Millet DB, Marshall JD. National spatiotemporal exposure surface for NO2: Monthly scaling of a satellite-derived land-use regression, 2000–2010. *Environmental Science & Technology*. 2015;49(20):12297–12305. Panel D: Percentage in Poverty, US Census 2000.

- socioeconomic measures from the US Census American Community Survey at the census tract level,
- modeled NO_2 air pollution estimates at the census block level,
- violent crime density across 30 m grid cells, and
- satellite derived measures of greenness (Normalized Difference Vegetation Index) across 250 m grid cells

To create such measures, home addresses have been georeferenced and saved as a spatial data set of points, and then the GIS spatial join tool is used to link the points to the administrative boundaries and grid cells. Creating a 30 m and 250 m grids for the metropolitan area provides researchers flexibility to create measures at different scales (Figure 8.3, Panel A). Creating surfaces representing exposures within various buffer distances around 30 m grid points is more efficient than creating individual overlapping buffers around the 350,000 addresses in the CHOP data. Exposure surfaces such as violent crime density can be created and efficiently stored as rasters (Figure 8.3, Panel B). Multiple grid cells may be used to create relevant attributes that are more stable, especially given that the address georeferencing techniques may commonly result in location inaccuracies of approximately 30 m, and the 30 m grid cell is smaller than typical house lots in Philadelphia.

A key consideration in developing this approach to geospatial linkage is protection of patients' privacy. Different project team groups have access only to data needed for their assigned tasks (Figure 8.4). CHOP staff link patient health data to addresses. A small group of Drexel University PBD researchers has access to address locations (but no corresponding health data) to link home locations to administrative boundaries and grid points. A larger team based at Drexel's UHC have no access to patient information, but are engaged in working to prepare environmental and social data aggregated to administrative units and grid cells, that can later be linked to by administrative boundary IDs or grid cell IDs. For statistical analyses, the CHOP team will then create deidentified data sets with both health outcomes and environmental and social measures, for use without sharing personal or geographic identifiers.

In this longitudinal study with health data for the period 2005 to 2016, it is important to consider the time periods associated with environmental data. Surfaces from many time periods and many types of exposures can be brought together using GIS software to create new attributes for home address, administrative areas, or grid cell features. For data sets available annually such as traffic density, exposure surfaces are created separately for each year. In other measures such as land use, data is expected to represent conditions over multiple years and is updated less frequently. Data

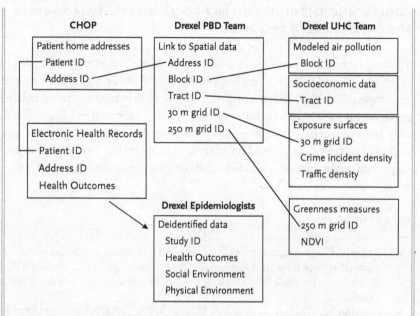

Figure 8.4 A multidisciplinary team approach facilitates processing large amounts of data while protecting patient confidentiality.

available at finer time scales—such as daily air pollution measurements or biweekly Normalized Difference Vegetation Index data—are linked to specific analytical data sets when needed for investigating hypothesis associated with these time scales.

The PBD project presents many data management challenges, but it is also an opportunity to bring together a diverse group of researchers with a broad range of expertise to leverage the power of EHRs, spatial data sets, and the latest computer technology. This study is part of the Pediatric Big Health Data initiative funded by the State of Pennsylvania and led by the Children's Hospital of Philadelphia, University of Pennsylvania, and the UHC at Drexel University.

However, access to potentially sensitive geographically identifiable data in combination with personal health information from clinical records is subject to confidentiality rules and restrictions.[20,43] Use and access to such data requires procedures for secure data sharing across teams, agencies, and sectors.[44,45] In addition, much useful content within EHRs is in free-text format (e.g., scanned medical reports), which adds an additional layer of complexity to effectively extracting and using EHR data. Incomplete, variably formatted, or inconsistent clinical data, particularly for repositories drawing from multiple clinical entities, make data cleaning and quality checking challenging.[46]

CONCLUDING THOUGHTS ON MANAGING DIVERSE DATA SOURCES FOR URBAN HEALTH RESEARCH

Working from the smallest data elements to efforts combining the multiple types of data needed for urban health research, we have highlighted several challenges. The place-based nature of urban health investigations creates opportunities while also requiring attention to the protection of confidentiality and the complexity of hierarchical data structures. In the next chapter, we turn our attention to the data analysis strategies that can be used to leverage high quality data to provide both descriptive and causal information.

REFERENCES

1. Reibel M. Geographic information systems and spatial data processing in demography: A review. *Population Research and Policy Review*. 2007;26(5–6):601–618.
2. Kennedy H. *The ESRI Press Dictionary of GIS Terminology*. Redlands, CA: ESRI Press; 2001.
3. Johnson SB, Whitney G, McAuliffe M, et al. Using global unique identifiers to link autism collections. *Journal of the American Medical Informatics Association*. 2010;17(6):689–695.
4. Chen X, Fann YC, McAuliffe M, Vismer D, Yang R. Checking questionable entry of personally identifiable information encrypted by one-way hash transformation. *JMIR Medical Informatics*. 2017;5(1):e2.
5. Monroe EE, Nelson MN. Say "yes" to metric measure. In: Goldston MJ, ed. *Stepping Up To Science and Math: Exploring the Natural Connections*. Arlington, Virginia: NSTA Press; 2009:3.
6. Rodopoulou S, Samoli E, Analitis A, Atkinson RW, de'Donato FK, Katsouyanni K. Searching for the best modeling specification for assessing the effects of temperature and humidity on health: A time series analysis in three European cities. *International Journal of Biometeorology*. 2015;59(11):1585–1596.
7. Son J-Y, Gouveia N, Bravo MA, de Freitas CU, Bell ML. The impact of temperature on mortality in a subtropical city: Effects of cold, heat, and heat waves in São Paulo, Brazil. *International Journal of Biometeorology*. 2016;60(1):113–121.
8. Weinberger KR. *Spatial and Temporal Distribution of Tree Pollen in New York City: Linking Aeroallergen Measurements to Health*. New York: Columbia University; 2015.
9. Osborne NJ, Alcock I, Wheeler BW, et al. Pollen exposure and hospitalization due to asthma exacerbations: Daily time series in a European city. *International Journal of Biometeorology*. 2017;61(10):1837–1848.
10. Jariwala S, Toh J, Shum M, et al. The association between asthma-related emergency department visits and pollen and mold spore concentrations in the Bronx, 2001–2008. *Journal of Asthma*. 2014;51(1):79–83.
11. Sharkey P, Schwartz AE, Ellen IG, Lacoe J. High stakes in the classroom, high stakes on the street: The effects of community violence on students' standardized test performance. *Sociological Science*. 2014;1:199–220.
12. Grønmo R, Berre A-J, Solheim I, Hoff H, Lantz K. DISGIS: An interoperability framework for GIS—using the ISO/TC 211 model-based approach. Paper

presented at: 4th Spatial Global Data Infrastructure Conference, Cape Town, South Africa; 2000.

13. Lee ES, Forthofer RN. *Analyzing Complex Survey Data, Vol. 71.* Thousand Oaks, CA: SAGE; 2005.

14. Rundle AG, Sheehan DM, Quinn JW, et al. Using GPS data to study neighborhood walkability and physical activity. *American Journal of Preventive Medicine.* 2016;50(3):e65–e72.

15. Freeman L, Neckerman K, Schwartz-Soicher O, et al. Neighborhood walkability and active travel (walking and cycling) in New York City. *Journal of Urban Health.* 2013;90(4):575–585.

16. Wickham H. Tidy data. *Journal of Statistical Software.* 2014;59(10):1–23.

17. Broman KW, Woo KH. Data organization in spreadsheets. *American Statistician.* 2018;72(1):2–10.

18. Codd EF. A relational model of data for large shared data banks. *Communications of the ACM.* 1970;13(6):377–387.

19. Lovasi GS, Grady S, Rundle A. Steps forward: Review and recommendations for research on walkability, physical activity and cardiovascular health. *Public Health Reviews.* 2012;33(2):484–506.

20. O'Keefe CM, Rubin DB. Individual privacy versus public good: Protecting confidentiality in health research. *Statistics in Medicine.* 2015;34(23):3081–3103.

21. De Wolf VA. Issues in accessing and sharing confidential survey and social science data. *Data Science Journal.* 2003;2:66–74.

22. Chaudhry B, Wang J, Wu S, et al. Systematic review: Impact of health information technology on quality, efficiency, and costs of medical care. *Annals of Internal Medicine.* 2006;144(10):742–752.

23. Roux AVD, Mair C. Neighborhoods and health. *Annals of the New York Academy of Sciences.* 2010;1186(1):125–145.

24. Institute of Medicine. *Capturing Social and Behavioral Domains in Electronic Health Records: Phase 1.* Washington, DC: National Academies Press; 2014.

25. Laranjo L, Rodrigues D, Pereira AM, Ribeiro RT, Boavida JM. Use of electronic health records and geographic information systems in public health surveillance of type 2 diabetes: A feasibility study. *JMIR Public Health and Surveillance.* 2016;2(1):e12.

26. Casey JA, Curriero FC, Cosgrove SE, Nachman KE, Schwartz BS. High-density livestock operations, crop field application of manure, and risk of community-associated methicillin-resistant *Staphylococcus aureus* infection in Pennsylvania. *JAMA Internal Medicine.* 2013;173(21):1980.

27. Gutilla MJ, Davidson AJ, Daley MF, Anderson GB, Marshall JA, Magzamen S. Data for community health assessment in rural Colorado. *Journal of Public Health Management and Practice.* 2017;23:S53–S62.

28. Zhang Y, Baicker K, Newhouse JP. Geographic variation in the quality of prescribing. *New England Journal of Medicine.* 2010;363(21):1985–1988.

29. Beck AF, Sandel MT, Ryan PH, Kahn RS. Mapping neighborhood health geomarkers to clinical care decisions to promote equity in child health. *Health Affairs.* 2017;36(6):999–1005.

30. Stahler GJ, Mennis J, Cotlar R, Baron DA. The influence of neighborhood environment on treatment continuity and rehospitalization in dually diagnosed patients discharged from acute inpatient care. *American Journal of Psychiatry.* 2009;166(11):1258–1268.

31.   Goldstein BA, Navar AM, Pencina MJ, Ioannidis JP. Opportunities and challenges in developing risk prediction models with electronic health records data: A systematic review. *JAMIA*. 2017;24(1):198–208.

32.   Tomayko EJ, Flood TL, Tandias A, Hanrahan LP. Linking electronic health records with community-level data to understand childhood obesity risk. *Pediatric Obesity*. 2015;10(6):436–441.

33.   Boscarino J, Kirchner HL, Pitcavage J, et al. Factors associated with opioid overdose: A 10-year retrospective study of patients in a large integrated health care system. *Substance Abuse and Rehabilitation*. 2016;7:131–141.

34.   Kind AJH, Jencks S, Brock J, et al. Neighborhood socioeconomic disadvantage and 30-day rehospitalization. *Annals of Internal Medicine*. 2014;161(11):765–774.

35.   Gabert R, Thomson B, Gakidou E, Roth G. Identifying high-risk neighborhoods using electronic medical records: A population-based approach for targeting diabetes prevention and treatment interventions. *PLoS ONE*. 2016;11(7):e0159227.

36.   Lee AC, Maheswaran R. The health benefits of urban green spaces: A review of the evidence. *Journal of Public Health*. 2011;33(2):212–222.

37.   Casey J, James P, Rudolph K, Wu C-D, Schwartz B. Greenness and birth outcomes in a range of Pennsylvania communities. *International Journal of Environmental Research and Public Health*. 2016;13(3):311.

38.   Carroll-Scott A, Henson RM, Kolker J, Purtle J. The role of nonprofit hospitals in identifying and addressing health inequities in cities. *Health Affairs*. 2017;36(6):1102–1109.

39.   Schinasi LH, Auchincloss AH, Forrest CB, Diez Roux AV. Using electronic health record data for environmental and place based population health research: A systematic review. *Annals of Epidemiology*. 2018;28(7):493–502.

40.   Fiechtner L, Sharifi M, Sequist T, et al. Food environments and childhood weight status: Effects of neighborhood median income. *Childhood Obesity*. 2015;11(3):260–268.

41.   Kenyon C, Maltenfort M, Hubbard R, et al. Practice variability in asthma diagnosis in young children in a large pediatric primary care network. Paper presented at: Pediatric Academic Societies (PAS) Meeting, 2019; Baltimore MD.

42.   Bechle MJ, Millet DB, Marshall JD. National spatiotemporal exposure surface for NO2: Monthly scaling of a satellite-derived land-use regression, 2000–2010. *Environmental Science & Technology*. 2015;49(20):12297–12305.

43.   Centers for Medicare and Medicaid Services. The Health Insurance Portability and Accountability Act of 1996 (HIPAA). 1996; https://aspe.hhs.gov/report/health-insurance-portability-and-accountability-act-1996.

44.   Wartenberg D, Thompson WD. Privacy versus public health: The impact of current confidentiality rules. *American Journal of Public Health*. 2010;100(3):407–412.

45.   VanWey LK, Rindfuss RR, Gutmann MP, Entwisle B, Balk DL. Confidentiality and Spatially Explicit data: Concerns and Challenges. *Proceedings of the National Academy of Sciences*. 2005;102(43):15337–15342.

46.   Botsis T, Hartvigsen G, Chen F, Weng C. Secondary use of EHR: Data quality issues and informatics opportunities. *AMIA Joint Summits on Translational Science Proceedings*. 2010;2010:1–5.

CHAPTER 9

Analysis Strategies for Relating the Urban Environment to Health

GINA S. LOVASI

A wide range of analysis tools are potentially useful within urban health research, depending on the research question and the nature of the data to be used. While comprehensive guidance on these is beyond the scope of this toolkit, throughout this chapter we highlight example studies and approaches, referencing more detailed resources that can be consulted for further information and recommendations for using these design and analytic strategies well.

DESCRIPTIVE, CAUSAL INFERENCE, AND EVALUATION-RELATED ANALYSES GOALS

Following the typology introduced in Chapter 1, we will review briefly descriptive, etiologic, and evaluation goals that analyses may be designed to address and then consider commonly encountered issues resulting from the place-based nature of urban health research.

Multivariable Descriptive Analyses: Attention to Characterizing the Underlying Population and Drivers of Inequity

An important role of descriptive urban health research is to provide new insights into the health-relevant realities and associations seen within the urban environment. Quantifying and visualizing trends across space and

Gina S. Lovasi, *Analysis Strategies for Relating the Urban Environment to Health* In: *Urban Public Health.* Edited by: Gina S. Lovasi, Ana V. Diez Roux, and Jennifer Kolker, Oxford University Press (2021). © Oxford University Press 2021. DOI: 10.1093/oso/9780190885304.003.0009.

time may highlight emerging reasons for concern, as well as bright spots with better than expected health, which might be examined for innovation.[1] These approaches are complementary to place-based qualitative research methods in Chapter 6 and of mapping health outcomes alone discussed in Chapter 7.

Accounting for geographically-based sampling weights (mentioned in Chapter 8) to approximate what would be estimated for the full underlying population is particularly central to many analyses aiming to describe environments and health in a specific urban setting.

Given the commitment within the field urban health—and public health more broadly—to taking understanding and addressing health inequities, descriptive data can be especially useful to highlight how such inequities arise and vary. In the spirit of bringing inequality to the foreground, stratification across important population groups can be an important part of descriptive analyses. For example, in a brief developed by the Drexel Urban Health Collaborative in collaboration with the Philadelphia Department of Public Health Greater,[2] an association between alcohol outlet density and violence was noted across poverty strata, as shown in Figure 9.1. The higher density of stores selling alcohol in high-poverty neighborhoods is revealed as a potential contributor to the higher rates of violent incidents, yet the association of alcohol outlet density with violence persists even within neighborhood poverty strata.

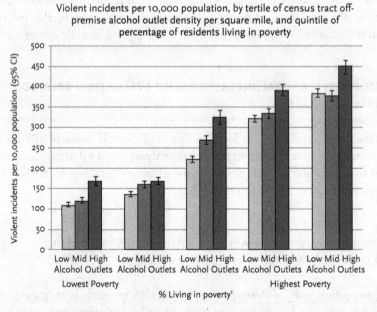

Figure 9.1 Association of alcohol outlets and poverty with violence.[3]
Source: Drexel University Urban Health Collaborative. Data brief: Alcohol Outlets and violence in Philadelphia. January 24 2017; https://drexel.edu/uhc/resources/briefs/Alcohol-Outlets/.

Etiologic Research Addressing Causal Questions About How the Urban Environment Influences Health

The special challenge of using data to inform our understanding of causation has been given much attention in fields of econometrics and epidemiology, among others. Identifying causation in neighborhood-scale health studies has been particularly recognized as challenging.[4] Whether making the most of available data sources or strategically designing a new study, there is value in considering questions embedded in cause and effect scenarios. Causal questions that might arise in our quest to improve urban health, such as moving from the descriptive question "Do residents of more walkable neighborhoods have higher levels of objectively measured physical activity?" to the causal question "If zoning changes were made to allow a neighborhood to become more walkable, would the resultant increase in walkability cause an increase in objectively measured physical activity of residents?" Certainly, one way to address these questions is to implement and evaluate such a change.

Evaluation Brings Attention to Multiple Health-Relevant Consequences of a Changing Urban Environment

Evaluation projects in urban health may address social, physical, policy or other changes with potential to affect the health of urban residents. While this may importantly yield causal evidence on how a specific change affects a specific health outcome, evaluation goals are often broader. There may be attention to analyses all along the multiple pathways from implementation of the change being evaluated to residents' quality of life. Anticipated benefits, co-benefits, and unintended adverse consequences may all feature in evaluation analyses. In addition, the complex systems approaches discussed in Chapter 11 are well-suited to predicting the health trajectories into the future under a range of scenarios, including hypothetical action.

Having these goals in mind, we now turn to discussing common challenges in analyzing urban health data due to violations of common regression assumptions (independence and linearity), as well as the unmeasured or residual confounding that can cloud our view of environmental influences on health. While general analysis guidance is provided in detail by other sources,[5,6] we note a range of strategies and examples especially relevant to urban health.

ACCOUNTING FOR MULTILEVEL AND SPATIAL STRUCTURE

Standard analysis tools such as linear regression assume that the outcomes to be analyzed are independent. Where individual health status is our outcome, we may assume that (beyond measures predictors) knowing how close two individuals are to each other does not tell us how similar their health will be. Yet if individuals influence the behavior and experience of their neighbors, we will expect spatially proximate observations to have similar health status (resulting in a form of nonindependence also labeled *spatial autocorrelation*). Likewise, analyses of rates across geographic units may violate the independence assumption if adjacent units are more likely to have similar health outcomes even after accounting for measured predictor variables.

Wrongly treating data as independent may result in incorrect standard errors, confidence intervals, and *P*-values. Fortunately, there are multiple options to account analytically for various forms of nonindependence.

One data commonly occurring in urban health research is two-level data, such as data on individuals nested within neighborhoods. Analysis options include generalized estimating equations (GEE),[7] multilevel models (MLM),[8] or even ignoring spatial clustering.[9] Within these options marginal model and random effects models can be implemented using either GEE or MLM, and their relative merits are an active topic of discussion in public health.[10–12] Choosing an analytic approach may depend on whether nonindependence is mainly considered as a nuisance or whether there is interest in modeling and describing resulting correlations, as well as on how data were sampled.[13]

Models assuming independence or a two-level structure do not account for other forms of spatial correlation. Extensions can include using more complex structures within MLM, such as three-level structures accounting for individuals nested within neighborhoods nested within cities. There are also multiple frequentist and Bayesian geospatial modeling approaches to more fully account for spatial autocorrelation.[14] Of particular interest for both descriptive and causally informative analyses is geographically weighted regression, which can be used to explore and map variation in the strength of associations. An example relevant to describing health inequities spatially explored how race and poverty disparities in coronary heart disease mortality vary across the United States.[15]

TRANSFORMATION OF URBAN ENVIRONMENT VARIABLES TO ADDRESS NONLINEARITY OR COLLINEARITY

While in clinical health research there is often a focus on dichotomous independent variables related to treatment or the presence of signs and symptoms, independent variables describing the urban environment commonly include continuous measures across a gradient. Examples include intensity of harmful environmental exposures (e.g., ambient air pollution) or health-promoting qualities of the environment (e.g., walkability). These have potential both to have nonlinear associations with health and to be strongly correlated. Correlations between multiple environmental characteristics (multicollinearity) can cause issues for convergence of regression models and interpretability of results.

Exploring Nonlinearity

The relationship of urban environment characteristics with health is potentially nonlinear, with floor or ceiling effects as well as nonmonotonic patterns. Dichotomizing or categorizing such variables or forcing a linear fit risks oversimplification and overlooking associations.

In discussing transformation of continuous variables, an important distinction is between linear and nonlinear transformations. Linear transformation or "scaling" approaches can be used to improve interpretability, such as use of a z-score transformation to anchor coefficient interpretation to the observed standard deviation. Nonlinear transformations such as a log-transformation, however, have uses ranging from reducing the influence of extreme values (outliers), more closely approximating normality or other distributional assumptions, and changing the shape of a modeled association to more nearly approximate linearity.

When the slope of an environment–health association is different across the range of the environment variable, nonlinear transformations of the environment variable may improve model fit. In addition, more flexible modeling strategies such as splines allow for graphical exploration of nonlinear associations, such as the sigmoidal and "j-shaped" curves shown in Figure 9.2, from an urban health study of the impact of greenspace and walkability on objectively measured physical activity.[16]

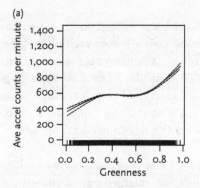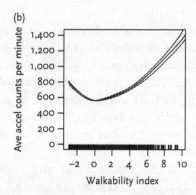

Figure 9.2 Example of a nonlinear association of place characteristics with physical activity. The outcome shown on the y-axis represents objectively measured physical activity, shown here as varying non-linearly in settings with more greenness and higher walkability.
Source: James P, Hart JE, Hipp JA, et al. GPS-based exposure to greenness and walkability and accelerometry-based physical activity. *Cancer Epidemiology, Biomarkers & Prevention.* 2017;26(4):525–532.

In addition to nonlinear associations between an environment character-istic and health, nonlinear patterns can arise in the changes in health out-comes seen over time. Indeed, if health outcomes are expected to continue a linear rate of change, observing a departure from that linear trend may be informative. Consider an example from an effort to catalogue legislative changes relevant to health in New York City[17] and link those changes to mor-tality trends over time.[18] Since mortality had already been decreasing in the early 1990s prior to the legislative changes of interest including smoke-free legislation initiated in 2002, observing a continuation of that trend would not signal any additional benefits from the legislation. All-cause mortality rates were modeled over time using a Joinpoint analysis, showing accelerating declines starting in 1993 (Figure 9.3A). Additional analyses then considered cause-specific mortality trends (Figure 9.3B), showing an accelerated decline in atherosclerotic cardiovascular disease starting in 2002 for men and in 2006 for women, whereas less preventable brain and nervous system cancers declined at a constant rate (Figure 9.3C).

Data Reduction: Constructing Variables and Modeling Approaches to Address Multicollinearity

In assessments of the environment relevant to health, multiple variables may provide complementary pieces of information relevant to the same underlying concept. Several methods are available for bringing this information together to construct one or more new variables.

Perhaps the simplest approaches use a prespecified formula for combining multiple variables, such as a count of dichotomous indicators or a sum of z-scored variables (e.g., for operationalizing the concept of walkability[19,20] or deprivation[21]).

Several approaches offer more empirical ways to extract one or more com-posite variables (labeled "factors" or "components") from multiple original variables (referred to as "items" or "features"). Common approaches include principal component or factor analyses. Of particular interest are the emerg-ing variants of these approaches, such as supervised principal components analysis (see Box 9.1),[22] which allows the extraction of components to be informed by what is most correlated with the health-relevant outcome of interest.

Another approach that can provide insight into how the items are working together is item response theory,[23] which has emerged out of educational testing. Multiple items are combined to assess some underlying ability or un-derlying continuous construct. Items themselves are distinguished in degree of difficulty or severity, as well as how informative they are in revealing the underlying gradient.

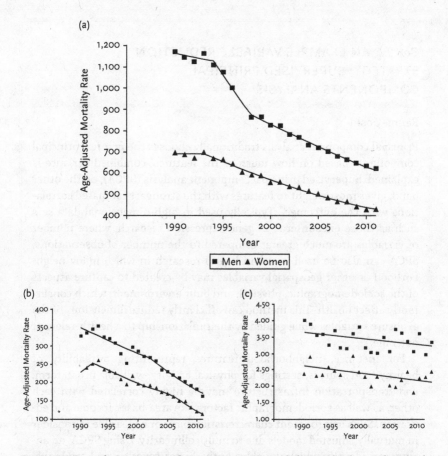

Figure 9.3 Example Joinpoint analysis examining city-wide longitudinal mortality trends. Panels display sex-stratified mortality rates adjusted for age in New York City for (A) all-cause, (B) atherosclerotic cardiovascular disease, and (C) brain and nervous system cancers; years with a change in slope were identified empirically using a Joinpoint analysis.[24]
Source: Ong P, Lovasi GS, Madsen A, Van Wye G, Demmer RT. Evaluating the effectiveness of New York City health policy initiatives in reducing cardiovascular disease mortality, 1990–2011. *American Journal of Epidemiology.* 2017;186(5):555–563.

Finally, the case of longitudinal data that include measures of the environment across multiple years may warrant the use of specialized tools such as latent trajectory analysis. Especially for built environment characteristics that are relatively stable, measures of the environment from adjacent years will be quite correlated. Latent trajectory analysis shifts our attention from each separate measurement toward the patterned time trends that can be compared across urban areas, showing in parallel, convergent, or divergent trajectories.[25,26]

There are also additional methods well-suited to address multicollinearity when distinct contributions of each environmental measure are of interest, including several arising in the realm of machine learning. For example, least

Box 9.1 AN EXAMPLE VARIABLE REDUCTION STRATEGY: SUPERVISED PRINCIPAL COMPONENTS ANALYSIS

Rennie Joshi

Principal component analysis traditionally chooses the first few principal components based on how much of the features' combined variance is explained. Supervised principal component analysis (SPCA), on the other hand, gives most weight to features with the strongest estimated correlations with the outcome.[27] Typically used in high-dimensional data sets such as those encountered in gene expression research, where number of variables are much greater compared to the number of observations, SPCA can also be used in urban health research in which many neighborhood or other geospatial variables may be created to capture aspects of the sociodemographic, physical, and built environment, which concurrently affect health. This method can efficiently reduce dimensions of the exposure variables while guided by their relationship to a health-relevant outcome.

For instance, neighborhood features representing availability of healthy food sources, settings for physical activity, walkable urban form, and transportation infrastructure may be highly correlated with each other, as well as sociodemographic factors like area-based income and education. Such environment characteristics may not be feasible to consider in mutually adjusted models due to multicollinearity. Using SPCA, an analyst can identify which variables both cluster together and are highly related to an outcome such as cardiovascular health score.

An SPCA can be conducted using the R package *superpc*, which currently supports survival analysis and linear regression analysis. According to Bair and colleagues,[27] the following steps are conducted to complete the SPCA:

1. Standard regression coefficients are first calculated for each variable.
2. Construct a reduced data matrix consisting of only those features whose univariate coefficients exceeding a certain absolute threshold, estimated by cross-validation using a test dataset.
3. Use the first few components in a regression model to evaluate the association with the outcome.

There are several known limitations of SPCA. Further development in the method is needed for situations where the outcome is jointly dependent on a set of predictor variables, not all of which have an independent association with the outcome.[28] Similarly, the SPCA would not work well if all variables marginally predict the outcome, but some of these are independent of the outcome given the rest of the predictors.[28]

Currently, SPCA functions well when considering a linear relationship between the exposures and the outcome, but methodologic development leveraging other approaches such as partial-least squares regression may be required to accommodate nonlinear forms.

absolute shrinkage and selection operator (LASSO) regression has been previously used in urban health research.[29–31] For many predictor variables that contribute little to explaining the variance of the outcome, the LASSO regression coefficient will be set to zero. This serves to guide attention toward an empirically selected subset of predictor variables (i.e., features) with nonzero coefficients, without the drawbacks of stepwise variable selection approaches.

DESIGN AND ANALYTIC STRATEGIES TO REDUCE CONFOUNDING IN STUDIES OF ENVIRONMENTAL INFLUENCE ON HEALTH

Confounding bias is a key reason why correlation does not always equal causation. This potential bias commonly arises in our etiologic and evaluation studies of urban environmental influence on health when an underlying factor influences both exposures to the urban environment and health.

What causes might contribute to our exposure to urban environments? First, we do not expect that people all have equal chances of living in harmful or health-promoting circumstances. In particular, harmful exposures may be disproportionately located close to socially disadvantaged communities, based on a legacy of structural discrimination highlighted in the extensive environmental justice literature.[32] Second, health-supportive aspects of the urban environment may be more likely to become available and be maintained in areas with concentrated wealth or social capital. And, finally, at the individual level, the choice of where to live and where to spend time within one's neighborhood depends on economic resources, social ties and obligations, and to some degree on lifestyle-related preferences. Drawing from the fields of psychology, vignettes or related experimental studies can be used to understand in how people express preferences about contrasting environments. While classic versions include written representations and schematic visual depictions, emerging technologies allow for such studies to use a more immersive environment (e.g., virtual reality).[33] Importantly, however, clinical health outcomes and their risk factors may themselves contribute to relocation,[34,35] making previous health status a possible common prior cause.

Why do such causes distort our understanding of environmental influences on health? Economic and social circumstances at the community and individual level, as well as personal lifestyle preferences, affect health through multiple pathways. This can result geographic concentration of environmental hazards and health burdens in the same areas, but with only part of the correlation due to the specific environmental hazard being investigated. For example, if the same communities experience elevated exposure to harmful air pollution, low availability of opportunities for physical activity, ongoing financial hardships, and higher rates of premature mortality, we will find it challenging to disentangle the effects of any one cause of mortality. Underlying social disadvantage may be confounding our understanding of how any specific harmful exposure contributes to worse health outcomes.

Various strategies can be used to statistically control for potential confounding, including restriction, stratification, matching, and statistical adjustment.[36] Yet, statistical adjustment and stratification can only be helpful in eliminating specific biases if the common prior cause has been identified and measured.

To control for both measured and unmeasured confounding, we can consider a powerful study design strategy: randomization.

Randomization and Pseudorandomization to Create Groups With Similar Characteristics and Health Risk

Randomized controlled trials are often considered to be the gold standard for addressing causal questions.[37] In such trials, units (usually individuals for human health studies, although for urban health, these may be geographic areas) are randomly allocated to intervention or control groups. The data are then analyzed based on an intent-to-treat approach to identify the causal effect of treatment.

A very helpful aspect of randomizing units to treatment groups is that we know the groups are only different due to chance. The likelihood of chance leading to large differences across groups is high if only a few units have been randomized, but as the sample size increases, we have a strong expectation for the groups to be similar in all health-relevant experiences except for the intervention being studied.

However, randomized controlled trials are resource-intensive and for some causal questions may be infeasible, unethical, or unacceptable. Even when randomization is not an option, the analogy to such a trial may still have relevance to data analyses harnessing existing variation, with such natural experiments guiding us toward a clear causal question and a convincing answer.[36,38] Natural experiments are shaped by chance events or political, economic, and social changes, and such pseudorandomizing events or conditions then affect who experiences the potential cause of health under investigation. Many clever natural experiments have originated from policy changes,[39] seemingly arbitrary rules, such as birthdate thresholds for school enrollment,[40,41] or from natural[42] or man-made[42-44] disasters.

One way to achieve an abrupt change in urban context is for a household to relocate. Randomized relocation opportunities have been harnessed to study environment-related influences on health (see Box 9.2). Even when not randomized in the context of a trial, household relocation can be considered as

---

Box 9.2 RANDOMIZED RELOCATION TRIALS AS A SOURCE OF VARIATION IN EXPOSURE TO URBAN CONTEXTS

One form of randomized studies relevant to urban health are relocation experiments, which feature the random assignment of people or households to move to a new home address. This has commonly occurred among disadvantaged groups such as public housing residents, whose residential choices are otherwise highly constrained. For causal questions about how the urban environment affects health, such relocation experiments provide an opportunity to harness abrupt changes to the environment.

The Move to Opportunity study[45] is an especially well-known example. This study was in the context of a program that provided housing vouchers on the basis of randomization, allowing some households to move to areas with higher socioeconomic status. Physical and mental health outcomes, although not the only or even the primary target of the intervention, have been monitored over times in families who did and did not receive a voucher.

In addition to providing novel findings, this study has fostered debate and resultant articulation of the types of questions such trials can and cannot address. First, the relevance of the results to our understanding of a voucher program are clear ("What if we provided vouchers to some households to expand their housing options?"). However, thinking about housing as part of a complex system (see Chapter 11) suggests that scaling up to universally providing vouchers to low-income families would change the nature of the intervention and, potentially, its health consequences. Second, randomized relocation studies also capture some aspects of how people respond to a change in their environment. However, such a relocation-based design bundles together many aspects of the physical and social environment that change at once. The relocation changes multiple potentially health-relevant exposures simultaneously, including not only the neighborhood but also proximity to existing social networks.[46]

In conclusion, there may be multiple potential explanations for the observed effects of relocation on health, and these remain difficult to disentangle despite the strong randomized study design to limit confounding bias.

part of a natural experiment if there is a strong determinant of relocation that is not otherwise health-relevant.[47] When multiple determinants predict relocation decisions, analytic strategies such as propensity score matching can be used (in this case matching on the propensity to relocate).[48]

Beyond relocation, place-based changes can be considered in randomized trials and natural experiments. Box 9.3 describes an example evaluation of

---

Box 9.3 PHILADELPHIA'S EXPERIMENT FOR GREENING

In 1995, a local neighborhood association, the New Kensington Community Development Corporation, decided to collaborate with the Philadelphia Horticulture Society to clean, green and maintain, a handful of vacant lots at the request of local residents. Impressed with the positive impact of just a few greened lots, this effort was continued, resulting in the greening of about 700 lots by 2002. The effort was simple, low-cost, and community-driven. While greened lots were diligently maintained for years after program initiation, many wondered whether there was any true benefit to lot greening. In 2008, University of Pennsylvania launched a quasi-experimental study to assess the impact of greening, including a sample of over 4,000 lots that were cleaned and greened via the endeavor, now called the Philadelphia LandCare program. The study reported that greening vacant lots had some impact on reducing local crime and improving certain health outcomes. However, a limitation of this study was that the chosen lots were not randomly assigned to be greened.

To provide stronger causal evidence on the health effects of vacant-lot remediation, funding from the Centers for Disease Control and the National Institutes of Health was pursued to conduct a three-year randomized controlled trial of vacant-lot greening in Philadelphia. There were 541 vacant lots randomly selected across the city, and they were randomly assigned into three groups:

1. full cleaning, greening, and maintenance;
2. just cleaning and maintenance; and
3. no intervention (control).

This allowed assessment of whether greening itself was a factor in reducing crime and improving health in communities. Consistent with the previously nonrandomized study, the trial found that those living near the remediated lots (whether fully greened or just cleaned) were less concerned about their personal safety and more often used outside spaces for relaxing and socializing, as compared with residents living near the control lots. Crime data analysis showed a reduction in gun assaults as well as in shootings that led to serious injury or death in the areas receiving vacant-lot remediation.

Gentrification of the area in which lots were chosen for intervention played a role in affecting the perceptions of the benefits of lot greening among residents. Ethnographic observations showed tensions arose among those who lived in already gentrifying neighborhoods, as they felt that lot remediation was tied to the increased construction of row homes and property tax increases in that area. However, individuals residing in more economically distressed neighborhoods had no such negative perception of greening lots, indicating that any future greening efforts must take into consideration the existing socioeconomic landscape of the area.

Changes in mental and physical health were also observed in the trial. A small sample of 12 individuals residing near two of the lots—one fully greened and one control lot—was asked to participate in a walking and stress study. Participants wore heart monitors to measure changes in heart rate during a walk around their neighborhood. Those who walked in neighborhoods with greened lots showed a significant decrease in heart rate when in view of lot greenery, whereas those near in the control group saw an increase in heart rate when walking past blighted lots. In larger survey, residents near all three lot types were asked to answer questions about their mental health status before and after the lots were remediated. Individuals residing near fully greened lots showed a 42% reduction in feeling depressed and a 51% reduction in feelings of worthlessness as compared to those living near lots that received no remediation. Together, these findings suggest the relevance of psychosocial stress and mental health to explaining the influence of vacant lot remediation on health.

This randomized control trial showed promising evidence of positive impacts to vacant lot remediation. Since the study in Philadelphia, similar efforts have been replicated in cities across the country, providing more scientific evidence on lot-greening as a strategy to improve urban health outcomes.

Adapted by Vaishnavi Vaidya from MacDonald, Branas, and Stokes.[28]

greening vacant lots in Philadelphia, showing subsequent improvements in perceived safety and gun violence. Several natural experiments have been conducted for transportation system improvements, with included health-relevant outcomes ranging from physical activity[49] to community violence.[50] As natural experiments, these transportation changes were not themselves investigator-controlled, nor were they designed exclusively for health improvement. Other natural experiments relevant to health behavior and social interactions in urban environment include studies of physical activity program sites,[51] upgrades to park spaces,[52] or the creation of new residential communities.[53,54]

For both randomized trials and natural experiments, an intent-to-treat analysis approach is recommended to limit bias.[55,56] This requires comparing health outcomes across groups created on the basis of the randomization or pseudorandomization (groups that are presumably balanced with respect to potential health risks). While analysts are often tempted to explore subgroup analyses, doing so risks reintroduction of biases typical of traditional observational studies (including not only confounding bias but also statistical inference challenges due to multiple testing).

Longitudinal Approaches to Explore Causation by Making Within-Unit or Cross-Group Comparisons

Concerns about confounding in observational studies can be ameliorated by focusing on longitudinal comparisons of the same individual or geographic unit over time as conditions change.[38] For example, a study investigated how bar and restaurant smoking bans affected individual-level smoking behavior within a longitudinal cohort study.[57] Individuals were more likely to quit smoking after the area where they lived implemented a ban on smoking in restaurants and bars, after controlling for all stable characteristics of the individual using fixed effects.[58] The key strength for such within-unit comparisons is that even unmeasured time-stable characteristics are held controlled.

When there is a single, abrupt change to an urban environment, a difference-in-difference[36] approach can also be considered. This relies on having measurements of the outcome before and after the change in both the affected (i.e., "intervention" community) and unaffected (i.e., "control" community) contexts. If the difference between before and after in the intervention community suggests a benefit, that could be due to more general improvements in the health of urban residents over time. However, if the improvements outpace improvements seen in one or more control communities, we would have more confidence that the intervention of interest caused those improvements. For example, when the city of Philadelphia implemented a soda tax, a short-term evaluation study[59] used a difference-in-difference approach to see whether beverage consumption was different before and after the tax went into effect in Philadelphia, as compared with the difference in the same time period from nearby cities used as a control group. Reported daily regular soda consumption declined in Philadelphia after the tax, but consumption did not decreased in the control cities.

Even without data on control communities, longitudinal observations can help in the evaluation of a change to the urban environment. However, comparisons relying only on outcomes before versus after will be challenging to interpret. More frequent observations can help to strengthen our causal inference. For example, multiple observations prior to the change can be used to inform our expectation for what would have happened over time in the absence of the intervention. In interrupted time-series analysis (a specific example of a technique more generally called regression discontinuity),[36] the focus is on whether the observations just following the intervention "jump" away from what would be expected based on the pre-intervention trend. Likewise, we can consider whether an acceleration or deceleration of the trends is observed before intervention (as shown in Figure 9.3). Finally, with multiple communities receiving interventions at different times, the availability of frequent observations over time provides a basis for approaches such as a stepped wedge design.[60]

CLOSING THOUGHTS ON ANALYSIS OPTIONS

In considering the types of analyses that provide insight into urban health patterns and processes, we note common issues including violations of standard assumptions about independence and linearity, as well as confounding bias.

Efforts to analyze the highly varied data that are relevant to urban health benefit from having diverse teams, and in particular the approaches discussed in this chapter draw from sociological, demographic, epidemiological, biostatistical, and econometric traditions. We underscore that no single approach is optimal for all urban health questions. Different approaches can be used for their complementary strengths. By evaluating the consistency of observed data with our expectations, we can build a case that may turn out to bolster or add nuance to our original hypotheses. Importantly, however, the weight of evidence may instead favor competing hypotheses. Analytic sophistication introduced in rigorously distinguishing between competing explanations needs to be balanced with transparency and with meeting the needs of non-academic audiences as noted in Part IV.

REFERENCES

1.   Foley R, Kistemann T. Blue space geographies: Enabling health in place. *Health & Place*. 2015;35:157–165.
2.   Joseph S GB, Nadji A, Sestito S, Carroll-Scott A. Community violence profile: Eastern North Philadelphia. Drexel University Urban Health Collaborative. 2018; https://drexel.edu/uhc/resources/briefs/Community-Violence-Profile-Eastern-North-Philadelphia/.
3.   Drexel University Urban Health Collaborative. Data Brief: Alcohol Outlets and Violence in Philadelphia. 2017; https://drexel.edu/uhc/resources/briefs/Alcohol-Outlets/. Accessed June 25, 2020.

4.   Oakes JM. The (mis)estimation of neighborhood effects: Causal inference for a practicable social epidemiology. *Social Science & Medicine*. 2004;58(10): 1929–1952.

5.   Panik M. *Regression Modeling: Methods, Theory, and Computation with SAS*. Boca Raton, FL: Chapman and Hall/CRC; 2009.

6.   Gelman A, Hill J. *Data Analysis Using Regression and Multilevel/Hierarchical Models*. Cambridge, UK: Cambridge University Press; 2006.

7.   Hubbard AE, Ahern J, Fleischer NL, et al. To GEE or not to GEE. *Epidemiology*. 2010;21(4):467–474.

8.   Diez-Roux AV. Multilevel analysis in public health research. *Annual Review of Public Health*. 2000;21(1):171–192.

9.   Clarke P. When can group level clustering be ignored? Multilevel models versus single-level models with sparse data. *Journal of Epidemiology & Community Health*. 2008;62(8):752–758.

10. Snijders TAB, Bosker RJ. *Multilevel Analysis: An Introduction to Basic and Advanced Multilevel Modeling*. 2nd ed. Thousand Oaks, CA: SAGE; 2012.

11. Subramanian S, O'Malley AJ. Modeling neighborhood effects: The futility of comparing mixed and marginal approaches. *Epidemiology*. 2010;21(4):475–478.

12. Hubbard AE, Ahern J, Fleischer NL, et al. To GEE or not to GEE: Comparing population average and mixed models for estimating the associations between neighborhood risk factors and health. *Epidemiology*. 2010;21(4):467–474.

13. Lovasi GS, Fink DS, Mooney SJ, Link BG. Model-based and design-based inference goals frame how to account for neighborhood clustering in studies of health in overlapping context types. *SSM—Population Health*. 2017;3:600–608.

14. Auchincloss AH, Gebreab SY, Mair C, Diez Roux AV. A review of spatial methods in epidemiology, 2000–2010. *Annual Review of Public Health*. 2012;33(1):107–122.

15. Gebreab SY, Diez Roux AV. Exploring racial disparities in CHD mortality between Blacks and Whites across the United States: A geographically weighted regression approach. *Health & Place*. 2012;18(5):1006–1014.

16. James P, Hart JE, Hipp JA, et al. GPS-based exposure to greenness and walkability and accelerometry-based physical activity. *Cancer Epidemiology, Biomarkers & Prevention*. 2017;26(4):525–532.

17. Rhodes-Bratton B, Fingerhut L, Demmer RT, Colgrove J, Wang YC, Lovasi GS. Cataloging the Bloomberg era: New York City legislation relevant to cardiovascular risk factors. *Cities & Health*. 2018;1(2):125–138.

18. Ong P, Lovasi GS, Madsen A, Van Wye G, Demmer RT. Evaluating the effectiveness of New York City health policy initiatives in reducing cardiovascular disease mortality, 1990–2011. *American Journal of Epidemiology*. 2017;186(5): 555–563.

19. Frank LD, Schmid TL, Sallis JF, Chapman J, Saelens BE. Linking objectively measured physical activity with objectively measured urban form: Findings from SMARTRAQ. *American Journal of Preventative Medicine*. 2005;28(2 Suppl 2):117–125.

20. Neckerman KM, Lovasi GS, Davies S, et al. Disparities in urban neighborhood conditions: Evidence from GIS measures and field observation in New York City. *Journal of Public Health Policy*. 2009;30(Suppl 1):S264–285.

21. Christine PJ, Auchincloss AH, Bertoni AG, et al. Longitudinal associations between neighborhood physical and social environments and incident type 2 diabetes mellitus: The multi-ethnic study of atherosclerosis (MESA). *JAMA Internal Medicine*. 2015;175(8):1311–1320.

22. Barshan E, Ghodsi A, Azimifar Z, Jahromi MZ. Supervised principal component analysis: Visualization, classification and regression on subspaces and submanifolds. *Pattern Recognition*. 2011;44(7):1357–1371.

23. Lord FM. *Applications of Item Response Theory to Practical Testing Problems*. New York: Routledge; 2012.

24. Ong P, Lovasi GS, Madsen A, Van Wye G, Demmer RT. Evaluating the effectiveness of New York City health policy initiatives in reducing cardiovascular disease mortality, 1990–2011. *American Journal of Epidemiology*. 2017;186(5):555–563.

25. McCall PL, Land KC, Parker KF. Heterogeneity in the rise and decline of city-level homicide rates, 1976–2005: A latent trajectory analysis. *Social Science Research*. 2011;40(1):363–378.

26. An L, Tsou MH, Spitzberg BH, Gupta DK, Gawron JM. Latent trajectory models for space-time analysis: An application in deciphering spatial panel data. *Geographical Analysis*. 2016;48(3):314–336.

27. Bair E, Hastie T, Paul D, Tibshirani R. Prediction by supervised principal components. *Journal of the American Statistical Association*. 2006;101(473):119–137.

28. MacDonald J, Branas C, Stokes R. *Changing Places: The Science and Art of New Urban Planning*. Princeton, NJ: Princeton University Press; 2019.

29 Hou F, Wu Z. Racial diversity, minority concentration, and trust in Canadian urban neighborhoods. *Social Science Research*. 2009;38(3):693–716.

30. Cilluffo G, Ferrante G, Fasola S, et al. Associations of greenness, greyness and air pollution exposure with children's health: A cross-sectional study in Southern Italy. *Environmental Health*. 2018;17(1):86.

31. Mooney SJ, Joshi S, Cerdá M, Kennedy GJ, Beard JR, Rundle AG. Contextual correlates of physical activity among older adults: A Neighborhood Environment-Wide Association Study (NE-WAS). *Cancer Epidemiology, Biomarkers & Prevention*. 2017;26(4):495–504.

32. Hall MHP, Balogh SB. Environmental justice in the urban environment. In: Hall MHP, Balogh SP, eds. *Understanding Urban Ecology*. Cham, Switzerland: Springer International; 2019:287–303.

33. Patterson Z, Darbani JM, Rezaei A, Zacharias J, Yazdizadeh A. Comparing text-only and virtual reality discrete choice experiments of neighbourhood choice. *Landscape and Urban Planning*. 2017;157:63–74.

34. Lovasi GS, Richardson JM, Rodriguez CJ, et al. Residential relocation by older adults in response to incident cardiovascular health events: A case-crossover analysis. *Journal of Environmental and Public Health*. 2014;2014:951971.

35. Plantinga AJ, Bernell S. The association between urban sprawl and obesity: Is it a two-way street? *Journal of Regional Science*. 2007;47(5):857–879.

36. Angrist JD, Pischke J-S. *Mostly Harmless Econometrics: An Empiricist's Companion*. Princeton, NJ: Princeton University Press; 2009.

37. Berk RA. Randomized experiments as the bronze standard. *Journal of Experimental Criminology*. 2005;1(4):417–433.

38. Lovasi GS, Mooney SJ, Muennig P, DiMaggio C. Cause and context: Place-based approaches to investigate how environments affect mental health. *Social Psychiatry and Psychiatric Epidemiology*. 2016;51(12):1571–1579.

39. Costello EJ, Compton SN, Keeler G, Angold A. Relationships between poverty and psychopathology: A natural experiment. *JAMA*. 2003;290(15):2023–2029.

40. Glymour MM, Kawachi I, Jencks CS, Berkman LF. Does childhood schooling affect old age memory or mental status? Using state schooling laws as natural experiments. *Journal of Epidemiology and Community Health*. 2008;62(6):532–537.

41. Malkin JD, Broder MS, Keeler E. Do longer postpartum stays reduce newborn readmissions? Analysis using instrumental variables. *Health Services Research.* 2000;35(5 Pt 2):1071–1091.

42. King S, Laplante DP. The effects of prenatal maternal stress on children's cognitive development: Project Ice Storm. *Stress.* 2005;8(1):35–45.

43. Susser E, Hoek HW, Brown A. Neurodevelopmental disorders after prenatal famine: The story of the Dutch Famine Study. *American Journal of Epidemiology.* 1998;147(3):213–216.

44. Lauderdale DS. Birth outcomes for Arabic-named women in California before and after September 11. *Demography.* 2006;43(1):185–201.

45. Leventhal T, Brooks-Gunn J. Moving to opportunity: An experimental study of neighborhood effects on mental health. *American Journal of Public Health.* 2003;93(9):1576–1582.

46. Lovasi GS, Adams J, Bearman P. Social support, sex and food: A chapter on social networks and health. In: Bird C, Conrad P, Fremont M, Timmermans S, eds. *Handbook for Medical Sociology.* Nashville, TN: Vanderbilt University Press; 2010:75–91.

47. Angrist JD, Imbens GW, Rubin DB. Identification of causal effects using instrumental variables. *Journal of the American Statistical Association.* 1996;91(434):444–455.

48. Stuart EA. Developing practical recommendations for the use of propensity scores: Discussion of "A critical appraisal of propensity score matching in the medical literature between 1996 and 2003" by Peter Austin. *Statistics in Medicine.* 2008;27(12):2062–2065; discussion 2066-2069.

49. MacDonald JM, Stokes RJ, Cohen DA, Kofner A, Ridgeway GK. The effect of light rail transit on body mass index and physical activity. *American Journal of Preventive Medicine.* 2010;39(2):105–112.

50. Cerdá M, Morenoff JD, Hansen BB, et al. Reducing violence by transforming neighborhoods: A natural experiment in Medellín, Colombia. *American Journal of Epidemiology.* 2012;175(10):1045–1053.

51. Fernandes AP, Andrade ACdS, Ramos CGC, et al. Leisure-time physical activity in the vicinity of Academias da Cidade Program in Belo Horizonte, Minas Gerais State, Brazil: The impact of a health promotion program on the community. *Cadernos de saude publica.* 2015;31:195–207.

52. Cohen DA, Golinelli D, Williamson S, Sehgal A, Marsh T, McKenzie TL. Effects of park improvements on park use and physical activity: Policy and programming implications. *American Journal of Preventive Medicine.* 2009;37(6):475–480.

53. Knuiman MW, Christian HE, Divitini ML, et al. A longitudinal analysis of the influence of the neighborhood built environment on walking for transportation: The RESIDE study. *American Journal of Epidemiology.* 2014;180(5):453–461.

54. Dunton GF, Intille SS, Wolch J, Pentz MA. Investigating the impact of a smart growth community on the contexts of children's physical activity using Ecological Momentary Assessment. *Health Place.* 2012;18(1):76–84.

55. Newell DJ. Intention-to-treat analysis: Implications for quantitative and qualitative research. *International Journal of Epidemiology.* 1992;21(5):837–841.

56. Lachin JL. Statistical considerations in the intent-to-treat principle. *Controlled Clinical Trials.* 2000;21(5):526.

57. Mayne SL, Auchincloss AH, Tabb LP, et al. Associations of bar and restaurant smoking bans with smoking behavior in the CARDIA Study: A 25-year study. *American Journal of Epidemiology.* 2018;187(6):1250–1258.

58. Allison PD. *Fixed Effects Regression Methods for Longitudinal Data Using SAS.* Cary, NC: SAS Institute; 2005.
59. Zhong Y, Auchincloss AH, Lee BK, Kanter GP. The short-term impacts of the Philadelphia Beverage Tax on beverage consumption. *American Journal of Preventive Medicine.* 2018;55(1):26–34.
60. Spiegelman D. Evaluating public health interventions: 2. Stepping up to routine public health evaluation with the stepped wedge design. *American Journal of Public Health.* 2016;106(3):453–457.

CHAPTER 10

What Do We Know About What Works?

Synthesizing the Evidence

GINA S. LOVASI AND ROSIE MAE HENSON

An assessment and synthesis of existing evidence can help urban health teams to build upon and leverage prior research. While there are excellent resources focused on the synthesis of evidence generally,[1,2] in the realm of urban health we are especially sensitive to the need to integrate place-based information and to anticipate the goal of communicating to multiple audiences, which we will turn to in the final chapters of this book (in Part IV).

WHAT CAN BE SYNTHESIZED

Evidence synthesis approaches provide a way to summarize and assess a body of evidence to inform both scholarship and practice. Evidence synthesis can help identify what is known and what remains unknown in urban health research. This is useful for academics who may want to know which research questions have been addressed, the rigor or quality of that evidence, and which questions remain to be answered. For practitioners, synthesis can provide a convenient summary of evidence and whether or how much consensus exists for certain exposures, policies, or interventions relevant for urban health.

Gina S. Lovasi and Rosie Mae Henson, *What Do We Know About What Works?* In: *Urban Public Health.* Edited by: Gina S. Lovasi, Ana V. Diez Roux, and Jennifer Kolker, Oxford University Press (2021). © Oxford University Press 2021. DOI: 10.1093/oso/9780190885304.003.0010.

GOALS FOR EVIDENCE SYNTHESIS

Goals and uses of evidence synthesis in urban health vary.

Often, starting from a question about the connection between some aspect of the urban environment with a specific health outcome, the aim may be to distill a narrowly defined set of relevant descriptive, etiologic, and evaluation findings. By distilling such findings, we may be better positioned to confirm or call into question a hypothesized relation and perhaps even the theory or framework from which that hypothesis arose. Where a relation is found, evidence synthesis strategies such as meta-analysis can be used to quantitatively estimate its magnitude. The relation and its magnitude can then be shared to inform relevant action to improve health in cities.

On the other hand, a proposed change to the urban environment may be the starting point for seeking evidence synthesis. A question about the full range of potential health effects for a change to the urban environment may prompt a health impact assessment (HIA), within which literature reviews may be used or produced. The role of HIAs in anticipating health effects in advance of an intervention is complementary to evaluations, as mentioned in Chapter 3. A useful typology of HIAs[3] distinguishes mandated, decision-support, advocacy, and community-led forms of HIA, with the latter types having more explicit attention to the role of values and judgments.

Finally, broader goals within evidence synthesis may include understanding multiple interrelated aspects of the urban context and the web of relations that link them to each other and to health outcomes. This can arise when using prior evidence as a basis for inputs to complex systems models, to be discussed in Chapter 11. The breadth of such efforts makes them also particularly well-suited to identifying gaps to be addressed by future research.

TYPES OF REVIEW: FORMALITY, FORMAT, AND BREADTH OF INCLUDED EVIDENCE

A diversity of review types have been defined that vary in the timeliness and formality of review process steps from scoping through analysis (see Table 10.1).[4] Trade-offs in selecting between these types arise because many urban health questions are at once time-sensitive and challenging to investigate, requiring attention to the strengths and weaknesses of various review types for any given situation.

Table 10.1 TYPES OF REVIEWS WITH STRENGTHS, LIMITATIONS, AND URBAN HEALTH EXAMPLES

Type of Review	Purpose	Main Advantages	Main Disadvantages	Example of Urban Health Question
Systematic review	To rigorously and comprehensively synthesize all evidence on a specific review question, usually guided by a standard process, and can include either a quantitative (e.g., meta-analysis) or qualitative assessment of quantitative evidence.	Transparent and trustworthy Comprehensive Replicable	Narrow in scope Time consuming to complete Restricted to inclusion of quantitative data	Have slum upgrading projects improved health and socio-economic outcomes?[25] How have complex systems approaches been used to understand drivers of mental health and to inform mental health policy?[6]
Qualitative systematic review/ meta-synthesis	To synthesize and interpret qualitative data across many studies to generate theories or hypotheses	Incorporates qualitative data as a source of evidence	Time consuming to complete, including time to adequately understand evidence and theory Limited only to high-quality qualitative studies Not readily replicable	What do cancer patients value about contact with nature?[7]
Mixed methods review	To synthesize evidence on at least two review questions that require the inclusion and assessment of both quantitative and qualitative data	Allows for assessment of both effectiveness and appropriateness Permits qualitative understanding of interventions Allows for inclusion of more diverse and heterogeneous evidence	Time consuming to complete Adds additional levels of complication to search and screening process, including no universally adopted methods for conducting Not readily replicable	How do small food stores differ in urban and rural areas?[8]

Review type	Purpose	Advantages	Disadvantages	Example question
Rapid review	To quickly and efficiently synthesize information on broad review questions, emerging topics, for updates to a previously completed review, or in response to an urgent policy or practice need	Completed quickly Utilizes rigorous and transparent methods Broader review question can be useful for policymakers	Introduces potential biases through simplification of review process Less comprehensive than systematic review	What items have been used in assessing neighborhood disorder and related concepts?[9]
Scoping review/ mapping review	To identify and characterize the nature, features, and extent of evidence, especially for a body of evidence that has not yet been systematically reviewed	Maps existing literature on topic that has not yet been reviewed	Time consuming Less structured or standard searching methods Broad scope may create large volume of citations and evidence to screen	What aspects of city size and urbanization have been linked with population health metrics?[10]
Umbrella review/ overview of reviews	To synthesize all available high-quality evidence on a topic into one accessible report, typically to inform decision making	Relatively rapid synthesis of high-quality evidence due to abbreviated searching and screening process	Requires expert to critically appraise systematic reviews Can only be completed for well-explored topics	What have previous reviews shown about how the built and natural environment impact health?[11]

Source: Adapted from Grant et al.[12] and Temple University Libraries.[13]

STEPS AND CONSIDERATIONS FOR CONDUCTING SYSTEMATIC REVIEWS RELEVANT TO URBAN HEALTH

To illustrate process using the relatively formal systematic reviews, we note the presence of well-established reporting guidelines such as the Preferred Reporting Items for Systematic Reviews and Meta-Analysis (PRISMA), which has been extended for equity-focused reviews.[14] Authorities in evidence synthesis such as the Cochrane Collaborative offer tools to facilitate systematic screening of titles, abstracts, and full text.[15]

Due to the interdisciplinary nature of many urban health inquiries, the range of databases searched may include fields beyond health—such as those focused on transportation[16]—as well as consideration of gray literature. Gray literature includes reports from city agencies or community organizations, as well as research reports that have not necessarily gone through peer review. Systematically accessing gray literature is challenging, although institutions such as the New York Academy of Medicine have undertaken efforts to facilitate searchable access to the gray literature.[17]

Following the search and screening to see which items meet the inclusion criteria, information is extracted from each piece of evidence and then synthesized in narrative format, through vote counting (i.e., how many of the included studies reported evidence in favor of the hypothesized relation) or more quantitatively using meta-analysis or meta-regression.

Beyond information abstraction, rating the quality of research evidence by the study design, quality, and completeness of reporting or by the risk of bias adds value to evidence synthesis projects by allowing for emphasis to be proportional to quality. Tools to appraise evidence quality are available, though attention and adaptation may be needed before use for urban health topics, as discussed in Box 10.1.

Key advantages of formal literature review strategies are the added assurances of transparency and comprehensiveness of the process (see Figure 10.1).

Additional Review Types and Motivations for Their Use

The general steps of search, appraisal, and analysis are shared between systematic reviews and other review types. Distinctions among these types may be found at the search phase, based on whether included evidence will be quantitative, qualitative, or both.[18] In addition, a limited timeline may encourage a less formal rapid review. Finally, the breadth of relevant evidence may point toward a scoping review or even use of previous reviews in an umbrella review, possibly for efficiency, either as an alternative to or in preparation for a systematic review.

APPRAISAL OF QUALITY AND RISK OF BIAS: TOOL ADAPTATION FOR URBAN HEALTH RESEARCH

Evidence synthesis often involves critical appraisal of study or evidence quality. Critical appraisal allows the reviewers to assess relevance, consistency, and potential bias of study results with respect to the questions guiding the review. Critical appraisal is most often applied to single studies, although there are also tools for appraising the strength of an overall body of evidence, such as the Grading of Recommendations Assessment, Development and Evaluation (GRADE) approach.[19]

Critical appraisal tools, often referred to as checklists, include aspects relevant to a specified study design. Some critical appraisal tools, however, including the MetaQat,[20] National Institute for Health and Care Excellence (NICE),[21] and Effective Public Health Practice Project (EPHPP)[22,23] checklists allow appraisal of multiple study designs within a single checklist. Among tools tailored to quality appraisal for randomized control trials, such as the Cochrane Risk of Bias 2.0 tool,[24] some can be used for several different trial designs, including cluster and cross-over designs that may be appropriate to place-based experimental studies. Urban health research, however, often relies on nonrandomized or observational study designs due to limited feasibility—practically, ethically, and financially—to randomize exposures and interventions.

Thus, it is particularly useful to note the range of tools that have been adapted to appraise the risk of bias in non-randomized and observational studies (see Table 10.2). For example, the ROBINS-I tool[25] was adapted from the Risk of Bias (RoB) 2.0 tool to provide a way to critically appraise non-randomized studies of interventions.[26] Domains to account for potential bias in observational studies include confounding, selection of participants into the study, and classification of exposures or interventions of interest. In addition to broadening the domains of appraisal, the ROBINS-I tool was developed to address a gap in available tools for observational studies. Although the Newcastle–Ottawa[27] and Downs–Black[28] tools for observational studies were available, the developers of ROBINS-I articulated a need for a tool that focused on internal validity—rather than external validity—and included a more comprehensive instructional manual.

Although many tools exist for critical appraisal, the dominance of tools for clinical settings may necessitate the adaption of an existing tool to better fit specific research questions in urban health. Guidance for such appraisal tool adaptation is available[29] and suggests the following steps:
1. Articulate the need for adaptation.
2. Identify items from existing quality appraisal tools, evidence reviews of sources of bias, or from a working-group of experts.
3. Pilot test the adapted tool.

Table 10.2 STUDY DESIGNS THAT CAN BE SYNTHESIZED WITH CORRESPONDING CRITICAL APPRAISAL TOOLS

Study Design	Critical Appraisal Tools
Randomized control trials	Cochrane Risk of Bias 2.0 (ROB 2.0)[30]
	Critical Appraisal Skills Program Randomized Controlled Trial Appraisal Tool (CASP RCT CAT)[31]
	The Consolidated Standards of Reporting Trials (CONSORT) Statement[32]
Nonrandomized control trials	Transparent Reporting of Evaluations with Nonrandomized Designs (TREND) Statement[33]
	The Methodological Index for Non-Randomized Studies (MINOR)[34]
Cohort studies	ROBINS-I Risk of Bias (for interventions)[35]
	ROBINS-E Risk of Bias (for exposures)[36]
	Newcastle-Ottawa Scale (NOS)[37]
	The STROBE Statement[38]
Case–control studies	Newcastle-Ottawa Scale (NOS)[37]
	The STROBE Statement
Cross-sectional (prevalence) studies	AXIS[39]
	The STROBE Statement[38]
Multiple study designs	MetaQat Meta-Tool[40]
	Effective Public Health Practice Project (EPHPP) Tool[41,42]
	National Institute for Health and Care Excellence (NICE) Checklist[43]
Systematic reviews	ROBIS Tool[44]
	Joanna Briggs Critical Appraisal for Systematic Reviews Checklist[45]
	AMSTAR-A Measurement Tool[46]

In particular, there are limitations and concerns regarding the use of critical appraisal tools that may systematically undervalue natural experiments in urban health and other studies of "complex interventions," as compared with more interventions administered within more tightly controlled laboratory or clinical settings.[47–50] Future development of tools may allow for better integration of innovative methodological and analytical techniques used by investigators to enhance study quality in the face of unique challenges of observational studies.[47]

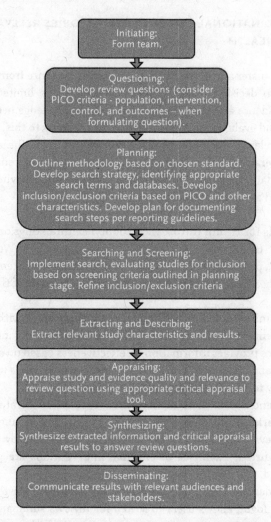

Figure 10.1 Systematic review process.

Some emerging directions that may increase the efficiency of reviews include the treatment of text as data and the analyses of citation patterns. Tools that treat text as data, such as natural language processing, have been used to analyze social media communications (e.g., Twitter) and can likewise be harnessed to understand patterns of response to urban health threats and potential solutions.[51,52]

This may have utility in streamlining the process of identifying topical coverage patterns and trends in consensus over time in the peer-reviewed literature[53-55] or in the prioritizing papers for inclusion in a review.[56] Such approaches could become helpful when synthesizing evidence to meet time sensitive needs of decision makers.

GLOBAL AND NATIONAL EVIDENCE REPOSITORIES RELEVANT TO URBAN HEALTH

Knowledge transfer and dissemination of existing evidence from the research community to decision makers, unfortunately, can be limited due to the volume of evidence and the time and specialized knowledge needed to identify, access, and evaluate all of this research. Responding to this, compilations of evidence relevant to urban health have been created. These are distinct from most literature reviews in that rather than resulting in a snapshot of the literature to date, they take the form of an ongoing and evolving resource to be maintained as new evidence emerges.

- What Works for Health (http://www.countyhealthrankings.org/roadmaps/what-works-for-health), with support from the Robert Wood Johnson Foundation, provides references and examples, ordering potential solutions to a given health challenge with respect to the strength of the underlying evidence.
- The Community Guide (http://thecommunityguide.org/), with key support from the Center for Disease Control and Prevention, is organized by topic. This resource provides information on effectiveness based on systematic review, costs and related economic aspects, and considerations when tailoring the strategy to a local setting or population group.
- The Compendium of Community-Based Prevention Strategies (http://healthyamericans.org/report/110/) from the Trust for America's Health and the New York Academy of Medicine is organized by the targeted health condition. Examples of effective interventions are provided and summarized.
- Health Evidence (http://healthevidence.org/) from McMaster University, with a free login, allows users to search for reviews summarizing the evidence for particular interventions on a given topic, with a rating of the review quality provided for quick reference.
- National Institute for Health and Care Excellence (NICE) evidence guidelines (https://www.nice.org.uk/) includes evidence-based recommendations to improve health and social care. Recommendations are developed by independent committees of professionals and lay members and are organized by conditions and disease topics as well as lifestyle and well-being topics.

CONCLUDING NOTE ON EVIDENCE SYNTHESIS FOR URBAN HEALTH

Evidence synthesis is a way to organize, assess, and summarize the state of evidence and is useful for understanding and communicating what is known in urban health, thus guiding future research and action. While methods development in the more formal systematic review and meta-analysis has been closely tied to clinical intervention studies, a broader range of natural experimental and observational evidence relevant to urban health can be included in reviews of various types.

When synthesizing, appraising, and disseminating evidence for urban health, attention is needed on how the evidence fits into the broader context of values and judgments and how research may need to be adapted to the local context as necessary.[57]

REFERENCES

1. Stroup D, Berlin J, Morton S, et al. Meta-analysis of observational studies in epidemiology: A proposal for reporting. *JAMA*. 2000;283(15):2008–2012.
2. Higgins J, Green S. *Cochrane Handbook for Systematic Reviews of Interventions*. Cochrane. 2009; http://www.training.cochrane.org/handbook. Accessed July 26, 2013.
3. Harris-Roxas B, Harris E. Differing forms, differing purposes: A typology of health impact assessment. *Environmental Impact Assessment Review*. 2011;31(4): 396–403.
4. Grant MJ, Booth A. A typology of reviews: An analysis of 14 review types and associated methodologies. *Health Information & Libraries Journal*. 2009;26(2): 91–108.
5. Turley R, Saith R, Bhan N, Rehfuess E, Carter B. Slum upgrading strategies involving physical environment and infrastructure interventions and their effects on health and socio-economic outcomes. *Cochrane Database of Systematic Reviews*. 2013;1:CD010067.
6. Langellier BA, Yang Y, Purtle J, Nelson KL, Stankov I, Roux AVD. Complex systems approaches to understand drivers of mental health and inform mental health policy: A systematic review. *Administration and Policy in Mental Health and Mental Health Services Research*. 2019;46(2):128–144.
7. Blaschke S. The role of nature in cancer patients' lives: A systematic review and qualitative meta-synthesis. *BMC Cancer*. 2017;17(1):370.
8. Pinard CA, Shanks CB, Harden SM, Yaroch AL. An integrative literature review of small food store research across urban and rural communities in the US. *Preventive Medicine Reports*. 2016;3:324–332.
9. Ndjila S, Lovasi GS, Fry D, Friche AA. Measuring neighborhood order and disorder: A rapid literature review. *Current Environmental Health Reports*. 2019;6(4):316–326.
10. McCulley EM, Mullachery P, Rodriguez D, Roux AD, Bilal U. Urban scaling of health outcomes: A protocol for a scoping review. *BMJ Open*. 2019;9(11): e031176.
11. Bird EL, Ige J, Pilkington P, Pinto A, Petrofsky C, Burgess-Allen J. Built and natural environment planning principles for promoting health: An umbrella. *BMC Public Health*. 2018;18(1):930.
12. Grant MJ, Booth A. A typology of reviews: An analysis of 14 review types and associated methodologies. *Health Information and Libraries Journal*. 2009;26(2): 91–108.

13. Temple University Libraries. Systematic reviews & other review types. 2018; http://guides.temple.edu/systematicreviews.

14. Welch V, Petticrew M, Petkovic J, et al. Extending the PRISMA statement to equity-focused systematic reviews (PRISMA-E 2012): Explanation and elaboration. *Journal of Development Effectiveness*. 2016;8(2):287–324.

15. McDonald S, Turner T. Transforming Cochrane. *Medical Journal of Australia*. 2016;204(1):6.

16. Daly JS. Transportation research thesaurus: TRID tool for better searches. *TR News*. 2019(319):33–34.

17. Mathews BS. Gray literature: Resources for locating unpublished research. *College & Research Libraries News*. 2019;65(3):125–129.

18. Dixon-Woods M, Agarwal S, Jones D, Young B, Sutton A. Synthesising qualitative and quantitative evidence: A review of possible methods. *Journal of Health Services Research & Policy*. 2005;10(1):45–53.

19. Guyatt GH, Oxman AD, Vist GE, et al. GRADE: An emerging consensus on rating quality of evidence and strength of recommendations. *BMJ*. 2008;336(7650): 924–926.

20. Rosella L, Bowman C, Pach B, Morgan S, Fitzpatrick T, Goel V. The development and validation of a meta-tool for quality appraisal of public health evidence: Meta Quality Appraisal Tool (MetaQAT). *Public Health*. 2016;136:57–65.

21. National Institute for Health Care Excellence. NICE Process and Methods Guides. *Methods for the Development of NICE Public Health Guidance* 2012; https://www.nice.org.uk/process/pmg4/chapter/introduction. Accessed June 25, 2020.

22. Thomas BH, Ciliska D, Dobbins M, Micucci S. A process for systematically reviewing the literature: Providing the research evidence for public health nursing interventions. *Worldviews on Evidence-Based Nursing*. 2004;1(3):176–184.

23. Armijo-Olivo S, Stiles CR, Hagen NA, Biondo PD, Cummings GG. Assessment of study quality for systematic reviews: A comparison of the Cochrane Collaboration Risk of Bias Tool and the Effective Public Health Practice Project Quality Assessment Tool: Methodological research. *Journal of Evaluation in Clinical Practice*. 2012;18(1):12–18.

24. Higgins J, Sterne J, Savović J, et al. A revised tool for assessing risk of bias in randomized trials. *Cochrane Database of Systematic Reviews*. 2016;10(Suppl 1): 29–31.

25. Sterne JA, Hernán MA, Reeves BC, et al. ROBINS-I: tool for assessing risk of bias in non-randomised studies of interventions. *BMJ*. 2016;355:i4919.

26. Sterne JA, Hernán MA, Reeves BC, et al. ROBINS-I: A tool for assessing risk of bias in non-randomised studies of interventions. *BMJ*. 2016;355:i4919.

27. Wells G, Shea B, O'connell D, et al. The Newcastle–Ottawa Scale (NOS) for Assessing the Quality Of Nonrandomized Studies in Meta-Analyses. 2016; http://www.ohri.ca/programs/clinical_epidemiology/oxford.asp.

28. Downs SH, Black N. The feasibility of creating a checklist for the assessment of the methodological quality both of randomised and non-randomised studies of health care interventions. *Journal of Epidemiology and Community Health*. 1998;52(6):377–384.

29. Whiting P, Wolff R, Mallett S, Simera I, Savović J. A proposed framework for developing quality assessment tools. *Systematic Reviews*. 2017;6(1):204.

30. Higgins J, Sterne J, Savović J, et al. A revised tool for assessing risk of bias in randomized trials. *Cochrane Database of Systematic Reviews*. 2016;10(Suppl 1): 29–31.

31. Critical Appraisal Skills Programme. CASP Randomised Controlled Trial Checklist. 2018; https://casp-uk.net/wp-content/uploads/2018/01/CASP-Randomised-Controlled-Trial-Checklist-2018.pdf.

32. Schulz KF, Altman DG, Moher D. CONSORT 2010 statement: Updated guidelines for reporting parallel group randomised trials. *BMC Medicine*. 2010;8(1):18.

33. Des Jarlais DC. TREND (transparent reporting of evaluations with nonrandomized designs). In: Moher D, Altman DG, Schulz KF, Simera I, Wager E, eds. *Guidelines for Reporting Health Research: A User's Manual*. Hoboken, NJ: Wiley; 2014:156–168.

34. Slim K, Nini E, Forestier D, Kwiatkowski F, Panis Y, Chipponi J. Methodological index for non-randomized studies (MINORS): Development and validation of a new instrument. *ANZ Journal of Surgery*. 2003;73(9):712–716.

35. Sterne JA, Hernán MA, Reeves BC, et al. ROBINS-I: tool for assessing risk of bias in non-randomised studies of interventions. *BMJ*. 2016;355:i4919.

36. Morgan R SJ, Higgins J, Thayer K, Schunemann H, Rooney A, Taylor K. A new instrument to assess Risk of Bias in Non-Randomised Studies of Exposures (ROBINS-E): Application to studies of environmental exposure. In. Abstracts of Global Evidence Summit, Cape Town, South Africa. *Cochrane Database of Systematic Reviews*. 2017.

37. Wells G, Shea B, O'connell D, et al. The Newcastle–Ottawa Scale (NOS) for Assessing the Quality Of Nonrandomized Studies in Meta-Analyses. 2016; http://www.ohri.ca/programs/clinical_epidemiology/oxford.asp.

38. Von Elm E, Altman DG, Egger M, Pocock SJ, Gøtzsche PC, Vandenbroucke JP. The Strengthening the Reporting of Observational Studies in Epidemiology (STROBE) statement: Guidelines for reporting observational studies. *Annals of Internal Medicine*. 2007;147(8):573–577.

39. Downes MJ, Brennan ML, Williams HC, Dean RS. Development of a critical appraisal tool to assess the quality of cross-sectional studies (AXIS). *BMJ Open*. 2016;6(12):e011458.

40. Rosella L, Bowman C, Pach B, Morgan S, Fitzpatrick T, Goel V. The development and validation of a meta-tool for quality appraisal of public health evidence: Meta Quality Appraisal Tool (MetaQAT). *Public Health*. 2016;136:57–65.

41. Thomas BH, Ciliska D, Dobbins M, Micucci S. A process for systematically reviewing the literature: Providing the research evidence for public health nursing interventions. *Worldviews on Evidence-Based Nursing*. 2004;1(3):176–184.

42. Armijo-Olivo S, Stiles CR, Hagen NA, Biondo PD, Cummings GG. Assessment of study quality for systematic reviews: A comparison of the Cochrane Collaboration Risk of Bias Tool and the Effective Public Health Practice Project Quality Assessment Tool: Methodological research. *Journal of Evaluation in Clinical Practice*. 2012;18(1):12–18.

43. National Institute for Health Care Excellence. NICE process and methods guides. In: *Methods for the Development of NICE Public Health Guidance*. London: National Institute for Health and Care Excellence (NICE); 2012.

44. Whiting P, Savovic J, Higgins JPT, et al. ROBIS: A new tool to assess risk of bias in systematic reviews was developed. *Recenti progressi in medicina*. 2018;109(9):421–431.

45. Porritt K, Gomersall J, Lockwood C. JBI's systematic reviews: Study selection and critical appraisal. *American Journal of Nursing*. 2014;114(6):47–52.

46. Shea BJ, Reeves BC, Wells G, et al. AMSTAR 2: A critical appraisal tool for systematic reviews that include randomised or non-randomised studies of healthcare interventions, or both. *BMJ.* 2017;358:j4008.

47. Humphreys DK, Panter J, Ogilvie D. Questioning the application of risk of bias tools in appraising evidence from natural experimental studies: Critical reflections on Benton et al., *IJBNPA* 2016. *International Journal of Behavioral Nutrition and Physical Activity.* 2017;14(1):49.

48. Movsisyan A, Melendez-Torres G, Montgomery P. Outcomes in systematic reviews of complex interventions never reached "high" GRADE ratings when compared with those of simple interventions. *Journal of Clinical Epidemiology.* 2016;78:22–33.

49. Movsisyan A, Melendez-Torres G, Montgomery P. Users identified challenges in applying GRADE to complex interventions and suggested an extension to GRADE. *Journal of Clinical Epidemiology.* 2016;70:191–199.

50. Ogilvie D, Egan M, Hamilton V, Petticrew M. Systematic reviews of health effects of social interventions: 2. Best available evidence: How low should you go? *Journal of Epidemiology & Community Health.* 2005;59(10):886–892.

51. Genes N, Chary M, Chason K. Analysis of Twitter users' sharing of official New York storm response messages. *Medicine 2.0.* 2014;3(1):e1.

52. Massey PM, Leader A, Yom-Tov E, Budenz A, Fisher K, Klassen AC. Applying multiple data collection tools to quantify human Papillomavirus vaccine communication on twitter. *Journal of Medical Internet Research.* 2016;18(12):e318.

53. Shwed U, Bearman PS. The temporal structure of scientific consensus formation. *American Sociological Review.* 2010;75(6):817–840.

54. Adams J, Light R. Scientific consensus, the law, and same sex parenting outcomes. *Social Science Research.* 2015;53:300–310.

55. Trinquart L, Galea S. Mapping epidemiology's past to inform its future: Metaknowledge analysis of epidemiologic topics in leading journals, 1974–2013. *American Journal of Epidemiology.* 2015;182(2):93–104.

56. Przybyła P, Brockmeier AJ, Kontonatsios G, et al. Prioritising references for systematic reviews with RobotAnalyst: A user study. *Research Synthesis Methods.* 2018;9(3):470–488.

57. Buffett C, Ciliska D, Thomas H. *Can I Use this Evidence in My Program Decision? Assessing Applicability and Transferability of Evidence.* Hamilton, ON: National Collaborating Centre for Methods and Tools; 2007.

CHAPTER 11

Systems Approaches to Urban Health

ANA V. DIEZ ROUX AND IVANA STANKOV

As we have reviewed in earlier chapters of this book, understanding the drivers of urban health and intervening effectively to promote health in cities requires us to consider factors defined at multiple levels of organization (e.g., individuals, neighborhoods, cities, states) that may interact with each other. It also requires us to consider the interconnections between people, neighborhoods and even cities. It requires us to keep in mind the possibility of feedbacks (e.g., individual behaviors affecting the environment and the environment, in turn, affecting behaviors). These are some of the cardinal features of systems.

There is a long tradition of conceptualizing cities as systems and using systems approaches such as simulation modeling to investigate the emergence and evolution of various characteristics of cities. Early work applying systems approaches to urban questions involved modeling the development, evolution, and decay of cities over time. For example, over 40 years ago, Forrester,[1] often described as one of the founders of system dynamics, used a growth model to generate the life cycle of an urban area from its founding through its decay 250 years later. He also used systems modeling to explore how various policies (related to employment, housing, and industry) might affect the evolution of a depressed city over the next 50 years. More recently, in his book *The New Science of Cities*, Batty[2] has argued that to understand cities we must view them as systems of networks and flows. He uses the concepts and tools of complex systems to discuss the structure of cities and how they function. Other work has used systems thinking to understand the links between the size of cities and various city properties including economic, social, and health-related features.[3]

Ana V. Diez Roux and Ivana Stankov, *Systems Approaches to Urban Health* In: *Urban Public Health*. Edited by: Gina S. Lovasi, Ana V. Diez Roux, and Jennifer Kolker, Oxford University Press (2021). © Oxford University Press 2021. DOI: 10.1093/oso/9780190885304.003.0011.

In the remainder of this chapter, we will review how the concepts and tools of systems approaches can be used to enhance our understanding of urban health and facilitate the identification of the most effective interventions to promote urban health. But first we review the key features of systems and illustrate why systems approaches are relevant to urban health.

KEY FEATURES OF SYSTEMS

In its simplest sense, a system is defined as "a regularly interacting or interdependent group of items forming a unified whole."[4] The systems most relevant to health are often characterized by (i) the presence of factors at multiple levels of organization (e.g., city level factors related to governance, neighborhood factors such as environmental or social characteristics, various institutions and their organizational characteristics, families, and individuals); (ii) heterogeneous units (e.g., individuals, institutions, neighborhoods); (iii) dependencies and interactions between units (e.g., norms being transmitted from person to person or neighborhoods close together in space influencing each other); and (iv) positive and negative feedbacks (e.g., environmental policies influencing residential segregation and segregation in turn reinforcing environmental policies).[5-7] Acting together, these factors and processes result in the emergence of patterns that may not be easily understandable or predictable if one is not cognizant of the functioning of the system as a whole. For example, they may lead to nonlinear effects, effects that are distant in space and time, or unexpected effects of interventions on the system (such as unintended consequences). When this happens—that is, when the behavior of the system is difficult to predict and cannot be fully comprehended without simulating its function—the system is referred to as a complex system. The features of complex systems are summarized in Box 11.1. Although we will use the more generic term *system* throughout this chapter, the systems we encounter in urban health are often complex systems.

Understanding the functioning of a system can be critical for identifying effective interventions, understanding details of how they work, or evaluating what their effects might be under different conditions. Systems approaches can be useful to determine potential policy impacts because the effect of a given intervention on the system may depend on the relationships and state of all other key system components. In addition, feedbacks and dependencies in the system can influence policy impacts and result in unanticipated effects. As a result, reductionist approaches that attempt to isolate the effect of a given factor while keeping all others constant may yield results that are unrealistic. This is why systems approaches are potentially so valuable to policy translation.

Box 11.1 WHAT IS A COMPLEX SYSTEM?

A system is defined as an interdependent and interacting set of items that form a unified whole.[4]

A complex system is a type of system in which the dynamic networks of interactions between components are such that the behavior of the system cannot be easily predicted. Simulation is necessary to understand the implications of these interactions for the behavior of the system and to predict what may happen as a result of the intervention on the system.

The term *complex adaptive system* is used to refer to complex systems that have the capacity to change and learn based on experience.

Key features of complex systems include

- the presence of units or factors at multiple levels of organization.
- heterogeneous or diverse interacting units.
- dependencies, that is units influencing each other.
- feedback loops (reinforcing or buffering).

As a result, complex systems often exhibit the following phenomena:

- Nonlinear effects (i.e., the absence of linear dose response relationships) and tipping points.
- Adaptation over time and memory (the past affects the future even after accounting for the present).
- Emergent properties (i.e., higher-level behaviors that result from the functioning of the system as a whole and cannot be easily reduced to the impact of individual and separate components).
- Sensitivity to initial conditions and conditional effects (i.e., the impact of an intervention depends on the state of other factors in the system).
- Effects of an intervention can be distant in space and time and difficult to predict (i.e., interventions can have unexpected consequences).
- Policy resistance (i.e., when an intervention fails to have the expected effect, instead remaining close to the status quo).

Separately from the long tradition of conceptualizing and modeling cities as systems, there has been increasing interest in applying the concepts and tools of systems thinking and systems analysis to population health problems.[5,6,8–10] Systems approaches go beyond the recognition that health is affected by distal factors or factors defined at multiple levels of organization, as has been the tradition in public health for a long time. They explicitly allow for dynamic processes including feedbacks as well as interdependencies and interactions between individuals and between individuals and environments over time. In going beyond the traditional emphasis on isolating the independent effect of specific factors to an understanding of the functioning of the system as a whole, the use of systems approaches implies a paradigm shift in the way in which population health is conceptualized, studied, and intervened on.

The study of infectious diseases (because of the contagious nature of many infections) has long embraced and incorporated some features of systems in analytical approaches such as the need to account for transmission from individual to individual and consequent dependencies. However, in the last few years, systems approaches have garnered attention in other areas of population health as well, including noncommunicable disease and health behaviors, mental health, drug and alcohol use, and violence.[10-16] Two important factors have contributed to this trend. One factor is the increasing frustration with traditional approaches used in population health research, essentially the randomized experiment and the use of observational data to approximate the randomized experiment. Although these strategies have yielded much useful information, there is a sense that they do not allow us to fully understand or identify the best way to act upon many big outstanding questions in population health.[5,6] A second major factor has been increasing availability of the tools necessary to build and simulate appropriate formal models of systems.[9,10,17-20]

In addition to capturing the dynamic processes (involving feedbacks, dependencies, and networks) that drive urban health, a major benefit of systems thinking for urban health is the ability to make explicit and explore the implications of the links between population health and environmental sustainability. As we discussed in Chapter 3, these relations underlie the planetary health approach, which has advocated for the need to document and leverage the health and environmental co-benefits of various urban policies. These co-benefits often involve reinforcing or balancing feedback loops.[21] Systems approaches can be used to investigate and make explicit these co-benefits and under what circumstances they can be maximized.

USING SYSTEMS APPROACHES TO ENGAGE STAKEHOLDERS: PARTICIPATORY GROUP MODEL BUILDING

An important application of systems thinking in urban health is the use of participatory approaches such as group model building (GMB) to develop and evaluate the implications of conceptual models of the systems that influence a particular urban health outcome. GMB, also known as community-based system dynamics, was developed in the 1980s as way of helping systems modelers elicit and structure the perspectives of diverse actors, so that these perspectives can inform the design of system dynamics models.[22] In GMB, a set of structured activities are used to engage participants (often stakeholders with little or no formal background in systems thinking or modeling) to develop a conceptual model of the system that is important to a particular problem or outcome (e.g., understanding how cities influence obesity) and then use this conceptual model to identify and explore the possible impact of interventions on the system (e.g., the plausible impact of a soda tax).[22]

GMB involves the use of carefully planned and evaluated activities that promote participation so that multiple perspectives can inform the products that are developed. Examples of commonly used activities include

1. "graphs over time" where participants create graphs showing anticipated changes in key factors over time under various conditions (e.g., status quo or if X were implemented) allowing participants to begin to think about relations between factors in a dynamic way;
2. "causal mapping" where participants are asked to create diagrams using a set of simple formal rules showing the relationships between factors, including feedbacks and various types of reinforcing or balancing loops resulting in the creation of a "causal loop diagram" representing the consensus of the group; and
3. "action ideas," involving the identification of leverage points and possible strategies for policy intervention that could be used to nudge the system in a specific direction (e.g., to reduce obesity) as well as a qualitative evaluation of the possible impact and feasibility based on participant knowledge.[23-25]

Recent years have seen a rise in the number of studies employing GMB to understand public health problems. Examples span primary care,[26] obesity,[27,28] tobacco control,[29] and, more recently, health effects of transportation and food purchasing in cities.[25]

Participatory approaches such as GMB have several uses and benefits. A primary goal is to provide input to researchers and systems modelers from a set of diverse stakeholders on the structure of system of interest. This involves identifying key factors, key relations, possible leverage points, and key possible actions or interventions on the system. This information can be used to inform the development of formal simulation models of the system. Depending on the modeling approach that will be used, the translation of GMB outputs into specific modeling decisions can be relatively straightforward or more indirect. For example, the causal loop diagrams often developed in GMB may be easier to translate into system dynamics models than into agent-based models (ABMs).

Aside from informing subsequent formal simulation efforts, GMB has several other goals that are just as important. These goals relate to facilitating communication, consensus-building, and learning among diverse actors.[30] The first, and perhaps most important, goal is *stakeholder engagement* in the development of a common conceptual understanding that can form the basis for future research or policy actions. This is invaluable to inform future research and policy translation efforts so that they are relevant, feasible, and impactful. Second, the experience of GMB can help *break down sectoral or disciplinary silos* by highlighting the interconnectedness of sectors and factors. For example, urban planners focused on roads and transportation systems may gain a deeper appreciation for the broad-reaching impacts of transportation policies. These could include relatively direct impacts on commuting behavior, such as the use of more active modes of transportation, which impact not only physical activity but also travel time and, by extension, free time, which, in turn, has implications for a range of behaviors including food purchasing and preparation. Finally, GMB can *build stakeholders' capacity* for systems thinking that can be useful in their daily practice and expand their understanding of the implications of their actions.[22] Gaining an appreciation for the complexity of urban systems and their interrelationship with health need not be overwhelming: on the contrary, it may crystalize opportunities for interdisciplinary collaboration and highlight novel actions with potentially lasting public health benefits. Box 11.2 describes the use of GMB in a

---

Box 11.2 USING PARTICIPATORY APPROACHES TO ENGAGE STAKEHOLDERS IN SYSTEMS THINKING FOR URBAN HEALTH

Participatory GMB has been applied to understand a range of urban health issues from the perspective of diverse actors and decision-makers. The Salud Urbana en América Latina (SALURBAL) Project, which involves collaborations between institutions across eight countries in Latin America and the United States is an example where GMB has been applied to understand the drivers of health in a multinational context. The SALURBAL project team[25] conducted three GMB workshops (one each in Peru, Brazil, and Guatemala) to better understand how food and transport systems impact health and environmental sustainability in Latin American cities and to identify policies that could improve these outcomes. To do this, the team convened food and transportation experts, including policymakers and academic researchers as well as private sector and civil society representatives.

During each workshop, participants created causal loop diagrams that highlighted important feedback structures. For example, participants across several workshops described how policies designed to combat the growing burden of obesity through disincentives on ultra-processed food (UPF) consumption, are often undermined by food industry lobbying and marketing efforts. Specifically, they illustrated within their causal loop

---

diagrams how policies raising the price of UPFs (i.e., through excise taxes) decrease purchasing and consumption of UPF by making these foods less affordable. In response to this, however, the food industry exerts its influence on governments by lobbying to weaken health promotion efforts while simultaneously increasing their own marketing of UPFs both to increase their appeal (e.g., through advertising campaigns promoting UPFs) and to reduce consumers' understanding of the low nutritional value of these foods (e.g., through misleading labels). These efforts in turn promote UPF consumption and undermine the effect of the initial policy,[25] an example of policy resistance.

Participants also identified two ways that cities can tackle the issue of congestion. The first is to invest more money into building freeways, and the second is by investing in public and active transportation infrastructure and programs to promote a shift to more active modes of transportation. They used these diagrams to think about (both intended and unintended) possible consequences of these interventions. These workshops gave participants insights into the dynamics relations affecting health outcomes in cities and the implications of these dynamics for policies.

GMB has also been used to understand local issues such as youth violence, a phenomenon that can unfold uniquely in each city and vary from one neighborhood to another. For example, Bridgewater and colleagues[31] used participatory GMB to help community residents in Boston capture their knowledge of youth violence in their communities, including the potential drivers of violent behavior and the institutions that influence it. In this study, community members were not just participants in the research; they were also involved in informing the design, execution, and evaluation of the project. By using this participatory approach, Bridgewater and his team quickly realized that, while community members were familiar with the violence in their communities, they knew little about the actions and motivations of those committing it. The team therefore invited gang members and violent offenders to share their experiences and knowledge. Bridgewater and colleagues found that for gang members, violence is intimately linked to identity and belonging and plays a dominant role in coping with threats to emotional well-being. It was also linked to trauma among those committing the violence. The feedback loop that was identified established a link between initial acts of violence, arising from a desire for belonging or a need to cope with emotional distress, and subsequent violent behavior that is further reinforced by "self-induced traumatization."[31p71] Community members, on the other hand, emphasized the far-reaching impact of violent acts in their neighborhoods and its contribution to traumatic stress within the community at large. Bridgewater subsequently used these findings to inform the development of a system dynamics model of youth violence in Boston.[31]

large international collaboration on urban health and the findings of a local project focused on understanding youth violence in Boston communities. An example of a causal loop diagram developed using this approach is shown in Chapter 3 of this book.

SIMULATING URBAN SYSTEMS: AGENT-BASED MODELS AND SYSTEM DYNAMICS MODELS

An important goal of systems approaches is the development of a formal simulation model that can be used to explore the functioning of a system and the plausible impact of various interventions on the system. The modeling can have two distinct goals.[10] One is furthering insight into mechanisms by integrating and exploring the implications of information that we have and by testing assumptions about hypothesized mechanisms. A second goal is predicting the plausible impact of interventions on the system under varying conditions. For example, Auchincloss and colleagues[11] used a systems model to show that dietary intake differences by income group could arise as a result of residential segregation and spatial differences in location of healthy food outlets even in the absence of preference differentials. The model developed was then used to explore the impact of various policies (price and education interventions) on income differences in diet.

Several types of formal simulation models exist including ABMs and systems dynamic models. These formal models involve the creation of virtual worlds, informed by empirical data, that can then be manipulated to better understand the implications for outcomes such as health of the various relations encoded in the model. It is important to emphasize that the extent to which conclusions derived from the model are valid in the real world depends on the extent to which the model appropriately captures the essential processes. The model is not the real world; it is merely our effort to mimic how it functions.[32] Because of this, simulation modeling will never replace rigorous observation, although it can help us understand the implications of several observed causal relations acting in concert. Next we briefly review the fundamental principles of two simulation approaches that are commonly used.

Agent-Based Models

ABMs explore the aggregate consequences of individual-level interactions between actors and their environment.[33] These actors, also referred to as "agents," may be organizations or people with characteristics that inform their decision-making and behavior. Agents' decision-making can be influenced by their own preferences, habits, and factors in their environment (e.g., their proximity to fast-food restaurants) as well as social factors (e.g., the behavior of other agents). Social influences can explicitly be represented as networks in ABMs. As such, network analysis techniques—which have been used to study a range of public health issues,[19] including but not limited to infectious disease transmission[34]—can also be used to visually describe and examine the relationships between agents in an ABM. For example, network analysis can be used to explore the influence of network position, which relates to an individual's level of connection relative to the connectedness of other members of their social network on health status.[35]

Agents in an ABM can also learn from past experiences and adapt their behavior in response to social and environmental signals. In turn, these individual-level decisions and behavior can lead to the emergence of novel and, at times, unexpected patterns at the collective or population-level.[36] For this reason, ABMs can be important tools for understanding how urban environments enable or constrain health-related behavior and how they structure health disparities in cities. Another important feature of these models is their ability to simulate scenarios of direct relevance to policy development and planning.[36] For example, ABMs provide a way of simulating and evaluating the potential effectiveness of large-scale, population-level interventions that may be prohibitively expensive or impractical to test experimentally in the real world.[36] They can also be used to provide insights into why a certain intervention may have been ineffective in achieving its intended aims.[36] Box 11.3 provides examples of the use of ABM to evaluate policy effects on diet and physical activity in urban areas.

System Dynamics Models

While ABMs consider how social and environmental influences impact the decision-making and behavior of individuals, system dynamics models focus on accumulations and flows of people, information or even physiological and health states, and how these change across different parts of a system.[20] For example, a system dynamics model can explore how patients accumulate and flow through a hospital's emergency room[37] or how people transition between different health states over time.[38] It is important to highlight that unlike ABMs, which focus on modeling the behavior of individual entities (e.g., individual people), system dynamics models concentrate only on collectives (e.g., entire populations). System dynamics models, much like ABMs, can be used to support policy planning by helping stakeholders better understand and predict the behavior of complex public health–relevant systems over time.[39] They can also be used to simulate different interventions and explore their potential health impacts.[20] By exploring how different types of interventions could affect the system, these models can also help decision makers learn a great deal about the system itself. For example, decision makers can get a better

Box 11.3 USING AGENT-BASED MODELS TO INVESTIGATE POLICY IMPACTS ON DIET AND WALKING BEHAVIOR

ABMs can be used to study a range of health behaviors. For example, Auchincloss and her team[11] were interested in understanding how neighborhood segregation can shape differences in dietary patterns among people of different income groups. They also wanted to understand whether changing household food preferences and the price of healthy foods would exacerbate or reduce income disparities in diet. To do this, they developed an ABM where households were segregated by income (i.e., people with similar income tended to live in the same neighborhoods). Each household was assigned an income and a food preference, which could change over time, ranging from healthy to unhealthy. In the model, these households shopped for food at stores that sell healthy or unhealthy food at different price points. A given store could change the type of food it sold based on consumer demand. Using this model, Auchincloss found that lower-income households had more unhealthy diets than high-income households when healthy food outlets were concentrated in high-income neighborhoods, while unhealthy food stores concentrated in predominantly low-income areas. Corresponding dietary differences persisted even when both income groups shared a preference for healthy food. Auchincloss found that a way to potentially overcome these dietary differences caused by segregation would be to increase the strength of households' preferences for healthy food and to simultaneously reduce the price of healthy food.

Another area where ABM has been applied is in the study of walking behavior. For example, Yang and colleagues[40] developed an ABM to explore how neighborhood safety and the distribution of workplaces, grocery stores, and social spaces in a city impacted levels of walking at the population level. In this model, the agents are people with a diverse set of personal characteristics such as gender, income, dog ownership, attitude toward walking, which can change over time based their own walking experiences and those of their friends or other members of their social network. People can decide whether to walk to work, for leisure, or to meet their basic needs. The way they make these decisions is influenced by their own personal characteristics and preferences, the behavior within their social network, as well as the safety and aesthetics of the neighborhoods they will travel through as part of their journey. Using this simple model, Yang found that people with lower incomes tend to walk more than high-income individuals but only when low-income residents live in or close to areas with high land use mix (i.e., areas where there are many different types of work, leisure, and basic needs destinations). These patterns are not evident, however, when low-income neighborhoods are unsafe.

Box 11.4 USING SYSTEM DYNAMIC MODELS TO EVALUATE THE SOCIETAL COSTS AND BENEFITS OF COMMUTER BICYCLING IN AUCKLAND, NEW ZEALAND

Faced with a long-standing decline in bicycling and increasing rates of car use, Macmillan and a group of researchers from New Zealand[41] developed a system dynamics model that allowed them to test the health and social impact of four policies that sought to promote bicycle ridership. These policies included

1. a regional cycle network that included new on-road bicycle lanes, shared bicycle and pedestrian footpaths, and shared bus and bicycle infrastructure;
2. a network of separated bicycle lanes on each side of every main road;
3. traffic-calming measures that reduced the speed limit of local streets such as planting trees or narrowing streets; and
4. a combination of policies 2 and 3.

Using their model, they simulated the impact of these policies on a range of outcomes including injury, physical activity, fuel costs, air pollution, and carbon emissions over a 40-year period.

Macmillian and his team found that the benefits of these policies—namely, the increases in bicycling—decreases with air pollution and carbon emissions, as well as declines in all-cause mortality attributable to increases in physical activity, outweighed the harms (i.e., increases in the total number of bike injuries and fatalities) for each of the four policy scenarios. The most effective way of increasing commuter bicycling was the combination of segregated bike lanes and with speed-reduction strategies on local streets (policy 4).

understanding of potential time delays and unintended consequences that may be associated with certain types of interventions. Box 11.4 provides an example of the use of systems dynamic models to evaluate the societal costs and benefits of commuter bicycling in Auckland, New Zealand.

CHALLENGES AND OPPORTUNITIES FOR SYSTEMS APPROACHES TO URBAN HEALTH

The use of systems approaches provides important opportunities in urban health to broaden our thinking, integrate different types of evidence, understand the implications of this integrated evidence, identify new actions or policies, improve our inferences regarding both etiology and policy impact, engage diverse stakeholders, and integrate health with environmental outcomes in an explicit, realistic and rigorous manner. In this section we discuss these challenges and opportunities in more detail with a special focus on urban health applications.

Developing Dynamic Conceptual Models of Urban Health

One major benefit of applying systems approaches to urban health problems (perhaps the most important benefit) is the development of conceptual models of the processes leading to health in urban settings that explicitly incorporate dynamic relations (i.e., dependencies and feedbacks) as appropriate to the context and problem at hand. These models must move beyond generic depictions to very specific conceptualizations relevant to a given health problem or research question. The development of these models may involve input from stakeholders as well as scientists. Figure 11.1 shows two examples of diagrams of two dynamic conceptual models used in systems modeling of urban health problems.

A major challenge in developing these dynamic conceptual models is setting the bounds and including only the elements fundamental to understanding the process at hand. It is important to remember that a systems model (or a complex systems model) is not necessarily a very complicated model. Intelligent abstraction is key if these models are to be useful in advancing knowledge. It is also important to recognize that often many aspects of these models can be investigated using traditional approaches (i.e., formal simulation of a system is not always necessary). The dynamic conceptual model serves to place findings in context regardless of whether formal simulation follows. Moreover, as we will review in more detail in the next section, the process of developing these models often starkly illuminates where knowledge about the underlying processes is thin or absent and points to new directions for inquiry. The knowledge gained about components of the dynamic model using traditional approaches can then be used to refine the conceptual model and inform formal simulation of the system in the future.

Asking Different, More Nuanced, and More Policy Relevant Questions

The use of systems approaches also has implications for the types of questions that we ask and, ultimately, for the types of policies that we may identify as important to improving health in cities. For example, a traditional urban health question might be "Are neighborhood characteristics independently

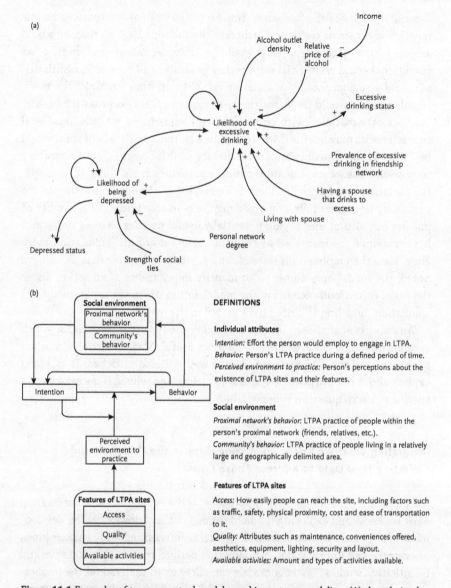

Figure 11.1 Examples of two conceptual models used in systems modeling: (A) the relation between depression and alcohol misuse among urban older adults and (B) Drivers of population patterns of leisure-time physical activity in urban areas. The arrows in both figures represent causal relationships either between variables or how a variable causes changes in its own state over time. In (A), the (+) signs represents positive relationships which signal that the variables move in the same direction (i.e., increases in one lead to increases in another variable, or decreases in one, lead to decreases in the other). Negative relationships are represented by a (–) sign. This implies an inverse relationship between a pair of variables, which means that the variable change in opposite directions (i.e., if one increases, it causes the other to decrease, and vice versa).[42,43]

Source: Panel A: Stankov I, Yang Y, Langellier BA, Purtle J, Nelson KL, Diez Roux AV. Depression and alcohol misuse among older adults: Exploring mechanisms and policy impacts using agent-based modelling. *Social Psychiatry and Psychiatric Epidemiology.* 2019;54(10):1243–1253. Panel B:. Garcia LM, Roux AVD, Martins AC, Yang Y, Florindo AA. Exploring the emergence and evolution of population patterns of leisure-time physical activity through agent-based modelling. *International Journal of Behavioral Nutrition and Physical Activity.* 2018;15(1):112. Abbreviation: LTPA, leisure-time physical activity.

associated with health after accounting for the individual-level socioeconomic position and race of residents?" whereas the related question that we would answer with a systems approach would be "To what extent (and under what conditions) could residential segregation generate, and reinforce, health disparities by socioeconomic position or race?" In another example, the traditional question would be "Is proximity to supermarkets (as proxy for healthy food access) associated with better diet after adjustment for individual-level characteristics of residents?" whereas a more systems oriented question would be "What is the plausible impact on dietary health inequalities of a strategy to subsidize the location of supermarkets in certain areas under various spatial patterning scenarios?"[11] These different kinds of questions allow for the possibility not only of directly assessing the plausible impact of a number of policies but also of identifying potentially useful policies that we might not have imagined (or identified as relevant) before doing the simulation modeling. Here the emphasis on *plausible* and *potential* is key, because as we have noted, the model only allows us to identify implications of an action under the set of conditions encoded in the model. Often the insights obtained from simulation modeling still need to be tested in the real world.

An important challenge is also identifying the type of questions for which systems modeling is needed or can be most useful. Many questions in urban health can and should be answered using traditional approaches. Thus, being explicit about the purpose of systems modeling and why it is necessary for a specific research question is important.

Integrating What We Know, Identifying Gaps in the Evidence, and Collecting New Data to Address Those Gaps

An important benefit of systems approaches is the explicit focus on integrating what we know and exploring the implications of this knowledge. The development of a formal systems simulation model requires integrating various kinds of evidence and information, including that derived from both qualitative and quantitative studies. Systems models can allow us to understand the implications and consequences of various pieces of quantitative and qualitative information in ways that we would not necessarily have predicted if we did not do the formal simulation. This is where the real value of systems modeling lies. In addition, the process of conceptualizing the dynamic model and then formalizing the simulation model often leads to the identification of important gaps in data or suggests new questions that can be answered using traditional approaches. The collection of new data and the responses to new questions can also subsequently serve to improve our understanding of how the system works and improve the validity of the simulation model for answering other questions.

The Tension Between Specificity and Generalizability

In applying systems modeling approaches to concrete research problems, there is often a tension between making the conceptual (and formal simulation) model general and abstract or specific and detailed. More general and abstract models have the advantage of being easier to explore and understand. They can also shed light on fundamental dynamics that may be important in many different contexts. In contrast, more specific and detailed models are tailored to specific contexts (e.g., to a specific city). They have the advantage of being very firmly connected to a real -world scenario but can often become very complicated and difficult to test, due to the simultaneous reliance on many assumptions. As a result, the conclusions that we draw from them can be of questionable utility in terms of generalizable knowledge generation. It is important to note that the goal of systems modeling is not necessarily detailed prediction but rather understanding of dynamics so that plausible policy impacts under different conditions can be understood. For this, abstract models are usually a good starting point and can be made more specific and tailored to a specific context as understanding advances.

Grounding Models in Reality: The Role of Data

Ensuring that both conceptual and simulation models are grounded in reality and are based on empirical observations as much as possible is a key challenge of systems approaches. Often, as we develop the model, we discover that there is much that we do not know about basic drivers of the system. Sometimes informed guesses are the best available starting point and model development informs future research and data collection efforts.

Nevertheless, for the conclusions of models to be meaningful, data and empirical observations must enter into the model development process in several different ways. These include (i) informing the magnitude and direction of the relations posited in the conceptual model and (ii) informing the rules and relations that govern agent actions (in an ABM) or stocks and flows (in a system dynamics model). Data can also be used in validating the model by comparing its behavior and output to real data that was not used to inform the parameters in the model. Sometimes there are no data for underlying key parameters (such as how attitude toward walking evolves in response to specific experiences). These parameters can be calibrated by comparing output to existing external data and tuning the parameter in question until a match is observed. Of course, the data used in calibration must be different from the data used to externally validate the model.

Communication and Policy Impact

Because of their complexity, systems models can sometimes be difficult to describe and communicate to others. The scientific community has developed helpful standards regarding scientific communication about these models in ways that allow replication and a full understanding of how and why decisions were made in their development.[36,44,45] However, communicating to the public and policymakers about these models remains very challenging. Here it is critical to emphasize that these models are most useful as tools to generate insight into causes or into possible impact of interventions. However, they should not be interpreted as detailed prediction models as they are often not designed with this purpose in mind.

CAVEATS AND CONCLUSION

Current interest in systems thinking in population health presents important opportunities for creative thinking in the area of urban health. Aside from the important contribution of encouraging the development of dynamic conceptual models of health in cities, systems approaches provide us with new analytical tools (specifically simulation modeling), which can be used to enhance insight and identify new areas for additional exploration using a range of analytical approaches. Systems thinking also provides formalized ways for urban health researchers to link to other disciplines interested in the functioning of cities and allows input from various stakeholders and communities in the formulation of conceptual models and in the interpretation of results of simulation modeling. Yet, to be truly transformative, these new approaches need to be employed to answer very specific questions that can yield new insights. Moving beyond metaphorical discussions of urban systems to concrete applications that yield new information will be key. At their best, the use of systems approaches will allow us to see and understand patterns and trends that researchers, communities, and policymakers would not otherwise notice. They may also allow us to identify new ideas for how to modify these patterns. Training in these approaches and the development of exemplar applications will be important.

Although broadly defined, "systems thinking" may be relevant to many urban health problems, it is important to remember that not all urban health questions will require or benefit from formal systems modeling. Identification of specific types of situations in which systems modeling may be most useful is important. Usually these will be situations where feedbacks and dependencies are strong, leading to emergent features that cannot be predicted unless the system as a whole is investigated. Modeling may also be especially informative when policy impacts are likely to vary depending on the state of other components of the system.

When used with scientific rigor, systems thinking and systems modeling may yield new insights into old problems, identify new important questions, and point to new kinds of data that need to be collected or analyzed to advance the goal of improving health in cities. Systems modeling will never replace traditional quantitative and qualitative empirical approaches in urban health research, but if integrated with other strategies, such models may advance our understanding of the determinants of urban health as well as enhance our ability to intervene to improve health and reduce health inequalities in urban settings.

REFERENCES

1. Forrester J. *Urban Dynamics*. Boston: Pegasus Communications; 1969.
2. Batty M. *The New Science of Cities*. Boston: MIT Press; 2014.
3. Bettencourt LMA. The origins of scaling in cities. *Science*. 2013;340(6139): 1438–1441.
4. System. *Merriam-Webster Dictionary*. https://www.merriam-webster.com/dictionary/system. Accessed June 25, 2020.
5. Galea S, Hall C, Kaplan GA. Social epidemiology and complex system dynamic modelling as applied to health behaviour and drug use research. *International Journal on Drug Policy*. 2009;20(3):209–216.
6. Diez Roux AV. Complex systems thinking and current impasses in health disparities research. *American Journal of Public Health*. 2011;101(9):1627–1634.
7. Sterman JD. Learning from evidence in a complex world. *American Journal of Public Health*. 2006;96(3):505–514.
8. Pearce N, Merletti F. Complexity, simplicity, and epidemiology. *International Journal of Epidemiology*. 2006;35(3):515–519.
9. Auchincloss AH, Diez Roux AV. A new tool for epidemiology: The usefulness of dynamic-agent models in understanding place effects on health. *American Journal of Epidemiology*. 2008;168(1):1–8.
10. Cerda M, Keyes KM. Systems modeling to advance the promise of data science in epidemiology. *American Journal of Epidemiology*. 2019;188(5):862–865.
11. Auchincloss AH, Riolo RL, Brown DG, Cook J, Diez Roux AV. An agent-based model of income inequalities in diet in the context of residential segregation. *American Journal of Preventative Medicine*. 2011;40(3):303–311.
12. Yang Y, Diez Roux AV, Auchincloss AH, Rodriguez DA, Brown DG. A spatial agent-based model for the simulation of adults' daily walking within a city. *American Journal of Preventive Medicine*. 2011;40(3):353–361.
13. Cerda M, Tracy M, Ahern J, Galea S. Addressing population health and health inequalities: The role of fundamental causes. *American Journal of Public Health*. 2014;104(Suppl 4):S609–619.
14. Wakeland W, Nielsen A, Geissert P. Dynamic model of nonmedical opioid use trajectories and potential policy interventions. *American Journal of Drug and Alcohol Abuse*. 2015;41(6):508–518.

15. Cerdá M, Morenoff JD, Hansen BB, et al. Reducing violence by transforming neighborhoods: A natural experiment in Medellín, Colombia. *American Journal of Epidemiology.* 2012;175(10):1045–1053.

16. El-Sayed AM, Seemann L, Scarborough P, Galea S. Are network-based interventions a useful antiobesity strategy? An application of simulation models for causal inference in epidemiology. *American Journal of Epidemiology.*2013;178(2): 287–295.

17. Marshall B, Galea S. Formalizing the role of agent-based modelling in causal inference and epidemiology. *American Journal of Epidemiology.*2015;181(2):92–99.

18. Tracy M, Cerdá M, Keyes KM. Agent-based modeling in public health: Current applications and future directions. *Annual Review of Public Health.* 2018;39(1): 77–94.

19. Luke DA, Stamatakis KA. Systems science methods in public health: Dynamics, networks, and agents. *Annual Review of Public Health.* 2012;33:357–376.

20. Homer JB, Hirsch GB. System dynamics modeling for public health: Background and opportunities. *American Journal of Public Health.* 2006;96(3):452–458.

21. Pongsiri MJ, Gatzweiler FW, Bassi AM, Haines A, Demassieux F. The need for a systems approach to planetary health. *The Lancet Planetary Health.* 2017;1(7): e257–e259.

22. Hovmand PS. *Group model building and community-based system dynamics process.* In: Hovmand PS, *Community Based System Dynamics.* New York: Springer-Verlag; 2014:17–30.

23. Richardson GP, Andersen DF. Teamwork in group model-building. *System Dynamics Review.* 1995;11(2):113–137.

24. Vennix JAM. *Group Model Building: Facilitating Team Learning Using System Dynamics.* New York: Wiley; 1996.

25. Langellier BA, Kuhlberg JA, Ballard EA, et al. Using community-based system dynamics modeling to understand the complex systems that influence health in cities: The SALURBAL study. *Health & Place.* 2019;60:102215.

26. Homa L, Rose J, Hovmand PS, et al. A participatory model of the paradox of primary care. *Annals of Family Medicine.* 2015;13(5):456–465.

27. Nelson DA, Simenz CJ, O'Connor SP, et al. Using group model building to understand factors that influence childhood obesity in an urban environment. *Journal of Public Health Management and Practice.* 2015;21:S74–S78.

28. Skouteris H, Huang T, Millar L, et al. A systems approach to reducing maternal obesity: The Health in Preconception, Pregnancy and Postbirth (HIPPP) Collaborative. *Australian and New Zealand Journal of Obstetrics and Gynaecology.* 2015;55(4):397–400.

29. Cavana RY, Broatch FM, Clifford LV. A system dynamics pilot study to demonstrate the impact of border intervention on tobacco related activities in New Zealand. 2003; http://citeseerx.ist.psu.edu/viewdoc/download?doi=10.1.1.485 .6634&rep=rep1&type=pdf

30. Scott RJ, Cavana RY, Cameron D. Recent evidence on the effectiveness of group model building. *European Journal of Operational Research.* 2016;249(3):908–918.

31. Bridgewater K, Peterson S, McDevitt J, et al. A community-based systems learning approach to understanding youth violence in Boston. *Progress in Community Health Partnerships: Research, Education, and Action.* 2011;5(1):67–75.

32. Diez Roux A. The virtual epidemiologist: Promise and peril. *American Journal of Epidemiology.* 2015;81(2):100–102.

33. Bruch E, Atwell J. Agent-based models in empirical social research. *Sociological Methods & Research*. 2015;44(2):186–221.

34. Keeling MJ, Eames KT. Networks and epidemic models. *Journal of the Royal Society Interface*. 2005;2(4):295–307.

35. Liu S, Hachen D, Lizardo O, Poellabauer C, Striegel A, Milenković T. Network analysis of the NetHealth data: exploring co-evolution of individuals' social network positions and physical activities. *Applied Network Science*. 2018;3(1):45.

36. Hammond RA. Appendix A: Considerations and best practices in agent-based modeling to inform policy. In: Wallace R, Geller A, Ogawa V, eds. *Assessing the Use of Agent-Based Models for Tobacco Regulation* (pp. 161–193). Washington, DC: National Academies Press; 2015.

37. Lane D, Monefeldt C, Rosenhead J. Looking in the wrong place for healthcare improvements: A system dynamics study of an accident and emergency department. In: Macmillan P, ed. *Operational Research for Emergency Planning in Healthcare*. Vol. 2. London: Springer; 2016:92–121.

38. Meisel JD, Sarmiento OL, Olaya C, Lemoine PD, Valdivia JA, Zarama R. Towards a novel model for studying the nutritional stage dynamics of the Colombian population by age and socioeconomic status. *PLoS ONE*. 2018;13(2):e0191929.

39. Currie DJ, Smith C, Jagals P. The application of system dynamics modelling to environmental health decision-making and policy—a scoping review. *BMC Public Health*. 2018;18(1):402.

40. Yang Y, Diez Roux AV, Auchincloss AH, Rodriguez DA, Brown DG. A spatial agent-based model for the simulation of adults' daily walking within a city. *American Journal of Preventive Medicine*. 2011;40(3):353–361.

41. Macmillan A, Connor J, Witten K, Kearns R, Rees D, Woodward A. The societal costs and benefits of commuter bicycling: Simulating the effects of specific policies using system dynamics modeling. *Environmental Health Perspectives*. 2014;122(4):335–344.

42. Stankov I, Yang Y, Langellier BA, Purtle J, Nelson KL, Diez Roux AV. Depression and alcohol misuse among older adults: Exploring mechanisms and policy impacts using agent-based modelling. *Social Psychiatry and Psychiatric Epidemiology*. 2019;54(10):1243–1253.

43. Garcia LM, Roux AVD, Martins AC, Yang Y, Florindo AA. Exploring the emergence and evolution of population patterns of leisure-time physical activity through agent-based modelling. *International Journal of Behavioral Nutrition and Physical Activity* 2018;15(1):112.

44. Grimm V, Berger U, Bastiansen F, et al. A standard protocol for describing individual-based and agent-based models. *Ecological Modelling*. 2006;198(1–2): 115–126.

45. Grimm V, Berger U, DeAngelis DL, Polhill JG, Giske J, Railsback SF. The ODD protocol: A review and first update. *Ecological Modelling*. 2010;221(23):2760–2768.

PART IV

From Evidence into Action

We have dedicated the last part of this book to the people and processes needed to facilitate change in urban health, taking us out of our academic institutions and into the practical world of urban public health.

Chapter 12 discusses the "who" in public health—those sectors and stakeholders in all cities who are engaged in urban health—directly and indirectly. Chapter 13 focuses specifically on community engagement and how we build bridges between research and practice, and work with the very communities we are hoping to improve. Chapter 14 addresses policy as an instrument for change—the policy actions uniquely afforded to cities and the challenges they face. Finally, Chapter 15 provides a roadmap for dissemination of research into practice and how to engage multiple audiences in the translation and dissemination of urban public health research.

As we have discussed throughout this book, cities are unique places, with unique challenges to and opportunities for improving the health of the people they inhabit. As more and more of the population reside in cities, urban areas will have increasing power to understand and impact public health. Part IV provides a map for turning our evidence into action.

CHAPTER 12

Partnerships and Collaboration

An Urban Focus

JENNIFER KOLKER AND AMY CARROLL-SCOTT

BACKGROUND

As we have discussed throughout this book, there are both challenges and opportunities that face public health researchers and practitioners in urban environments. First, as has been discussed in Chapter 4, urban populations experience severe and pervasive racial and socioeconomic inequities both in the United States and globally. The persistence and sometimes even widening of these inequities suggest that traditional approaches to prevention and health-care delivery are not working and that the vast research on health inequities is not being successfully translated into effective solutions.

Ameliorating adverse social and environmental determinants of health in cities requires engagement and collaboration across multiple sectors. Often, it requires a level of imagination and innovation as those collaborators are defined. High population density and increased cultural diversity mean there is a broader range of stakeholders and perspectives near each other in cities than in less urban contexts. Making positive, measurable impact on urban health requires collaboration, engagement, understanding and problem-solving at all levels of urban systems.

Understanding, developing, and implementing effective interventions related to the determinants of health requires drawing data and expertise from a variety of perspectives that go beyond traditional public health including city planning, education, employment, housing, and other social and economic

Jennifer Kolker and Amy Carroll-Scott, *Partnerships and Collaboration* In: *Urban Public Health*. Edited by:
Gina S. Lovasi, Ana V. Diez Roux, and Jennifer Kolker, Oxford University Press (2021). © Oxford University Press 2021.
DOI: 10.1093/oso/9780190885304.003.0012.

fields. Together with traditional public health, teams that bridge these perspectives can bring together a growing range of tools for building evidence using both existing and newly available data relevant to developing and refining innovative strategies for action.

Improving population health locally also requires taking seriously the questions posed by communities, health-care providers, and public health agencies who have a stake in improving population health outcomes, so that urban health work is relevant to their needs. It requires partnering with a broad range of stakeholders who understand the local needs, causes, and actions that may be most impactful, along with those who understand, most critically, the best way to develop and implement health-promoting policies and interventions so that they maximize their effectiveness in a setting.

URBAN PUBLIC HEALTH ACTORS

So, who are the actors in urban public health? They are the sectors and individuals that have the interest, power, and ability to transform cities to inform and improve the health of their populations. We offer next a broad inventory of the actors who play a role in turning public health research into action in cities. While much of this discussion is focused on the United States, the range of partnerships and stakeholders required to create change in urban public health is universal. What is critical to keep in mind is that the range of players in public health is broad, with little or no boundaries. As our definitions of public health have expanded, so too has our list of stakeholders, and over time, we have broadened our thinking to include parts of government and nongovernment (including private sector, industry, and nonprofit organizations) that are not directly connected to health (see Table 12.1). As we focus on the social determinants of health in cities, our definition must broaden even more to include those that influence social determinants.

Community Residents and Leaders

The first actors in urban health are the communities who are affected by the health issues being addressed. Community has "historically been left out of health improvement efforts even though it is supposed to be the beneficiary of those efforts."[1] Community itself is composed of many different types and levels of actors. The first and most obvious actors in this sphere are the community members themselves. When a community is defined geographically,

Table 12.1 URBAN PUBLIC HEALTH ACTORS

Sector	Urban Public Health Actors
Government	
Public Health	Local health departments
	Boards of health
	Behavioral health agencies
	Public health care delivery
Nonpublic health	Public Safety (police, fire, emergency response)
	Schools
	Streets/traffic/infrastructure
	Child welfare
	Social services-housing support
	Urban development, commerce, economic development Basic city services-trash, water
Health Care System	Hospitals/health systems
	Federally qualified health centers/safety net providers
	Public hospitals
	Insurers
Nongovernment organizations	Public health organizations
	Advocacy organizations
	Thought leaders
	School organizations
Funders	Local community and corporate foundations
	National/regional foundations investing in urban health
Academia	Public health and other relevant disciplines

its members are its residents. Community can also be defined based on history, culture, and/or values, even if members don't share the same geographic identify.

Other important community actors are grassroots leaders, meaning residents who take on leadership positions on behalf of and alongside their neighbors to serve the needs of their own community. Examples of neighborhood organizations include neighborhood civic associations, spiritual communities, or other resident-led organizations that provide leadership for urban neighborhoods. This also includes parent-engagement organizations for schools (e.g., home-school associations or parent–teacher organizations). In addition, every neighborhood also has informal organizations that serve the various and often specialty needs of its residents. These organizations often don't have a bricks-and-mortar address, operating as an informal network of residents; however, long-standing grassroots organizations may become formalized as a nonprofit organization. Some examples include local volunteer associations, neighborhood watch groups, resident-led issue-based advocacy organizations (e.g., violence prevention, community-supported agriculture), or social groups such as exercise or walking groups, book clubs, and bowling leagues. Chapter 13 is devoted specifically to the engagement of communities at all levels in urban public health.

Governmental Public Health: Local Health Agencies/Departments

Government is at the core of urban public health because government bears the ultimate responsibility and authority for protecting the health of city residents. Most cities have governmental public health authority; in most US cities, that authority rests with a local health department. Most city health departments are governed in some way by a local board of health, which is designated by law for overseeing local public health policy, services or programs. The reach and power of boards of health vary by city and the state in which they reside, but all have some role in overseeing public health in their jurisdiction.

The National Association of City and County Health Officials (NACCHO) completes a National Profile of Local Health Departments every few years with a rich array of data on services, governance, policy engagement, and other areas of interest to local public health. NACCHO defines "large" health departments as those serving jurisdictions of 500,000 people or more.[2]

According to the Big Cities Health Coalition, as of 2016, in the United States alone, nearly 62 million people, or one in five Americans, live in a city served by a local health department. Health departments in US cities provide a range of services from policy development, chronic disease prevention, communicable disease control, lead prevention and control, tobacco prevention/control, environmental health services, and some direct primary care services and screening. While each health department is organized differently and with some variation in the scope and depth of what they provide, all bear essential responsibility for core public health responsibilities—the 10 Essential Public Health Services (see Table 12.2)—in in their jurisdictions and act as the hub of governmental public health activity in their cities.[3] In cities across the globe, local ministries of health and other local health authorities provide similar public health functions in their jurisdictions.

An oft-used quote by health leaders states "If you've seen one health department, you've seen one health department." Organization and jurisdiction of health departments varies greatly and can be complicated by the crossing of city and county lines. While all required to perform the essential public health services, health departments vary greatly on the scope of activities they engage in and the priorities they set for their jurisdiction. This variation is informed in part by size, urbanicity, relationship to the state or higher level of

Table 12.2 ESSENTIAL PUBLIC HEALTH SERVICES

The 10 essential public health services describe the public health activities that all health departments in the United States should undertake:

1. Monitor health status to identify and solve community health problems
2. Diagnose and investigate health problems and health hazards in the community
3. Inform, educate, and empower people about health issues
4. Mobilize community partnerships and action to identify and solve health problems
5. Develop policies and plans that support individual and community health efforts
6. Enforce laws and regulations that protect health and ensure safety
7. Link people to needed personal health services and assure the provision of health care when otherwise unavailable
8. Assure competent public and personal health care workforce
9. Evaluate effectiveness, accessibility, and quality of personal and population-based health services
10. Research for new insights and innovative solutions to health problems

Source: Center for State Tribal Local and Territorial Support.[1]

government, and the political and legislative context. Table 12.3 shows the range of primary prevention activities performed by local health departments by size and urbanicity.

Approximately 50% of large (>500,000 population) US cities are also governed by a local board of health. Boards of health play a governance role with health departments and help to shape public health policy in the cities they serve. Like health departments, boards of health activities vary across cities, but most enact, revise, recommend, or review public health regulations; advise, recommend, or establish public health policies; and recommend community public health priorities. Boards of health are usually appointed by the chief executive (mayor) and their role is usually set by either the city in which they operate or by state statute.

Local Government-Agencies Beyond Public Health

The governmental role in public health is not limited to the local health department or public health authority. It is hard to find a government agency in any urban area that does not have some impact on the social and environmental determinants of health. All actions taken by cities, whether directly connected to health care or not, will have an impact on the health of its residents.

Public safety—police, fire, and emergency services—play an obvious and critical role in urban public health. Public safety acts as a core public health partner in emergency preparedness and response, working closely with public health agencies in responding to natural disasters and disease outbreaks.

Table 12.3 POPULATION-BASED PRIMARY PREVENTION SERVICES PROVIDED DIRECTLY IN THE PAST YEAR BY LOCAL HEALTH DEPARTMENT CHARACTERISTICS

| | | Size of Population Served (%) | | | | Degree of Urbanization (%) | | |
	All LHDs	Small (<50,000)	Medium (50,000– 499,999)	Large (500,000+)		Urban	Suburban	Rural
Nutrition	74	70	81	85		69	79	75
Tobacco	74	72	77	86		70	76	79
Physical activity	60	55	68	73		59	61	61
Chronic disease programs	57	50	65	79		59	57	52
Unintended pregnancy	51	46	56	66		42	58	51
Injury	42	38	49	51		39	45	45
Substance abuse	34	31	36	43		33	33	35
Violence	22	19	25	36		21	24	19
Mental illness	17	15	19	31		19	16	16

n = 1,672 to 1,886.
Source: National Association of County and City Health Officials.[1]
Abbreviation: LHD, local health department.

Public safety addresses issues of violence and substance misuse and as those issues continue to pervade cities, their public health role has increased. As we have seen in the opioid epidemic, police administering of naloxone has been vital in preventing overdose and saving lives, and the intersection and collaboration between public health and criminal justice is critical in addressing gun violence in cities. It is important to note that policing strategies and community relations overall can affect the ability of the criminal justice system to engage in public health in ways that support—rather than stress—urban residents.

City departments that manage streets, housing, and inspection and licensing of development are an integral part of urban public health by developing bike lanes and ensuring pedestrian safety, maintaining safe housing and physical infrastructure and air and water quality, and addressing the other urban environmental determinants of health.

Finally, local government actors in health include those agencies providing basic city services such as trash collection, provision of safe water, and investment in economic development and the myriad of governmental safety net agencies and programs that may vary by city and country but that provide food, shelter, and other supportive services for people living in cities.

Hospitals, Health Systems, and Health-Care Providers

Hospitals and health-care systems have an obvious role to play in urban health and are increasingly engaging in local collaborative partnerships to address population health. In the United States, nonprofit hospitals have always been required to perform some type of community benefit activity in their jurisdiction to maintain their tax-exempt status. Prior to 2008, that requirement was largely met with the provision of some select community services and the provision of charity care to uninsured patients. Since 2014, the Affordable Care Act requires hospitals to conduct a community health needs assessment every three years, in which each hospital evaluates the health needs of the community it serves and an implementation plan annually in which they propose plans to address those needs. While the depth and quality of these community health needs assessments may vary across hospitals and health systems, the requirement that they be conducted at least every three years provides a framework for health-care engagement more broadly in urban public health.

Federal Qualified Health Centers have long been the safety-net provider of care for the uninsured in all parts of the United States and play a critical role in most US cities in the provision of primary health care and behavioral health services as well in public health functions such as chronic disease prevention. Urban hospitals and health-care systems are also important research partners; hospitals are increasingly using their own data to better understand population health and are collaborating with external partners such as academia and governmental public health in understanding and using data to improve urban health.

Education and School Health

Educators and health professionals working within educational settings have unique access to and investment in child health both for its own sake and for the role that health plays in laying a foundation for academic achievement and the critical role that education plays in health later in life with the established knowledge that adults with higher educational attainment lead healthier and longer lives. School systems are public health partners at a range of levels—with a research eye to learn about child health; as a place to connect children and their families to the health-care system through vaccination campaigns, obesity screenings, and sexually transmitted disease screening and treatment; and as an economic and health safety net for school-age children, through provision of federally funded meals, basic health care and mental health services, and health education.

Other Nongovernment Organizations

While government bears the ultimate responsibility for public health, the actual practice of public health is done by many nongovernmental health and social service organizations. In some jurisdictions, these organizations are under contract from city government; others are more independent. Nongovernmental organizations (NGOs) can range from large, multiservice organizations with substantial budgets to smaller, community-based organizations. Community-based organizations encompass a range of public and nonprofit entities that represent a community or a segment of a community and are engaged in meeting human, educational, environmental, or public safety needs. Examples include health and social service organizations, advocacy organizations, and community health centers. Leaders of NGOs are often major actors in urban health.

Academic Public Health and Other Relevant Academic Disciplines

Academic public health researchers and educators must collaborate with those who are on the front lines of public health practice, including policymakers and government entities, health-care delivery systems, NGOs, and communities themselves. Relationships between academia and public health practice are critical in training of future practitioners, developing research agendas that benefit cities, and in the translation and dissemination of that research to public health practitioners (discussed in more detail in Chapter 15).

Urban Planners, Architects, and Other Design Professionals

The relationship between urban health and urban planning is long-standing, although it has ebbed and flowed in recent decades in the United States. These connections between the health sciences and urban planning and architecture have recently been revived, particularly in regard to transportation and physical activity.[4] Other points of common interest include stress, sleep quality, and climate resilience. Urban health has increasingly turned to planning and design for support in solving urban health problems, and a 2013 report by the American Planning Association on healthy plan-making describes case studies and recommendations for incorporating public health into urban planning:

> Today, as public health concerns increasingly center on chronic disease and safety, specialists and city planners realize they cannot afford to operate in isolation any longer. Decisions that leaders have made regarding land use, urban design, and transportation have impacted local air quality, water quality and supply, traffic safety, physical activity, and exposure to contaminated industrial sites (i.e., brownfields). These decisions are linked to some of the most intractable public health problems, including adult and childhood obesity, inactivity, cancer, respiratory problems, and environmental justice.[5]

Box 3.1 in Chapter 3 of this volume further discusses the links between urban planning and urban health.

Business and Industry

As economic engines in a city, business and industry play a role in urban health. Some have direct connections—health insurers, pharma, and other industries that are actively engaged in urban health. At the same time, large employers have a direct impact on health through their economic impacts on the city as a whole as well as through their direct impacts on the health of workers via work conditions as well as through workplace policies (e.g., around tobacco and wellness). As economic drivers in cities, business and industry play an important role in economic development, job creation, and other economic measure that impact health.

MULTISECTOR COLLABORATION

As we discussed in Chapter 1, a multisectoral approach to health is one of the elements distinguishing urban health as a field. Identification of sectors and partners is necessary but not sufficient for improving urban public health. Urban public health practice requires the ongoing building and maintaining of relationships between sectors and partners and using necessary partnerships to advance urban health goals.

The World Health Organization has defined a healthy city as a "process, not an outcome," further emphasizing the key role that partnership and collaboration plays in advancing urban health.[6] The WHO Healthy Cities Approach emphasizes the need to work in collaboration across different sectors and organizations, with an emphasis on equity, participatory governance and solidarity, and intersectoral collaboration to address the social determinants of health.

The need for multisectoral collaboration and partnership in public health—and, particularly, urban public health—has gained traction in recent years. Public Health 3.0, a new framework for public health put forth by the Centers for Disease Control and Prevention (see Figure 12.1), emphasizes the need to "engage multiple sectors and community partners to improve health."[7] As DeSalvo et al.[7] state in their Public Health 3.0 Call to Action:

> To solve the fundamental challenges of population health, we must address the full range of factors that influence a person's overall health and well-being. Education, safe environments, housing, transportation, economic development, access to healthy foods—these are the major social determinants of health, comprising the conditions in which people are born, live, work, and age.

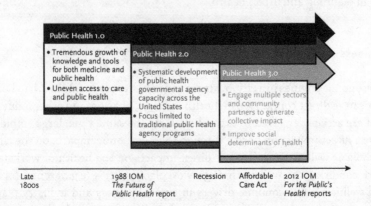

Figure 12.1 Evolution of public health practice.

Source: DeSalvo KB, Wang YC, Harris A, Auerbach J, Koo D, O'Carroll P. Public health 3.0: A call to action for public health to meet the challenges of the 21st century. *Preventing Chronic Disease.* 2017;14:170017.

Community Planning Processes for Health

There are many examples of community planning processes for health. the Mobilizing for Action through Planning and Partnerships (MAPP),[8] is a community-driven strategic planning process for improving community health developed by NACCHO and has been adapted and used in many cities to bring together stakeholders to address public health. City health departments that have undergone public health accreditation have had to engage in a Community Health Improvement Plan (CHIP) process,[9] bringing together stakeholders to set health priorities for their jurisdictions. As mentioned earlier, the community health needs assessment requirement of the Affordable Care Act engages nonprofit hospitals with communities in cities in determining their health needs.[10] Promise Neighborhoods, a US Department of Education program, is a place-based initiative that provides children and youth access to schools and systems of family and community support in distressed communities in the United States.[11] Saurabh Salud Urbana en América Latina (SALURBAL)'s Urban Health in Latin America is a five-year project launched in April 2017. The Drexel University Dornsife School of Public Health and partners throughout Latin America and in the United States are working together to study how urban environments and urban policies impact the health of city residents throughout Latin America. Their findings will inform policies and interventions to create healthier, more equitable, and more sustainable cities worldwide.[12] The Big Cities Health Coalition brings together the United States' largest urban areas to share data and policy challenges.

Collaborations and partnerships often arise out of specific health goals. The Vision Zero Network, is a collaboration of US cities to with the goals of eliminating all traffic fatalities and severe injuries, through collaboration between government, community organizations, and city residents. First implemented in Sweden in the 1990s, Vision Zero has proved successful across Europe and is increasing its presence in the United States, with over 40 cities designated as Vision Zero communities.[13] C40 is a network of 94 cities across the globe working collaborating to drive sustainable action around climate change.[14]

CONCLUSION

Developing and maintaining partnerships for urban health is not an easy task. Working within and outside of multiple sectors takes time, deliberate effort, and a commitment to engagement. Practicing urban public health is a team effort. Successful partnerships—whether narrow or broad—are built on trust between all actors and respect for different sectors and perspectives and have mutual benefit for all involved. Ultimately, successful partnerships and collaboration are built upon a shared vision and goal—improving the health of the city—and not the benefit of a particular research agenda, stakeholder, or organization.

REFERENCES

1. National Institutes of Health. *Principles of Community Engagement: Executive Summary.* 2nd ed. 2011; https://www.atsdr.cdc.gov/communityengagement/pce_execsummary.html.
2. National Association of County City Health Officials. National profile of local health departments, United States, 2016, restricted-use level 2 data. Inter-University Consortium for Political and Social Research. 2018; https://doi.org/10.3886/ICPSR37145.v1
3. Center for State Tribal Local and Territorial Support. The Public Health System & the 10 Essential Public Health Services. Centers for Disease Control and Prevention. Last updated June 26, 2018; https://www.cdc.gov/publichealth-gateway/publichealthservices/essentialhealthservices.html.
4. Handy SL, Boarnet MG, Ewing R, Killingsworth RE. How the built environment affects physical activity: Views from urban planning. *American Journal of Preventative Medicine.* 2002;23(2 Suppl):64–73.
5. Ricklin A, Kushner N. Integrating health into the comprehensive planning process: An analysis of seven case studies and recommendations for change. American Planning Association. 2013; https://www.planning.org/publications/document/9148247/. Accessed June 25, 2020.
6. World Health Organization. What is a healthy city? WHO European Healthy Cities Network. http://www.euro.who.int/en/health-topics/environment-and-health/urban-health/who-european-healthy-cities-network/what-is-a-healthy-city. Accessed June 25, 2020.
7. DeSalvo KB, Wang YC, Harris A, Auerbach J, Koo D, O'Carroll P. Public health 3.0: A call to action for public health to meet the challenges of the 21st century. *Preventing Chronic Disease.* 2017;14:170017.
8. National Association of County and City Health Officials. Mobilizing for Action through Planning and Partnerships (MAPP). 2001; https://www.naccho.org/programs/public-health-infrastructure/performance-improvement/community-health-assessment/mapp.
9. Bender K, Kronstadt J, Wilcox R, Lee TP. Overview of the public health accreditation board. *Journal of Public Health Management and Practice.* 2014;20(1):4–6.
10. Lundeer E, Liu EC. 501 (c)(3) hospitals: Proposed IRS rules under § 9007 of the Affordable Care Act. Congressional Research Service. July 27, 2012; https://www.naccho.org/uploads/downloadable-resources/501c3-Hospitals-Proposed-IRS-Rules-under-9007-of-the-Affordable-Care-Act-2.pdf.
11. US Department of Education Office of Innovation and Improvement. Promise Neighborhoods https://www2.ed.gov/programs/promiseneighborhoods/index.html. Accessed June 25, 2020.
12. LAC-Urban Health. Salud Urbana En America Latina (SALURBAL) Project. https://drexel.edu/lac/salurbal/overview/. Accessed June 25, 2020.
13. Vision Zero Network. What is the Vision Zero Network? 2018; https://visionzeronetwork.org/about/vision-zero-network/. Accessed June 25, 2020.
14. C40 Cities. https://www.c40.org/. Accessed June 25, 2020.

CHAPTER 13

Community Engagement and Participatory Approaches for Urban Health

AMY CARROLL-SCOTT

INTRODUCTION

The urban communities experiencing intergenerational health inequities also experience underlying social inequities that create barriers to optimal health and to contributing to solutions. In addition, urban health research struggles to recruit and retain study participants from these same populations due to feelings of mistrust and disenfranchisement from research and medical establishments.[1-3] As a result, research that does not partner with community residents and trusted leaders when recruiting from vulnerable urban populations experiences challenges regarding representation and validity. In addition, it is well-established that community actors are frequently not included in research dissemination,[4] nor do they seek, understand, or trust the public health research literature when taking action.[3,5,6] Therefore, urban health research that does not partner with communities and community-based practitioners (as well as policymakers, as argued in Chapter 14) lacks an avenue for translation of findings into changes in practice, program, and policy development and social change. Without this translation, research will not result in health improvements to urban communities.

This chapter describes the biggest challenges facing equitable, collaborative work between researchers and community actors in urban health research

Amy Carroll-Scott, *Community Engagement and Participatory Approaches for Urban Health* In: *Urban Public Health*. Edited by: Gina S. Lovasi, Ana V. Diez Roux, and Jennifer Kolker, Oxford University Press (2021). © Oxford University Press 2021. DOI: 10.1093/oso/9780190885304.003.0013.

and practice. We also draw from scientific literature and community voices to outline practical solutions to these challenges to improve the health of urban communities.

COMMUNITY PARTNERSHIP CHALLENGES

The challenges commonly facing community partnerships include a history of mistrust, limited capacity for partnership on both sides, and community research exhaustion.

History of Mistrust

Before public health researchers partner with community actors for the benefit of conducting urban health research and practitioners partner with community actors for the benefit of intervention planning, they need to understand the history of mistrust that may precede their current partnership. There is a long-established and well-known history of ethical abuses in health research, particularly research conducted with socioeconomically disadvantaged or minority populations. The most well-known example was the Tuskegee Syphilis Study, which denied syphilis treatment to its Black male participants, even after it became available.[7] The continuing legacy of this history cannot be overemphasized. It has contributed to the belief among US Black communities that Black genocide is possible and that researchers and public health authorities cannot be trusted.[8,9] This history, combined with the failure of the promises of opportunity and equality envisioned by the civil rights movement, has led to a social context of conspiracy theories in Black communities, including those positing that AIDS and drug abuse were promoted by the government as a form of Black genocide.[9] Recent increases in anti-immigrant rhetoric and US Department of Homeland Security's Immigration and Customs Enforcement agency raids have spread similar fear and mistrust among urban immigrant groups that have had direct effects on immigrant health-care access and health status.[10] Beyond a challenge for partnership that arises particularly for minority populations, mistrust itself can have negative consequences, as mistrust of the medical establishment has been shown to lead to worse health outcomes.[1]

Box 13.1 illustrates perspectives from a community leader, which addresses how important past experience and mistrust is when determining if a new partnership is worthwhile.

Box 13.1 PERSPECTIVE OF A COMMUNITY RESIDENT AND LEADER

Bettye Ferguson

Collaborations and partnerships for urban health may appear daunting in the eyes of the local neighborhood residents whom over the years have lost trust in the process due to lack of inclusion and transparency. Within urban areas researchers must keep in mind the people who reside there who are below the income median may share similarities pertaining to health and a host of other related risk factors that need to be addressed.

When approaching collaborations for urban health from the community's perspective, a stakeholder representing local institutions, hospitals, or other agencies may have good intentions and legitimate concern, but if their ideas and planning is done from the beginning without community input, the project is doomed to failure. The initial team should ask itself from the start when attempting to meet the community's needs: What will it take to make the project go smoother, who should we contact to help us when trying to reach project goals, and how and when will we share data once they have been collected? The most important part is to keep an open relationship with these partnerships.

In the eyes of local nonprofit groups or residents from any urban community, there can be advantages of positive research collaborations over the years. The ideal collaboration occurs when goals are created and met that bridge research and the betterment of the community. The collaboration is strengthened when all parties' expectations are met with respect to inclusion, transparency, and shared funding, and result in programs that meet the community's main goal of developing a healthier community. A well-planned collaboration between researchers and grassroots organizations helps both parties. This process, in short, allows the grassroots organizations to participate and also gives them a leg up with capacity building to help further their sustained efforts to strengthen their local communities.

Of course, as important as they are, collaborations or partnerships may stumble and disappoint. This is especially true when the collaboration lacks a shared plan or goal. An unplanned project can have negative effects when one party shows that they are only concerned about their goals, power, prestige, privileges or money gained to achieve the results they are looking for. It does damage to all parties when partnerships are not inclusive; now others question your motives and begin to pull away from the table. When information is not shared openly, a community can be blind-sided by hidden agendas. This is especially hurtful due to unequal voice with those standing on the pillar, insensitive to needs within a society of people who expect to be treated with respect no matter how they factor into the picture.

Equitable and respectful collaborations and partnerships for urban health is an ideal way to make progress on urban communities' struggles to understand and improve their community's health.

Research Evidence Is Not Necessarily Relevant to Community Context and Needs

Since community research largely still exists within an academic paradigm, it is typically driven by a priori research questions responsive to disease-focused funding agendas.[11-16] Researchers and community leaders are often attracted to research for different reasons;[17] community members and organizations are more interested in how data can describe risks and assets useful to improving community health rather than merely answering basic science questions or demonstrating methodological innovation. Also, community members do not think of their health in terms of specific disease categories, the predominant model for health research funding, as individuals' construction of their own health is much more contextual and nuanced by nature.[18,19] Further, urban health data and research results are commonly reported at geographic levels that are easier for researchers to gather (e.g., postal codes) but not at the levels at which residents form identities, organize, and advocate for change (e.g., neighborhoods, schools, police precincts, legislative districts). What this means is that community actors have fundamentally different research questions they would ask about their community's health but are left out of the process of formulating them.[20,21]

Limited Capacity for Partnership

The most commonly cited barrier to effective community–researcher collaboration is the lack of research capacity in communities and the community-based organizations (CBOs) that serve them. Not understanding research terminology or processes can alienate community members and CBO representatives.[13,15] It also limits the ability of communities to effectively influence research design and utilize results for social change.[13,15,17] Yet there is a recognized need for CBOs to use data to assess their community's health needs, adopt and evaluate evidence-based programs, and effectively advocate for the individuals and communities they serve.[11,22] Thus, throughout urban health research and practice, there is a need to strengthen CBO capacity to make it possible for these partnerships to be equitable. Otherwise, differences between partners in understanding research terminology and methods introduces yet another power differential.

Engaging with community actors can also be challenging for investigators. Variability exists in investigator experience with community engagement approaches and their capacity for incorporating this into their research design. This may mean a lack of capacity in the individual researcher's community engagement knowledge and skills, such as knowledge about the community (e.g., history, priorities), ability to share project tasks with CBO partners, and ability to communicate results to nonscientific audiences.[23] Capacity may also refer to the environment created by the researcher's institution for facilitating community engagement. Policies and processes vary in how well they support sharing study activities or financial resources with CBO partners.[24] Currently, there are no comprehensive, standardized measure to assess a researcher's community engagement capacity[25]; therefore, many researchers likely are unsure about the knowledge and skills they need to effectively engage communities as partners in their research. As a result, some researchers avoid community engagement in research, and some of those who do attempt to conduct it lack sufficient knowledge and skills and may unintentionally perpetuate issues of distrust and discord between community and academia.[26]

Community Research Exhaustion

Urban populations that experience social and health inequities are also the same populations that are most vulnerable to *respondent burden*, or "a subjective . . . perception by the subject of psychological, physical, and/or economic hardships associated with participation in the research process. (p. 17)"[27] Community advocates have argued that a *community-level research exhaustion* occurs when their neighborhood or population experiences frequent and duplicative research without any tangible benefit back to them, such as reporting back of results, translation of results to meet community data needs, or use of results to create community health improvements.[28] These experiences are especially intense in proximity to research institutions like higher education and hospital institutions, which may build their reputations conducting research that makes community members feel like guinea pigs.[29] Indeed, research institutions frequently promote their accomplishments such as large grants received, faculty promotions, and other accolades, which can be negatively received by surrounding urban neighborhoods. They see it as another way in which these institutions continue to advance their power and privilege and accrue resources that are not shared with surrounding communities.

Researchers and practitioners who enter into urban communities without an appreciation of the history and context as previously outlined and experienced in unique ways in each community will be hindered in building community research partnerships. What follows are several solutions to addressing these challenges and investing in the systems needed to strengthen partnerships between community actors and urban health researchers and practitioners to create sustainable community impacts.

Acknowledging and Addressing Mistrust

A study of CBOs and their university-based researcher collaborators found that although both groups of interviewees agreed that there was an important historical impact of race, power, and privilege on research collaborations, only the community leaders described the need to acknowledge it when creating a partnership.[16] They felt that to partner researchers and CBOs need to have the difficult conversations that are essential for overcoming often negative historical legacies of prior relationships between resource-rich research institutions and urban communities. While there are not a lot of models for how to effectively conduct such conversations in public health, urban health researchers and practitioners can find guidance from such tools from other fields such as education. For example, the Pacific Educational Group, focused on achieving racial equity in education, developed their Courageous Conversation™ protocol for effectively engaging, sustaining, and deepening interracial dialogue in education.[30]

Another solution is for researchers to employ culturally sensitive approaches. One approach is *cultural competence*, which arose out of medical provider training to solve the problem of cultural, linguistic, literacy, and other barriers to effective communication with patients.[31] Although contemporary cultural competence standards emphasizes active listening and regular assessments of patient population assets and needs,[32] cultural competence has been criticized for relying on and contributing to generalizations, stereotyping, and assumptions of culture as uniform and unchanging.[33] Indeed, how could a provider know all relevant expectations and dynamics within a particular culture or, more realistically, across the many different cultures and subcultures they encounter, particularly in diverse urban contexts?

A more effective solution to hearing and responding to mistrust between researchers and disenfranchised communities is a *cultural humility* approach, or a willingness to suspend what you know, or what you think you know, about a person or a group of people based on generalizations about their culture.[34] It shifts the focus to self-awareness and listening, acknowledging that one's own perspective may be impeded by assumptions and biases. What this looks like in practice is that rather than learning to identify and respond to sets of culturally specific traits (stereotyping), a culturally humble and culturally collaborative researcher listens and explores similarities and differences between their own and community partners'/study participants' priorities, goals, capacities, and approaches.[35] As with cultural competence, it acknowledges that culture provides the framework through which someone understands themselves and their experiences. The core difference is that cultural humility attempts to understand individuals' cultural and personal framework through respect and listening and not through emphasis on public health professionals' own confidence in retaining knowledge about the cultural backgrounds of the patients or community members they work with.

This means spending time for partners to get to know each other and what each hopes to get out of the partnership, whether it relates to a research project, public health program planning activity, or advocacy project. Ideally this process occurs unbounded by the scope of a specific prespecified project so that it fosters a more general understanding of what each partner brings to the table to best align activities undertaken together. But if this process happens as a result of funding already gained or a project already started, it is still important to take the time to engage in it.

Community-Engaged Research

This potential for major mismatches in researcher and community contexts, interests, and capacities argues for the importance of community actor engagement in urban health research. There is a long tradition of community-engaged research (CEnR) and planning, the goal of which is to engage organizations and individuals in research and the development of solutions that address their own well-being.[36–38] CEnR has been recognized as an essential component of translational and dissemination and implementation research,[39] particularly as patients participate in clinical implementation and community stakeholders participate in developing, improving, and replicating effective community-based interventions.[40,41] CBOs are necessary partners in this research, as they play a vital role in providing trusted access to community members and assets and are leaders in addressing health disparities, disease prevention, and the social determinants of health in their communities.[42,43]

Benefits to the research from community-engaged approaches have been demonstrated in the literature and address many of the challenges highlighted in this chapter. Benefits to the research include development of buy-in and trust with community partners, improved participant recruitment and/or retention, productive conflict resolution between research stakeholders, increased quality and outcomes of research, increased sustainability of project goals, and identification and achievement of actions that result from research, including systems change.[44-46] Community engagement can also enhance the development, testing, implementation, and dissemination of effective interventions into practice.[47] There are potentially other benefits conferred upon community partners as a result of participation, including the creation of research jobs for community members in current and future research projects, increases in community stakeholders' research self-efficacy and skills, increases in community stakeholders' perceptions of the value of data and research to their organizational mission, and improvements to CBOs' organizational networks.[11,28,48]

The ideal research project for a new CEnR partnership is a community health assessment, particularly one that assesses a balance of assets and needs in urban communities.[11,49] A community health assessment can provide the foundation for a longer-term cycle of research, planning, implementation, and evaluation to observe and measure the longer-term community health improvements created by policy or programmatic interventions, as guided by the Institute of Medicine's framework for collaborative public health action by communities.[50] In addition, a community health assessment requires diverse community stakeholders to work together to collectively plan and implement research that will have immediate benefit to community planning and advocacy efforts. Such a collaborative undertaking can also lead to an effective sustainability plan, as such a cycle would necessitate roles and benefits for diverse community stakeholders such as CBOs, providers, researchers, and government agencies. Furthermore, in the United States, the Affordable Care Act requirement for nonprofit hospitals to conduct a community health needs assessment every three years in collaboration with community stakeholders and their local health department creates additional opportunities for these urban health actors to collaborate to document health inequities and plan for an implementation plan that would promote health equity.[51,52]

Box 13.2 illustrates the importance of equitable research partnerships from the perspective of a leader in a large, community-based, nonprofit organization.

Practical Participatory Approaches

But what does CEnR actually look like in urban communities? Community-based participatory research anchors the most participatory end of the community engagement continuum, arguing for the engagement of community actors in all phases of research, from planning to data collection,

Jannette Diaz

In 2017, Congreso and Drexel University's Dornsife School of Public Health collaborated on a community-based project that focused on documenting and increasing awareness about community violence experienced by Latino residents in Eastern North Philadelphia. The goal of this project was to use existing data from multiple agencies to improve understanding and narrate the extent of the issues facing the residents of this community to create a user-friendly resource for community based organizations and community members to find information that can support anti-violence efforts. The data, including disparities, risk factors, consequences, and assets, were compiled and a website was developed, called Neighborhoods United Against Violence, https://www.nuavnow.org/. The website will continue to help community residents and organizations research community resources for years to come and provides links to valuable community resources and organizations.

Throughout 2018 and 2019, staff from Congreso also worked with a Doctor of Public Health candidate from the Dornsife School of Public Health to compile research for a dissertation. The research focused on the role of cardiovascular disease knowledge and psychosocial factors for cardiovascular disease perception within the HIV/AIDS community and is one of the first studies of this type with this population. Participants from Congreso's HIV/AIDS program, or "Esfuerzo" as it is called (meaning "strength" in Spanish), were involved in qualitative interviews, which revealed information that has since supported Congreso in understanding how to best meet the needs of these particular clients. The information gathered is also of particular significance to the Congreso Health Center, a federally qualified health center that manages the health care of many of the Esfuerzo clients. The information gained in this study will not only be useful to Congreso in the future but may also support programs and health-care providers treating a similar population in other areas of the country.

BENEFITS OF CBO–RESEARCHER PARTNERSHIP

Typically, nonprofit organizations want to grow and change with the communities they serve, and as they evolve over time, they must acknowledge that they need to be a learning organization, often needing robust data and research. This can be difficult for an agency with restricted funding sources and specific, program-focused grants. Congreso and Drexel have been able to address this issue by creating a partnership in which Drexel seeks funding for research and Congreso identifies projects and subjects for the proposed research. Congreso has over 40 years of experience working with the Eastern North Philadelphia Latino population and can gain entrance into the target population easily as a result of a long-standing history of providing excellent social services.

Over the past two years, Congreso has gone through a Theory of Change process, in pursuit of more efficient and impactful services. The partnership forged with Drexel's School of Public Health has strengthened and supported Congreso's efforts to gain a better understanding of individual and community assets and needs. It has enhanced curiosity, increased questioning, and informed program enhancements to create impactful services. It also allows for data-informed conversations with funders as the organization seeks to increase funding for innovative services.

data analysis, dissemination, and the creation and achievement of action that results from research.[53,54] Understanding that this is the ideal goal but that it is not achievable in all community-based research and planning contexts, what we outline here are tips for how to include community actors in each phase of research and planning, so that researcher–community partnerships can plan for those phases of research which can be equitably and effectively shared.

Participatory research design. When community actors are involved in research design, project scope is defined only after a planning process that engages community actors and any other multisector partners (e.g., government agencies, policymakers, health-care system, business). In this context, the lead agency for subsequent funding proposals is carefully agreed upon and is not necessarily the academic, provider, or governmental partner. If a lot of the work will occur at a CBO and it is feasible for the CBO to be the lead agency (based on funder requirements and the CBO's fiscal and administrative infrastructure), then this should be considered. Wherever the leadership and fiscal oversight roles are formally, a participatory approach to research design means that decisions are made more collectively by partners rather than in a traditional academic researcher-led model.

In this approach, the research questions that drive the study design and data collection methods are developed with input from all interested partners so that everyone benefits from the research. Community partners can shape research questions to yield data most useful for community health planning and advocacy. Academic partners can ensure scientific rigor and identify how the study can be designed to contribute to generalizable knowledge.

Besides the documented improved research outcomes of CEnR, there are also practical advantages of a participatory research design process. First, each partners' capacity and readiness to take on specific research activities are discussed openly, and so CBO capacity-building activities (e.g., staff training on survey administration), researcher capacity-building activities (e.g., researcher training on history of research partnerships in this community), or co-capacity building activities (e.g., development of a dissemination plan) can be incorporated into the timeline and budget. This improves grant conceptualization and writing, as it is not just the academic researcher's ideas about how the research should be realized in the community but is informed by the reality of community life. An example is selection of the best time of year for participant recruitment given other data collection efforts or competing activities in a community to limit participant burden and avoid research exhaustion. It will also lead to the engagement of research institutions' institutional review boards, community institutional review boards, and other research gatekeepers early in the process. Lastly, when research activities and new project hires are shared among partner organizations, it distributes resources more equitably, improves partner buy-in, and aligns better with collective interests and skill sets. This can inform a participatory and transparent budgeting process where those responsible for each research activity outline their costs and have voice in to the overall budget planning.

The memorandum of understanding is an important tool in the process of developing transparency, trust, and accountability in urban health partnerships. It is created to govern partnerships for which there are no contracts or in advance of an expected contract (as would accompany a grant subaward or consulting agreement) but are constructed in the same way as a contract. These can be treated as legally binding, as most research institutions do, or as a more informal agreement codifying decisions being made in the planning process for the roles and responsibilities of researcher and community actors. Memorandum of understanding content in the context of urban health research may include elements such as those shown in Table 13.1.

Participatory data collection. Including community actors in data collection is not a novel approach. However, CBOs have historically been engaged in data collection in roles related to study promotion, participant recruitment, provision of space for data collection, and linguistic/cultural translation of data collection instruments. Although these are valuable roles, CBO support of research they did not conceptualize is often not adequately funded, as researchers often assume mission or organizational alignment would allow for the extension of staff duties to include research activities. This is often not true. When the data collection plan is thought

Table 13.1 ELEMENTS TO INCLUDE IN A MEMORANDUM
OF UNDERSTANDING BETWEEN RESEARCH INSTITUTIONS
AND COMMUNITY-BASED ORGANIZATIONS

Consider including any of the following in a memorandum of understanding

Guiding principles for engagement or partnership (e.g., CEnR, CBPR)

Purpose of the partnership and/or project

Specific goals or aims of the shared project

Roles and responsibilities of each partner

Potential risks and benefits of each partner

Basic governing principles of the partnership

Financial arrangements, if relevant

Acknowledge any conflicts of interest

Other topics of importance to either partner

Abbreviations: CBPR, community-based participatory research; CEnR, community-engaged research.

through during a participatory planning process, the process will ensure that CBOs and other community actors take on the roles and responsibilities in the work that make the most sense for their organizational interests and capacities and are not automatically relegated to a supportive or underresourced role. If a CBO commits to a leadership role in collecting primary data, this includes funds for hiring new staff or training existing staff for data collection, data collection supervision, and research costs (e.g., participant incentives, transportation). Engaging CBO partners as leaders or critical partners in developing the data collection process will also ensure careful thought and awareness of context informs data collection protocols such as key experiential capacity of data collectors, data collector training, outreach, selection, recruitment, consent, safety, communication, and tracking response rates in oftentimes challenging data collection contexts. Indeed, a data collection workforce that is hired from among community residents and/or are staff of CBOs will be better able to articulate community benefits of the research and why they think participation is important.

CBO engagement in the data collection process addresses the challenge of data not being relevant to community contexts. Community input into the data collection process can ensure that data are aggregated or collected at the level required to lead to community change and that neighborhood boundaries are drawn appropriately. Community engagement can also ensure that data collection instruments are created to capture data points that represent the community experience, balance both risk and protective factors so as not to further stigmatize urban communities, and ensure that instructions and items are worded in a way that will engender trust and candidness rather than force random answers.

Participatory data collection can also address trust issues by improving community buy-in, creating infrastructure for problem-solving during recruitment and data collection, and ultimately increasing response rates among traditionally hard-to-reach urban populations.

Participatory data analysis. As with participatory research design and data collection, participatory data analysis is all about collective decision-making starting at the planning stage. The analytic team should be led by someone within the partnership who takes on the research guidance role (whether an academic researcher or other partner with required research experience). The analytic lead should thoughtfully hire staff from among the other partners and their networks and not just assume the only skilled analysts would come from academic partners. Whenever possible, CBO staff should be supported to conduct data analyses, or community members should be hired and trained to be member(s) of the analysis team. The required skill set should be clearly articulated in position description(s). For qualitative data analysis, formally trained analysts may particularly benefit from working alongside those with relevant lived experience (e.g., being a resident of the urban community being studied). For quantitative data analysis, more specialized training and experience are often needed. Roles that benefit from lived experience (see Table 13.2) are especially good for CBO partners. Many CBOs or other community actors also have analytic experience relevant to a CEnR study and can therefore be engaged in a variety of data analytic roles.[55,56] If data analysis will occur outside of an academic institution, then access to appropriate technology and software needs to be

Table 13.2 POTENTIAL ROLES AND TASKS IN PARTICIPATORY DATA ANALYSES

Role	Tasks
Qualitative analysis lead	Conduct formal analyses informed by theory and interacting with software
Qualitative analysis support	Aid in tasks such as identification of themes based on lived experience
Quantitative analysis lead	Data management and analyses using data analysis software
Quantitative analysis support	Data entry, input into data cleaning based on lived experience, conducting descriptive analyses
Analysis team	Data interpretation, reporting, and dissemination that incorporates insights from lived experience

considered in budgeting. Wherever the analytic team is based, teams should be trained together to create a co-learning experience. This is particularly important for coming to consensus on important thematic coding or quantitative data interpretation processes.[57]

Regardless of who is hired to conduct the data analysis, community perspectives should be incorporated into the data interpretation process. Uncovering facts regarding a community is not sufficient to draw conclusions. Analytic results must be interpreted to appreciate the practical significance of what has been learned and which results can be translated into shareable recommendations, conclusions, and action steps. Interpretations can be strengthened through active discussion between partners or even with the broader community during a community forum (a format further discussed as part of a dissemination strategy in Chapter 15).

The benefits of participatory data analysis planning are that the analytic plan will be feasible within the collective capacities of the partnership, will include multiple perspectives in results generation and interpretation, and will build partners' collective analytic and software-enabled capacity for analysis, all while maintaining scientific rigor.

Participatory dissemination and action. Participatory dissemination occurs when all partners are involved in translating results to be relevant to current urban health advocacy opportunities or community health planning processes. A participatory dissemination plan will ensure the right information gets into the hands of the right influencers or decision makers in the right way. In Chapter 15, we will discuss how dissemination products should be user-friendly, graphics-forward, and written in plain language, avoiding or defining scientific jargon terms. Another important component of participatory dissemination is the acknowledgement that the knowledge generated has been co-created. This means including community partners as co-authors and co-presenters, supporting community partners to attend scientific or practice-based conferences where results will be shared, and exploring equitable data-sharing processes such as open data portals.

Community involvement in generating and disseminating results most useful to their own needs is exactly what translation of research for community action in urban health looks like. It is thus important to think early in the project and partnership development about what kinds of actions community actors will wish to inform with the results of the research. These can vary greatly but are different from researcher dissemination priorities to scientific audiences. These can include using data or research results to

• Describe community health needs or disparities.
• Describe community health assets, or resilience factors.

- Raise their community members' or other constituents' awareness of health needs, disparities, and assets.
- Seek funding or report to existing funders.
- Identify program or service needs.
- Develop a new or expand/improve an existing program or service.
- Identify necessary policy changes.
- Engage in policy change or advocacy efforts.
- Mobilize leaders and residents around an issue.
- Identify additional stakeholders, allies, or partners.
- Identify further research needs.
- Develop an on-going collaboration or coalition.
- Develop a longer-term work plan.
- Develop a sustainability plan.

Research Institution Investment in Equitable and Sustainable Community Partnerships

Urban community mistrust of research institutions and government agencies could be partially mitigated by these institutions' investment in mechanisms for community engagement. This could include public-facing efforts such as hosting conferences or community forums on community engagement; increasing access to relevant academic conferences for community members[58]; providing seed grants for either community-engaged or community-led research or intervention development projects[28,59]; or supporting faculty, staff, and/or students to work collaboratively with community leaders and organizations on their research needs.[60] Academic institution–led community research capacity-building efforts such as Data & Democracy at UCLA have successfully improved CBOs' use of data and research for their own mission-aligned health advocacy and program planning.[11,49] Capacity-building programs not only demystify the research process and build trust between academic and community partners, but they are also necessary for building systems for community health planning, policy development, and sustainability from within the very urban communities needing and seeking health improvements.

Another solution is institutional investment in community engagement skill training for researchers and practitioners who enter into community settings. The Centers for Disease Control and Prevention and the National Institutes for Health's Clinical and Translational Science Awards Consortium developed nine principles of community engagement that can provide a good framework for such capacity building.[23,61] These principles include items to consider prior to beginning engagement (be clear, become knowledgable about the community), conditions necessary for engagement to occur (establish relationships, build trust, acknowledge that the community empowers itself), and perspectives to enable successful engagement (recognize partnership is necessary, respect the community and its diversity, build on community assets and build its capacity, be prepared to release control, sustain commitment over the long term). Online research training tools exist such as the Harvard Catalyst's Community-Engaged Research modules[62,63] on the Collaborative Institutional Training Initiative (CITI) website or the Community–Campus Partnerships for Health's community-based participatory research curriculum.[29] Such training is best provided in advance of community-engaged research development.

Institutions can also invest in building the capacity of its institutional review boards to understand the ethical implications of community-engaged research, such as requiring community-engaged research training for researchers proposing community-placed research, requiring input from reviewer(s) with community-lived experience and community-engagement expertise, and evaluating risks to communities versus individuals.[64] Some hospital and academic institutions have also supported the development of community research review boards of their surrounding communities in the belief that community member review of studies proposed to occur in their community will ensure the research maximizes benefits and minimizes risks to the community as a whole.[20,65]

THE IMPORTANCE OF COALITION-BUILDING FOR CROSS-SECTOR, PLACE-BASED, COLLECTIVE ACTION APPROACHES TO IMPROVING URBAN HEALTH

Chapters 1 and 3 outline the importance of multisectoral and systems approaches to improving urban health. The recognition of multisector collaboration, collective action, and place-based initiatives as critical to urban health has led to increasing calls to build the kinds of coalitions that can work across disciplines, viewpoints, and capacities. In this section, we discuss coalition-building strategies important for creating and sustaining the multisector, transdisciplinary partnerships necessary to advance this work.

Working effectively and collaboratively across sectors and with diverse individual and organizational stakeholders requires being aware of multi-institutional histories and issues of trust that can affect multilateral partnerships within coalitions. There are also historical tensions between hospitals and urban communities and many examples of collaboration failures between various coalition actors. As discussed previously for partnerships, coalitions need to provide supported time and resources to directly address these histories, work through tensions, gain trust, and sustain learning conversations. At the foundation of coalition trust is first working through differences in terminology and approaches to coalition structure and functioning and then allowing time to develop a common language and consensus-built processes. Another practical strategy for establishing trust and sustaining coalitions is to collectively develop and adhere to rules of engagement and self-governance, including decision-making processes, leadership terms and transitions, and clear grievance and conflict resolution processes.

A major challenge of coalitions is maintaining the morale and energy of members, especially if funding is uncertain or volatile. Transitioning from one small grant or project to another can be disruptive and jarring as goals and focus shift. A solution is to engage coalition members as champions from multiple sectors who see and can articulate the value and community benefits of this shared work with their organizations and networks. It is also important to develop a long-term plan (beyond individual projects) with partner buy-in and commitments and to focus on facilitating forward progress. This reinforces the value of the coalition to the collective and ensures that individual partners and their organizations are experiencing direct benefits.[66,67] This is how partnerships and coalitions are sustained. Besides regular meetings for accomplishing the shared work, regular convenings are needed that are more reflective in nature to highlight partner expertise, build consensus, and celebrate accomplishments.

Another major challenge of coalitions is that inconsistent participation disrupts momentum or changes identity and focus (what is often called "mission drift"). Thus, successful urban health coalitions spend time on long-term process and sustainability.[68] Most coalition work is project-based, where there is more work to do than time for critical self-reflection. Therefore, creating a coalition plan that secures long-term goals and commitment from individuals and organizations is key to sustaining the work of the coalition. This maintains engagement and "institutional knowledge" even with individual representative turnover. Some coalitions may even tap into member expertise or seek funding to evaluate effectiveness of the collaboration and look for ways to improve coalition functioning or outcomes. Sustainability is the capacity to endure, but that endurance may mean the coalition with the exact same members and commitments, or it may mean sustaining the structure and processes but the membership and focus changes over time. Indeed, urban communities change, and their health issues and needs change, and so sustainability may mean endurance and evolution over time.

Although it may at first appear a minor point, the importance of well-run meetings cannot be overemphasized when building an urban health coalition.

Meetings should be facilitated by someone with group process experience who is skilled at facilitation, establishing group norms for how meetings will be conducted, facilitating agreement on action items, and creating systems of accountability. It is also essential that this same or another member is effectively scheduling and sending reminders about action items in between meetings. Positions of power (i.e., chairs, co-chairs, principal investigators, co-principal investigators, and other positions with decision-making power) in urban health coalitions should be shared between research institutions and CBOs. Meetings should be held at regular intervals (such as a fixed time each month so that it is consistently on members' calendars) and should be held at locations and times accessible to all partners. If members are coming outside of their regular job, then meetings after work hours should be considered so that an entire group of members are not excluded. If parents or community members are included, then childcare and food can be offered to reduce participation barriers. A good meeting facilitator should ensure that all members have an opportunity to express their opinions and be heard. This means making sure there are no language barriers and offering interpretation services if needed, establishing ground rules and group norms around respect and listening such that quieter people have opportunities to speak and more vocal members do not dominate, and resolving conflicts as they occur. Well-run meetings distribute agendas ahead of time so that members can see what the focus of each meeting is and make sure they attend or send someone in their stead if there is an issue of particular relevance to their roles and responsibilities or decisions being made that they want to contribute to. It is important to document in meeting minutes decisions made and action items set and to establish ways for participation in decision-making outside of meetings if needed. This ensures all partners are involved to the extent they are interested in creating the important work of the coalition. A coalition model for urban health research and planning is one built on CEnR principles, where all members are equitably engaged in decision-making and the development of shared work.

Community Advisory Committees to Inform Research When More Equitable Models Are Not Feasible

While the community advisory committee model of community actor engagement in urban health is not as equitable of a model of engagement, in some urban contexts it may be the best avenue for community engagement and an improvement over no community engagement at all.[69] Therefore, we finish this section with some tips on dos and don'ts for engaging community advisory committees, many of which apply to other types of coalitions as well (Table 13.3).

Table 13.3 COMMUNITY ADVISORY BOARD TIPS

DON'T	DO
Rely solely on very busy individuals who occupy many different leadership positions and commitments	Choose a structure for advisory committee membership such as member selection, term commitments, and roles and responsibilities
Establish redundant or contradictory communication strategies	Inform and engage members through regular meetings and by sharing agendas, meeting minutes, and contact information of all members
Schedule inconsistent meetings or cancel meetings frequently: board members will not value the work if you show meetings are not important	Establish group norms and good meeting administration
Exclude important community actors	Ensure all members contribute to the project or partnership and are not just there to "rubber stamp" decisions already made
Manage meetings by allowing all speakers unlimited time to air their full thoughts and concerns	Ensure all members perceive value and receive professional or personal benefits from participation
Focus on the successes of the one or two most active committee members, ignoring partnership members who are less engaged	If one set of partners are receiving resources to be engaged in the process (e.g., salary support from a grant), then some sort of compensation should be considered for all partners
Take on tasks that do not align with established focus and structure	Strengthen connections between members and their organizations
	Celebrate successful project completion or completion of important components of the work. Reinforce members' role and commitments that helped to accomplish successes.

CONCLUSION: AN INTEGRATED VIEW OF COMMUNITY HEALTH ACTION IN URBAN CONTEXTS

Urban health research and planning is about recognizing the value of contributions from actors from many different sectors and with diverse viewpoints and experiences. Social determinants of health and health in all policies approaches to creating sustainable solutions to persistent urban health inequities, require urban health researchers, practitioners, and policymakers to embrace a coalition approach. This means embracing community engagement and coalition-building principles and practices. Regardless of the urban health partner, and especially among coalitions, there is a need to be explicit about power inequalities, terminology, and capacity differences and employ the community-engaged research design, translation, and action strategies discussed in this chapter to overcome them.

REFERENCES

1. Armstrong K, Rose A, Peters N, Long JA, McMurphy S, Shea JA. Distrust of the health care system and self-reported health in the United States. *Journal of General Internal Medicine.* 2006;21(4):292–297.
2. Corbie-Smith G, Thomas SB, St George DMM. Distrust, race, and research. *Archives of Internal Medicine.* 2002;162(21):2458–2463.
3. Holzer JK, Ellis L, Merritt MW. Why we need community engagement in medical research. *Journal of Investigative Medicine.* 2014;62(6):851–855.
4. Chen WS, Petitti DB, Enger S. Limitations and potential uses of census-based data on ethnicity in a diverse community. *Annals of Epidemiology.* 2004;14(5):339–345.
5. Waddell C. So much research evidence, so little dissemination and uptake: Mixing the useful with the pleasing. *Evidence-Based Mental Health.* 2001;4(1):3–5.
6. Worton SK, Loomis C, Pancer SM, Nelson G, Peters RD. Evidence to impact: A community knowledge mobilisation evaluation framework. *Gateways.* 2017;10:121–142.
7. Howell J. Race and U.S. medical experimentation: The case of Tuskegee. *Cadernos de Saúde Pública.* 2017;33(Suppl 1). doi:10.1590/0102-311x00168016.
8. Freimuth VS, Quinn SC, Thomas SB, Cole G, Zook E, Duncan T. African Americans' views on research and the Tuskegee Syphilis Study. *Social Science & Medicine* (1982). 2001;52(5):797–808.
9. Heller J. Rumors and realities: Making sense of HIV/AIDS conspiracy narratives and contemporary legends. *American Journal of public health.* 2015;105(1): e43–e50.
10. Hacker K, Chu J, Arsenault L, Marlin RP. Provider's perspectives on the impact of Immigration and Customs Enforcement (ICE) activity on immigrant health. *Journal of Health Care for the Poor and Underserved.* 2012;23(2):651–665.
11. Carroll-Scott A, Toy P, Wyn R, Zane JI, Wallace SP. Results from the Data & Democracy initiative to enhance community-based organization data and research capacity. *American Journal of Public Health.* 2012;102(7):1384–1391.
12. Horowitz CR, Robinson M, Seifer S. Community-based participatory research from the margin to the mainstream: Are researchers prepared? *Circulation.* 2009;119(19):2633–2642.
13. Israel BA, Schulz AJ, Parker EA, Becker AB. Review of community-based research: Assessing partnership approaches to improve public health. *Annual Review of Public Health.* 1998;19:173–202.
14. Seifer SD. Building and sustaining community-institutional partnerships for prevention research: Findings from a national collaborative. *Journal of Urban Health-Bulletin of the New York Academy of Medicine.* 2006;83(6):989–1003.
15. Tandon SD, Phillips K, Bordeaux BC, et al. A vision for progress in community health partnerships. *Progress in Community Health Partnerships: Research, Education, and Action.* 2007;1(1):11–30.

16. Wang KH, Ray NJ, Berg DN, et al. Using community-based participatory research and organizational diagnosis to characterize relationships between community leaders and academic researchers. *Preventive Medicine Reports.* 2017;7:180–186.

17. Bilodeau R, Gilmore J, Jones L, et al. Putting the "community" into community-based participatory research: A commentary. *American Journal of Preventive Medicine.* 2009;37(6 Suppl 1):S192–194.

18. Conrad P, Barker KK. The social construction of illness: Key insights and policy implications. *Journal of Health and Social Behavior.* 2010;51(1 Suppl):S67–S79.

19. Sontag S. *Illness as Metaphor and AIDS and Its Metaphors.* London: Penguin; 2002.

20. Martin del Campo F, Casado J, Spencer P, Strelnick H. The development of the Bronx Community Research Review Board: A pilot feasibility project for a model of community consultation. *Progress in Community Health Partnerships: Research, Education, and Action.* 2013;7(3):341–352.

21. Wolfson M, Wagoner KG, Rhodes SD, et al. Coproduction of research questions and research evidence in public health: The study to prevent teen drinking parties. *BioMed Research International.* 2017;2017. doi:10.1155/2017/3639596.

22. Hacker K, Tendulkar SA, Rideout C, et al. Community capacity building and sustainability: Outcomes of community-based participatory research. *Progress in Community Health Partnerships: Research, Education, and Action.* 2012;6(3): 349–360.

23. Shea CM, Young TL, Powell BJ, et al. Researcher readiness for participating in community-engaged dissemination and implementation research: A conceptual framework of core competencies. *Translational Behavioral Medicine.* 2017;7(3):393–404.

24. Cutforth N. The journey of a community-engaged scholar: An autoethnography. *Quest.* 2013;65(1):14–30.

25. Minkler M, Salvatore AL, Chang C. Participatory approaches for study design and analysis in dissemination and implementation research. In: Brownson RC, Colditz GA, eds. *Dissemination and Implementation Research in Health: Translating Science to Practice* (pp. 192–212). New York: Oxford University Press; 2012.

26. Scharff DP, Mathews KJ, Jackson P, Hoffsuemmer J, Martin E, Edwards D. More than Tuskegee: Understanding mistrust about research participation. *Journal of Health Care for the Poor and Underserved.* 2010;21(3):879–897.

27. Ulrich CM, Wallen GR, Feister A, Grady C. Respondent burden in clinical research: When are we asking too much of subjects? *IRB.* 2005;27(4):17–20.

28. Santilli A, Carroll-Scott A, Ickovics JR. Applying community organizing principles to assess health needs in New Haven, Connecticut. *American Journal of Public Health.* 2016;106(5):841–847.

29. The Examining Community–Institutional Partnerships for Prevention Research Group. *Developing And Sustaining Community-Based Participatory Research Partnerships: A Skill Building Curriculum.* 2006; www.cbprcurriculum.info

30. Singleton GE. *Courageous Conversations About Race: A Field Guide for Achieving Equity in Schools.* 2nd ed. Thousand Oaks, CA: Corwin; 2014.

31. Axtell SA, Avery M, Westra B. Incorporating cultural competence content into graduate nursing curricula through community-university collaboration. *Journal of Transcultural Nursing.* 2010;21(2):183–191.

32. US Department of Health and Human Services. National CLAS standards for culturally and linguistically appropriate services (CLAS) in health and health care. Last updated October 2, 2018; https://minorityhealth.hhs.gov/omh/browse.aspx?lvl=2&lvlid=53.

33. Beagan BL. A critique of cultural competence: Assumptions, limitations, and alternatives. In: Frisby CL, O'Donohue WT, Frisby CL, O'Donohue WT, eds. *Cultural Competence in Applied Psychology: An Evaluation of Current Status and Future Directions*. Cham, Switzerland: Springer; 2018:123–138.

34. Tervalon M, Murray-García J. Cultural humility versus cultural competence: A critical distinction in defining physician training outcomes in multicultural education. *Journal of Health Care for the Poor and Underserved*. 1998;9(2):117–125.

35. Yeager KA, Bauer-Wu S. Cultural humility: Essential foundation for clinical researchers. *Applied Nursing Research*. 2013;26(4):251–256.

36. Ahmed SM, Maurana C, Nelson D, Meister T, Young SN, Lucey P. Opening the black box: Conceptualizing community engagement from 109 community-academic partnership programs. *Progress in Community Health Partnerships: Research, Education, and Action*. 2016;10(1):51–61.

37. Isler MR, Corbie-Smith G. Practical steps to community engaged research: From inputs to outcomes. *The Journal of Law, Medicine & Ethics*. 2012;40(4):904–914.

38. Pearson CR, Duran B, Oetzel J, et al. Research for improved health: Variability and impact of structural characteristics in federally funded community engaged research. *Progress in Community Health Partnerships: Research, Education, and Action*. 2015;9(1):17–29.

39. Leshner AI, Terry S, Schultz AM, Liverman, CT, eds. *The CTSA Program at NIH: Opportunities for Advancing Clinical and Translational Research*. Washington, DC: National Academies Press; 2013.

40. Goodman MS, Sanders Thompson VL. The science of stakeholder engagement in research: Classification, implementation, and evaluation. *Translational Behavioral Medicine*. 2017;7(3):486–491.

41. Kost RG, Leinberger-jabari A, Evering TH, et al. Helping basic scientists engage with community partners to enrich and accelerate translational research. *Academic Medicine*. 2017;92(3):374–379.

42. Bloom T, Wagman J, Hernandez R, et al. Partnering with community-based organizations to reduce intimate partner violence. *Hispanic Journal of Behavioral Sciences*. 2009;31(2):244–257.

43. Minkler M. Linking science and policy through community-based participatory research to study and address health disparities. *American Journal of Public Health*. 2010;100(Suppl 1):S81–S87.

44. Agency for Healthcare Research and Quality. 2012 national healthcare disparities report. AHRQ publication no. 13-0003. May 2013; https://archive.ahrq.gov/research/findings/nhqrdr/nhdr12/index.html.

45. Jagosh J, Macaulay AC, Pluye P, et al. Uncovering the benefits of participatory research: Implications of a realist review for health research and practice. *Milbank Quarterly*. 2012;90(2):311–346.

46. Viswanathan M, Ammerman A, Eng E, et al. Community-based participatory research: Assessing the evidence. In: *AHRQ Evidence Report Summaries*. Rockville, MD: Agency for Healthcare Research and Quality; 1998–2005:99. https://www.ncbi.nlm.nih.gov/books/NBK11852/

47. Chambers DA, Azrin ST. Research and services partnerships: partnership: A fundamental component of dissemination and implementation research. *Psychiatric Services*. 2013;64(6):509–511.

48. Santilli A, Carroll-Scott A, Wong F, Ickovics J. Urban youths go 3000 miles: Engaging and supporting young residents to conduct neighborhood asset mapping. *American Journal of Public Health*. 2011;101(12):2207–2210.

49.   Otiniano AD, Carroll-Scott A, Toy P, Wallace SP. Supporting Latino communities' natural helpers: A case study of promotoras in a research capacity building course. *Journal of Immigrant and Minority Health.* 2012;14(4):657–663.

50.   Institute of Medicine. *The Future of the Public's Health in the 21st Century.* Washington, DC: National Academies Press; 2002.

51.   Carroll-Scott A, Henson RM. Leveraging nonprofit hospital community benefit dollars and community health needs assessment requirements for community health innovations. *Social Innovations Journal.* 2016;27.

52.   Carroll-Scott A, Henson RM, Kolker J, Purtle J. The role of nonprofit hospitals in identifying and addressing health inequities in cities. *Health Affairs (Millwood).* 2017;36(6):1102–1109.

53.   Israel BA, Coombe CM, Cheezum RR, et al. Community-based participatory research: A capacity-building approach for policy advocacy aimed at eliminating health disparities. *American Journal of Public Health.* 2010;100(11):2094–2102.

54.   Minkler M, Wallerstein N. *Community-Based Participatory Research for Health: From Process to Outcomes.* 2nd ed. San Francisco, CA: Jossey-Bass; 2008.

55.   Cashman SB, Adeky S, Allen AJ, et al. The power and the promise: Working with communities to analyze data, interpret findings, and get to outcomes. *American Journal of Public Health.* 2008;98(8):1407–1417.

56.   Humphries DL, Carroll-Scott A, Mitchell L, Tian T, Choudhury S, Fiellin DA. Assessing research activity and capacity of community-based organizations: Development and pilot testing of an instrument. *Progress in Community Health Partnerships: Research, Education, and Action.* 2014;8(4):421–432.

57.   Curry RM, Cunningham P. Co-learning in the community. *New Directions for Adult and Continuing Education.* 2000;87:73–82.

58.   Travers R, Wilson M, McKay C, et al. Increasing accessibility for community participants at academic conferences. *Progress in Community Health Partnerships: Research, Education, and Action.* 2008;2(3):257–264.

59.   Tendulkar SA, Chu J, Opp J, et al. A funding initiative for community-based participatory research: lessons from the Harvard Catalyst Seed Grants. *Progress in Community Health Partnerships: Research, Education, and Action.* 2011;5(1):35–44.

60.   Wells KB, Staunton A, Norris KC, et al. Building an academic-community partnered network for clinical services research: The Community Health Improvement Collaborative (CHIC). *Ethnicity & Disease.* 2006;16(1 Suppl 1): S3–S17.

61.   National Institutes of Health. *Principles of Community Engagement.* 2nd ed. 2011; https://www.atsdr.cdc.gov/communityengagement/pdf/PCE_Report_ 508_FINAL.pdf.

62.   MacDonald MA, Jacob C-A, Bierer BE, Opp, J, Winkler S. Introduction to community-based participatory research (CBPR). CITI Program. https://www. citiprogram.org. Accessed February 25, 2020.

63.   Kaberry J, Winkler S, Sengupta N, Bernstein H, Brugge D, Bierer BE. Ethical and practical considerations in community-engaged research (CEnR). CITI Program. https://www.citiprogram.org. Accessed February 25, 2020.

64.   Tamariz L, Medina H, Taylor J, Carrasquillo O, Kobetz E, Palacio A. Are research ethics committees prepared for community-based participatory research? *Journal of Empirical Research on Human Research Ethics.* 2015;10(5):488–495.

65.   Johnson JC, Hayden UT, Thomas N, et al. Building community participatory research coalitions from the ground up: The Philadelphia area research community coalition. *Progress in Community Health Partnerships.* 2009;3(1):61–72.

66. Khodyakov D, Mikesell L, Bromley E. Trust and the ethical conduct of community-engaged research. *European Journal for Person Centered Healthcare.* 2017;5(4):522–526.

67. Khodyakov D, Stockdale S, Jones F, et al. An exploration of the effect of community engagement in research on perceived outcomes of partnered mental health services projects. *Society and Mental Health.* 2011;1(3):185–199.

68. Israel BA, Krieger J, Vlahov D, et al. Challenges and facilitating factors in sustaining community-based participatory research partnerships: Lessons learned from the Detroit, New York City and Seattle Urban Research Centers. *Journal of Urban Health.* 2006;83(6):1022–1040.

69. Dubois JM, Bailey-Burch B, Bustillos D, et al. Ethical issues in mental health research: The case for community engagement. *Current Opinion in Psychiatry.* 2011;24(3):208–214.

CHAPTER 14

Policy in Urban Health

The Power of Cities to Translate Science into Action

JENNIFER KOLKER

POLICY DEFINED

What do we mean by *policy*? There are many definitions of policy, public policy, and health policy. Webster[1] defines policy as "A definite course or method of action selected from among alternatives and in light of given conditions to guide and determine present and future decisions." The Cambridge Dictionary[2] defines policy as "a set of ideas or a plan for action followed by a business, a government, a political party, or a group of people." The US Centers for Disease Control and Prevention[3] (CDC) states that "policy is a law, regulation, procedure, administrative action, incentive, or voluntary practice of governments and other institutions."

In some cases, however, policy is defined more narrowly to refer to the actions of government. For example, the Organization for Economic Development and Cooperation defines urban policy as

> a co-ordinated set of policy decisions to plan, finance, develop, run and sustain cities of all sizes, through a collaborative process in shared responsibility within and across all levels of government, and grounded in multi-stakeholder engagement of all relevant urban actors, including civil society and the private sector (p. 2).[4]

Broadly defined, policy can be divided into two overarching categories: public policy and organizational policy. *Public policy*, which includes laws and regulations that are passed by elected officials or government

Jennifer Kolker, *Policy in Urban Health* In: *Urban Public Health*. Edited by: Gina S. Lovasi, Ana V. Diez Roux, and Jennifer Kolker, Oxford University Press (2021). © Oxford University Press 2021.
DOI: 10.1093/oso/9780190885304.003.0014.

Table 14.1 FEATURES OF PUBLIC POLICY

Common Features of Public Policy
Policy is usually made in response to some sort of issue or problem that requires attention.
Policy is what the government chooses to do (actual) or not do (implied) about a particular issue or problem.
Policy might take the form of law, regulation, tax, or order that governs a particular issue or problem.
Policy is made by government on behalf of the "public" even if the ideas come from outside government or through the interaction of government and the public.

agencies. Once enacted, public policies may influence behavior of organizations and individuals. They can include constitutions, charters, statutes, codes, ordinances, resolutions, orders, agency regulations, and proclamations, as well as guidance documents—those documents that are created by governmental bodies that interpret laws and regulations. Public policy is simply what government (as represented by a range of public officials such as mayors, councilmembers, school officials, county supervisors, etc.) does or does not do about a problem that comes before them for consideration and possible action.

Organizational policies are those formal policies adopted by businesses and organizations to address how they operate and may impact their employees, members, people they serve, volunteers, or visitors on their property. Also known as *private policies*, organizational policies can have a significant impact on urban health if the size of the organization is large or if the organization is influential within health-relevant partnerships or coalitions.

Policies that affect health can encompass both government and nongovernment sectors. Health systems, private sector employers, associations, and accrediting agencies all have a role in setting health policy. At the city level, however, policies that impact health are most often made by government and those closely connected to government. For that reason, our discussion of policy moving forward will focus primarily on the governmental role in urban health policy. In this context, we adopt the Public Health Institute[5] policy definition:

> The term "policy" deserves special attention. While policy is often seen as synonymous with legislation, it describes a broad range of activities, and can be defined much more broadly as an agreement on issues, goals, or a course of action by the people with power to carry it out and enforce it. In this guide, 'policy' refers to public policy, which can be defined as the 'sum of government activities, whether acting directly or through agents,' that have an influence on residents and communities. Public policy has also been defined as "the actions

of government and the intentions that determine those actions," "political decisions for implementing programs to achieve societal goals," or simply 'whatever governments choose to do or not to do.'

POLICY AND PUBLIC HEALTH

The well-known Health Impact Pyramid created in Tom Friedan's *Framework for Public Health Action*,[6] describes those interventions that have the greatest impact on population health (Figure 14.1). While top of the pyramid actions (counseling and education and clinical interventions) have the smallest impact in terms of the number of people reached or the population impact of those actions, the bottom of the pyramid includes actions that have the greatest impact on improving health. Those factors—changing the context to make individuals' default decisions healthy and changing socioeconomic factors—are primarily affected through public policy. While many of these policies may be at the state or federal level, much can be accomplished through policies defined and implemented at the city level.

The Institute of Medicine (IOM), in their 2011 report *For the Public's Health: Revitalizing Law and Policy to Meet New Challenges*[7] addressed three categories of law and public policy pertinent to health:

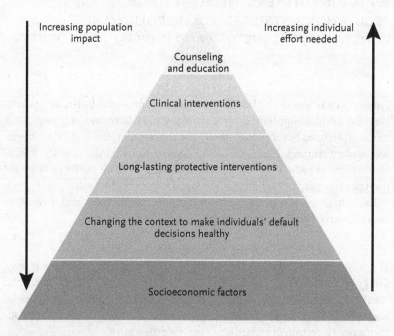

Figure 14.1 Health impact pyramid.[8]
Source: Frieden TR. The future of public health. *New England Journal of Medicine.* 2015;373(18):1748–1754.

1. Laws that establish the structure, function, and authority of government public health agencies at the federal, state, and local levels.
2. Statutes and other policies that are designed to achieve specific health objectives, for example, taxing tobacco products and requiring immunization for school entry.
3. Policies in other areas of government, such as education, transportation, land use planning, and agriculture, that have health effects. In this area, intersectoral strategies are necessary—non-health agencies can align with efforts to improve health by considering the health implications of their policies.

Relevant terms are defined in Box 14.1. The IOM goes on to describe the additional policy actions that public health practitioners may influence: the power to regulate (e.g., restaurant licensure and inspections), the power to tax and spend (e.g., beverage taxes), and the power to modify the built environment (e.g., urban development rules to encourage walking and biking; land use planning to limit proliferation of fast-food outlets and provide incentives for supermarkets).[7]

Box 14.1 INSTITUTE OF MEDICINE DEFINING LAWS, REGULATIONS, STATUTES, PUBLIC POLICY, AND CONSTITUTIONAL HISTORY AND JUDICIAL PRECEDENTS

PUBLIC POLICY

Public policy refers to the broad arena of positions, principles, and priorities that inform high-level decision making in all branches of government but is often used to refer collectively to laws, regulations and rules, executive agency strategic plans, executive agency guidance documents, executive orders, or judicial decisions and precedents. Many public policies are not laws but may help change norms and behaviors in health.

Each branch of government—executive, legislative, and judicial—makes contributions to public policy.

LAWS: STATUTES AND ORDINANCES

These are usually originated by the legislative branch of government (e.g., Congress, state senate or assembly, city council). Under the federal and most state constitutions, laws are not finalized until signed by the chief executive officer (e.g., president, governor, mayor). Laws require conformance to certain standards, norms, or procedures.

These are rules, procedures, and administrative codes often promulgated by the executive branch of government, such as federal or state agencies, to achieve specific objectives or discharge specific duties. These are applicable only within the jurisdiction or toward the purpose for which they are made. Laws authorize administrative agencies to promulgate regulations.

CONSTITUTIONAL HISTORY AND JUDICIAL PRECEDENTS

These refer to the judiciary's interpretation of the Constitution, laws, and regulations, including case law from prior judicial opinions.

Source: Institute of Medicine.[9]

POLICY AND CITIES: TOOLS TO IMPACT HEALTH

Our health is shaped by decisions made by those in power at all levels of government—in the United States, federal, provincial/state, and local. As discussed in Part I, the number of people living in cities is expected to grow, and as the number of people living in cities grows, so too does the power of cities to improve health. While we often think of policy at the federal and state level—in large part because of their level of power—cities have a range of options for policy creation (Figure 14.2; Tables 14.1 and 14.2). Local governments have the power to legislate, regulate, tax, issue executive orders, and—perhaps most important—distribute resources through budgeting to make change.

Who Makes Urban Health Policy?

In most cities, the local public health authority plays a central role in developing and implementing policies designed specifically to improve urban health. It can also play a role in coordinating and promoting policies in other sectors (such as education policy or social policy) that while not designed specifically to promote health can have significant health impacts. In the United States, the local health authorities are local health departments, usually charged with carrying out the public health functions within city government, working closely with other city agencies and nongovernmental partners and communities. In cities, the governmental policy players usually include a mayor or chief executive and some type of legislative or governing body (e.g., city council). As such, policy actors include all of the public

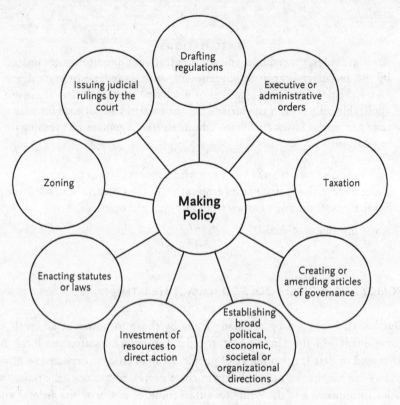

Figure 14.2 Types of public policy action affecting health in cities.

Table 14.2 URBAN POLICIES TO IMPROVE HEALTH

Examples of Urban Policies to Improve Health

Tobacco	Age restrictions on sale of tobacco products
	Density-based restriction on sales
Chronic disease prevention	Beverage taxes
	Regulation of salt
	Menu labeling
Substance use/misuse	Needle exchange
	Safe injection sites
	Limit on alcohol sales using density regulation
Lead	Landlord disclosure laws
Poverty reduction/antidiscrimination	Minimum wage legislation
	Bans on cashless stores
Pedestrian safety	Speed limits
	Bike lanes
	Walking lanes
Climate	Auto emission standards for city fleets
	Commercial air pollution regulations

Table 14.3 INVOLVEMENT IN POLICY AREAS BY SIZE OF POPULATION SERVED

		Size of Population Served (%)		
	All LHDs	Small (<50,000)	Medium (50,000 to 499,999)	Large (500,000+)
Tobacco, alcohol, or other drugs	74	72	78	81
Emergency preparedness and response	72	73	70	75
Infectious disease (e.g., vaccination)	68	66	68	79
Food safety	57	53	62	67
Obesity/chronic disease	55	48	62	67
Waste, water, or sanitation	43	40	47	46
Animal control or rabies	41	38	45	49
Education	34	33	35	40
Oral health	31	27	35	44
Injury or violence prevention	29	26	32	51
Mental health	27	22	36	40
Funding for access to health care	27	21	36	44
Safe and healthy housing	23	19	28	40
Body art	18	15	23	23
Land use	17	12	21	33
Affordable housing	11	8	13	21
Occupational health and safety	10	9	10	15
Criminal justice system	9	5	14	20
Labor	2	2	2	9
None	7	8	6	3

n = 1,872.
Source: National Profile of Local Health Determinants.[1]
Abbreviation: LHD, local health department.

health actors described in Chapter 12. Anyone who has the authority or capability to influence or determine decisions, actions, or behaviors and who wants to achieve a desired outcome or goal over time is a participant in the policy process.

The urban role in policymaking represents both great opportunity and significant challenges. City governments—and their partners—are close to the ground and the people they serve and so understanding and creating policy is much closer to affected communities than that at a state or federal level. Cities can play a role in the more formal policymaking roles of enacting legislation, but a city's policymaking power also comes from regulation, zoning, and taxation (within certain limits, as discussed later in this chapter), as well as establishing broad political, economic, social, and organization directions and investment of resources to effect change. Cities can act as policy laboratories—informing other cities both in their own countries and others. In the United States, we have seen with soda and other taxes the domino effect of urban health policies—when one city achieves success it often paves the way for others to act. Policy at the city level is usually quicker to enact from idea to implementation than at higher levels of government. External influences of lobbying and other political influence are generally focused on state and federal law and thus can be less constraining to local policymaking (although local advocacy from various groups for or against a policy can be fierce).

Cities have an opportunity and responsibility to design and implement policies that are specific to the urban environment. As discussed throughout this book, cities are characterized by population diversity and social inequalities that have major implications for health. Policy in cities, then, can ameliorate or exacerbate these inequities—focusing on the needs of the full city with attention to disparities within and between neighborhoods and population groups. Finally, cities have an opportunity to reduce health disparities and further health equity through policy actions at the local level.

In their book *The New Localism: How Cities Can Thrive in the Age of Populism*, Katz and Nowak (p. 1)[10] discuss how power has increasingly shifted to more local areas.

For generations, the locus and nature of power seemed settled, reflected in the vertical lines of political authority. National and state governments sat at the apex, writing laws, promulgating rules, distributing resources, and running the country. Cities and metropolitan regions—the places where the overwhelming majority of the population lives and where national wealth is disproportionately generated—resided at the bottom, often acting as administrative arms of higher levels of government more than as agents in charge of their own future.

This picture, hierarchically neat and textbook tidy, is radically changing. The location of power is shifting as a result of profound demographic, economic, and social forces. Power is drifting downward from the nation-state to cities and metropolitan communities, horizontally from government to networks of public, private, and civic actors, and globally along transnational circuits of capital, trade, and innovation.

In sum, power increasingly belongs to the problem solvers. And these problem solvers now congregate disproportionately at the local level, in cities and metropolitan areas across the globe.

The power of cities in making health policy exists around the globe. The World Health Organization's Healthy Cities Vision,[11] arising out of the healthy cities network, states:

Healthy cities are places that deliver for people and the planet. They engage the whole of society, encouraging the participation of all communities in the pursuit of peace and prosperity. Healthy cities lead by example in order to achieve change for the better, tackling inequalities and promoting good governance and leadership for health and well-being. Innovation, knowledge sharing, and health diplomacy are valued and nurtured in healthy cities.

What follows are some examples of areas of public health policy making in cities (see as well the typology discussed in Chapter 3). Just as we discussed in Chapter 12, this is not—and cannot—be all inclusive as all policy decision that happen in a city have the ability to have an impact on the health of those city residents. We provide here some examples of areas of known policy intervention in public health as well as those policy areas not traditionally viewed as public health policy but that have an effect on the social determinants of health (see Figure 14.3). Additionally, Box 14.2 discusses the role of leadership and governance in urban health.

Tobacco control is one of the major areas of health policy in cities. Local governments have the ability to raise the cost of tobacco products through tax and nontax mechanisms; promote and enforce restrictions at the point of sale; reduce or restrict the number, location, and density of tobacco retailers; and limit other advertising and point-of-sale activities. Cities have taken policy action to establish or increase licensing fees, ban flavored noncigarette tobacco products, create age requirements for tobacco clerks at retailers, create minimum age to purchase laws, and ban certain types of tobacco products. The growth in use of e-cigarettes has prompted new policy development geared at age of purchase and sale and other use requirements specific to e-cigarettes. The recent outbreak of vaping-related illnesses has led to additional city-initiated policy on nicotine regulation and age of sale limits.

In recent years, cities have created policy initiatives around obesity prevention. City-level policies aimed at obesity prevention include healthy food procurement policies in schools and government agencies, zoning to incentivize

Box 14.2 LEADERSHIP AND GOVERNANCE FOR URBAN HEALTH

Jo Ivey Bufford

The role of government is to protect the public interest, and unlike non-governmental entities, it can be held responsible to the public for its actions. In matters of health, most international agreements assume that governments have the ultimate responsibility for assuring the conditions in which people can be as healthy as they can be, but as we have learned more about the multiple determinants of health and the complex environments that influence health, it is increasingly clear that government alone cannot meet these responsibilities.

Governments must be able to work effectively with an increasing number of nongovernmental actors—civil society, business, professional associations, academia, donors, and residents and with regional and international organizations. The process of involving this expanded number of actors has led to the increasing use of the term *governance*. There are multiple definitions of this term, but most reflect, at the simplest level, the alignment of multiple actors and interests to promote collective action toward an agreed-upon goal. Although there are evolving international standards for effective government, *governance* is almost always local and context-specific, because local stakeholders vary and effective governance must reflect the ways in which all stakeholders interact in a particular set of societal circumstances to create effective programs and/or influence the outcomes of public policies.

Government's ability to lead, facilitate, or catalyze the governance process is critical, and, most important, government officials must have the political will to make the needed changes. Inclusiveness and the active engagement of communities affected by programs and policies in their formation, implementation, and evaluation is increasingly being emphasized as critical to effective governance. There are many models for such engagement, but the fact that communities have historically been missing stakeholders in the governance process means that the evidence from their lived experience of local conditions and societal circumstances is often missing, and this gap may have contributed to historical failures of programs and policies to be both effective and sustainable.

Sustainable Development Goal 11 in the UN SDGs and UN Habitat's New Urban Agenda have been accepted as elements of national policy for global economic and social development over the next 15 years. As a result, attention to the rate and process of urbanization worldwide and to cities as a level of government that may be uniquely suited to creating effective models of governance has increased dramatically. While all countries differ in the degree to which government responsibilities and authority are decentralized to local government, mayors of cities have become increasingly visible as global champions for health in areas like climate change, air and water pollution, children and youth, violence prevention, aging, and local economic development.

A HiAP approach to government and governance means that there is recognition that decisions made in sectors in addition to the traditional health-care sector (e.g., transportation, housing, land use, education, and economic development) can have positive or negative consequences for human health. To implement the approach, there must be the political will to assess health impacts of all policies and programs before decisions for action are made. As an increasing percentage of the world's population lives in cities, cities can truly be the drivers of global health through effective models for governance and the political will and commitment of urban leaders to act for health.

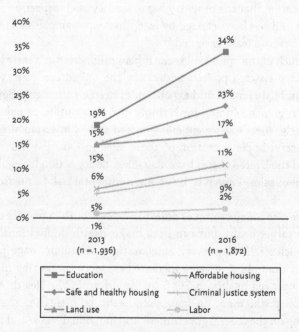

Figure 14.3 Involvement in policy areas related to social determinants of health over time.
Source: National Association of County City Health Officials. National profile of local health departments, United States, 2016, restricted-use level 2 data. Inter-University Consortium for Political and Social Research. 2018; https://doi.org/10.3886/ICPSR37145.v1.[12]

availability of healthy foods, and taxes to reduce intake of unhealthy foods, such as sugar sweetened beverages. In 2015, Berkeley, California, implemented a penny per ounce tax on sugar-sweetened beverages, the first city-level tax in the nation. As of 2017, six cities have sugar-sweetened beverage taxes: Berkley, California; Albany, California; Oakland, California; Chicago, Illinois (all of Cook County); Philadelphia, Pennsylvania; and Boulder, Colorado. City policies to increase physical activity include built environment policies such as creation of bike paths and greenspace to encourage outdoor activity, investment of public transportation infrastructure, and "complete streets" policies. Cities have also passed variations of menu-labeling laws, although there have been some issues with federal pre-emption depending upon what type of labeling is required.

Cities have long identified lead exposure as a public health issue and availed themselves of policy interventions to reduce lead poisoning in urban children. Some cities have laws that require landlords to ensure that properties rented to families with young children are lead safe,[13] and others require training for contractors remodeling housing with lead-based materials. Other cities have requirements for registering housing with lead paint and requirements for remediation. For example, in Philadelphia, landlords of properties built before 1978 with a new occupant aged six or less must provide a prospective tenant with certification that the property has passed a visual inspection for deteriorated paint and has been cleared by lead dust wipe samples or is free of any lead paint, before a lease is signed.[14]

While much of the opioid epidemic is being addressed at a state level, many US cities have enacted policies addressing the opioid epidemic, which have included establishment of and expansion of needle exchange programs; drug buy-back programs; funding for training and distribution of naloxone; and, more recently, steps toward establishing supervised injection sites, learning from successful implementation of these sites in Canadian cities. Cities in Canada and the United States have also taken policy action in regulating density of alcohol sales, known to be an environmental risk factor for excessive drinking.

There are also many examples of health-relevant urban policies that do not specifically target health but can have major health implications. Examples include policies related poverty amelioration. Minimum wage policies are an excellent example. Following increased evidence connecting higher living wages to improved health, in 2016 the American Public Health Association issued a policy statement on improving health by increasing the minimum wage, calling on the federal government and individual states and municipalities to consider increasing the minimum wage and indexing it to inflation and the cost of living.[15] Prior to 2012, only five localities in the United States had minimum wage legislation that differed from the state wage. As of early 2019, that number had risen to 41, and several other cities have declared intents to engage in a policy discussion around minimum wage. Most research in the literature demonstrates that increased minimum wage reduces poverty. More recent research published in *Health Affairs* showed some connection between higher wages and improved health,[16] although much more research in this area is needed.

Other urban policies that relate to economic development and commerce include investments in small businesses or business improvement districts, investments in universal prekindergarten, congestion pricing to reduce traffic and emissions, greening and vacant lot remediation, and programs and investments in improving urban housing. Internationally, improvements in sanitation and housing have had far-reaching public health impacts in cities. Housing and neighborhood interventions are important strategies to improve health in cities and reduce urban health inequities. Policies to ameliorate lead paint, asthma- related allergens, and conditions unhospitable to healthy living are important tools to improve the health of city residents, as well as local policies that disallow utility shutoffs in winter months.

Cities are emerging as major drivers of policies connected to climate change and sustainability. Over 90% of all urban areas are coastal, putting most cities at risk from flooding from rising sea levels and powerful storms.[17] As mentioned in Chapter 12, C40 Cities[17] is an international network of over 90 cities working on policy initiatives to address climate change and achieving the goals of the Paris Agreement. City policy initiatives include emissions standards for municipal fleets, congestion pricing, waste reduction/recycling, development of green space, and zoning regulations attached to new construction that encourages green building.

Health in All Policies

Improving urban health requires not only health-specific policies, but an eye to health in all policymaking. As discussed in Part I, urban factors that impact health are far more wide-reaching than those policies specific to health itself. Transportation, wages, zoning, food accessibility, housing, built environment, etc. all impact health and are all within the purview of urban policy. Policies to improve health in cities need to draw upon all the components of urban living. Taking a "health in all policies" (HiAP) approach, cities can improve the health of their residents through a broad approach to policy that extends into all aspects of the social, environmental, and economic determinants of health (see example in Box 14.3).

As discussed in Chapter 3, the CDC defines the HiAP approach as "a collaborative approach to improving the health of all people by incorporating health considerations into decision-making across sectors and policy areas."[5] The approach implies a recognition that a broad range of policies outside

Box 14.3 HEALTH EQUITY IN ALL URBAN POLICIES

Jason Corburn and Joseph S. Griffin.

Richmond is a working-class community of color in the San Francisco Bay Area with about 115,000 residents. In the early 2000s, Richmond was one of the poorest, most violent, and, by almost every measure, unhealthiest cities in the United States. Richmond is also one of the most ethnically diverse cities in the San Francisco Bay Area. In 2007, Richmond was the ninth most violent city in the United States, with 47 gun homicides per 100,000.

Yet, by 2017, many indicators of the social determinants of health had turned around. Richmond residents were reporting feeling safer and healthier, and they rated their community and city positively. Unemployment and gun homicides were at historic lows. This box briefly reviews how Richmond turned itself around from a violent and unhealthy population into a more equitable and healthier city.

After a series of toxic releases from the city's Chevron oil refinery, environmental justice groups mobilized and formed the Richmond Equitable Development Initiative. This coalition conducted "citizen science" to survey, measure, and document the environmental, social, economic, and health issues in Richmond, securing support from the California Endowment to integrate health into the city's General Plan Update Process,[18] the city's long-range development and policy "blueprint." What emerged was California's first ever Community Health and Wellness Element, or chapter, as part of a General Plan.[19] A series of place-based, low-cost actions were recommended, such as street painting and signal timing to improve intersection safety, converting abandoned tennis courts to futsal courts, and bringing mobile clinics to local schools.

Wanting to further institutionalize the health equity work, a group of community organizations, the county health department, the local school district, and city officials were organized into the Richmond Health Equity Partnership (RHEP) by University of California at Berkeley Professor Jason Corburn. The first task of the RHEP was to engage residents and city staff to describe what they thought were the key barriers to and opportunities for being healthy in Richmond. One result of this process was that the RHEP translated community narratives into a graphic of "cumulative stressors" and linked this to the biomedical research on *toxic stress*—or how prolonged adversity alters the body's cognitive and immune systems and contributes to some of the most prevalent diseases in Richmond, such as obesity, hypertension, diabetes, asthma, and poor mental health. The sources of community toxic stress were identified as structural racism, and reducing stressors required addressing structural discrimination and building structural competencies within government policies and decision-making processes.

In 2012, the RHEP used the toxic stress and structural racism frameworks to draft a HiAP strategy.[20] The HiAP strategy identified ways to reduce or eliminate toxic stressors through city agency decisions, budget allocations, and new partnerships with other institutions, according to six action areas: (i) governance and leadership, (ii) economic development and education, (iii) full-service and safe communities, (iv) residential and built environments, (v) environmental health and justice, and (vi) quality and accessible health homes and services. Each action area included short-term (one- to two-year) and medium-term (five-year) policy and programmatic strategies targeting one or more toxic stressors in Richmond and quantifiable indicators to track progress for both specific population groups and neighborhoods. After more than three years of collaborative work, the Richmond City Council passed the nation's first HiAP ordinance in 2014.

The multiple strategies within the HiAP Strategy and Ordinance provided a new health equity framework for all city agencies and demanded new partnerships between government and community-based organizations. An interdepartmental team, led by the City Manager's Office, was established to coordinate actions within and across city agencies as well as strengthen ties between the city, community groups, and county government. A series of health equity–focused policies emerged from these intracity and city–community partnerships. For example, a living wage ordinance was adopted in June 2014 that mandated $15 per hour and adjusted the rate annually based on the regional Consumer Price Index. A city program called Richmond BUILD refocused its efforts to train young people, many formerly incarcerated, in building-trade skills. These same skills were contracted by the city in its partnership with the nonprofit Grid Alternatives to offer subsidized and free solar power and home energy efficiency upgrades to low-income residents.

While the transformation is ongoing and incomplete, we offer the following principles that contributed to today's successes: (i) develop a long-range plan, co-drafted with residents, not for them; (ii) develop a health equity strategy explicitly framed around structural racism and toxic stress to ensure that you address the root causes of poor health; (iii) put youth, undocumented residents, former felons, and other highly marginalized groups at the center, not margins, of the work; (iv) ensure that residents benefit economically, such as through employment, and politically, from strategies; (v) institutionalize health equity through the law and municipal budgets to avoid overburdening nonprofits and relying on private foundations; (vi) embrace urban acupuncture, or focused interventions that support the most vulnerable population groups and places that also catalyze city-wide and population-level improvements; and (vii) do not expect to get it all right the first time: learn-by-doing, measure impacts along the way, and adjust interventions as new knowledge emerges.

Adapted from Coburn et al.[21]

of the traditional health care sector can have important health impacts. Examples of these policies include social, economic, and educational policy. These policies are, of course, of great relevance to urban areas. In urban settings, other critically important policies include transportation policies and other urban planning policies such as zoning, street design, cycling policies, and mobility policies including strategies like congestion pricing and vehicle use restrictions.

Some are moving even further in this thinking from HiAP to "health in all decisions," recognizing that there are decisions made every day in communities that can have an impact—positive or negative—on health.

CHALLENGES TO POLICYMAKING

While cities are engaged in policy innovation to improve public health, they face multiple jurisdictional and political challenges to their policymaking power.

Jurisdiction and Authority

When discussing the role of cities as policymaking bodies, two factors are critical to understanding a city's potential policy scope and reach. The first relates to constraints imposed by geographic and administrative boundaries. Cities do not exist in a vacuum and are attached to other jurisdictions. They are also nested within larger regions. But although urban health problems do not respect geographic or administrative boundaries, there are clear jurisdictional boundaries for policymaking purposes.

For example, if a city enacts a restaurant smoking ban, what happens with those communities who live on the edge of the city limits—will patrons travel over the border to a business outside of the city limits? What, then, is the impact of that policy? If a city enacts policy to limit emissions to improve air quality, what do they do about the airport that lies just outside of their border? Transportation policy is particularly complex since transportation systems cross urban boundaries and provide critical infrastructure for economic and job development both in cities and in close-ring suburbs.

Second, many cities have defined legal power and authority based upon the state or province in which they reside and their own constitutions or charters. Cities in the United States are generally governed by a legislative body and a chief executive, but the reach of authority can vary based on the degree of local control.

Home Rule and Dillon Rule

The power that cities have to make policy is rooted in the level of autonomy they have within the state in which they reside. The US Constitution makes no mention of local government or authority and reserves key governing power for the states. Local governments in the United States fall under two general governing principles: *Home Rule* or *Dillon Rule*.[22] Home Rule grants cities governing and legislative authority over matters not addressed by the state, giving those cities greater control and policy authority. Dillon Rule operates in the opposite form, giving cities only the legislative power that is granted to them by the state. The degree of governance power and policy autonomy in Dillon Rule states depends upon the state itself, with states giving more or less control to their cities. Home Rule is provided for in certain state constitutions, either by default or if the city itself has enacted Home Rule legislation, and some states provide for Home Rule only for cities of a certain size. Finally, many states apply some combination of Dillon and Home Rule to their cities, adding greater variation—and sometimes confusion—to their governance power.

Pre-emption

There is no greater challenge to policy at the local level than pre-emption. Pre-emption occurs when a higher level of government (usually state or federal) limits the authority of a lower level of government (usually a city) over a particular issue. Pre-emption has been a challenge for many health policies in the United States—particularly recently in tobacco regulation, food-labeling laws, firearm regulation, and other tax policy mechanisms aimed at improving population health. While the Institute of Medicine recommended[7] that federal and state policymakers "should set minimum standards . . . allowing states and localities to further protect the health and safety of their inhabitants," and "should avoid language that hinders public health action," many states have, in fact, done just the opposite. The number of pre-emption bills passed by states has increased in recent years in the United States. More than half of all states now explicitly disallow local efforts to address minimum wage policy, and almost half pre-empt cities from enacting paid leave policy. States have also passed as pre-emption laws that limit city efforts on the environment, firearms, and LGBTQ and other forms of discrimination.[23]

There are two types of pre-emption, express and implied. Express pre-emption occurs when a law or regulation explicitly limits the power of lower government; implied pre-emption occurs when a court finds pre-emption to exist even if not explicitly stated. Once pre-emption is determined, it is usually impossible to change. The federal government has broad pre-emption powers, and those powers have been used to limit policy action in public health. State pre-emption can affect the city's ability (or lack thereof) to tax or regulate since most cities are granted taxation powers by the state. The ways in which a city can be pre-empted by the state can vary depending upon its governance structure and how much Home Rule authority they have. Pre-emption can either be *floor pre-emption*—establishing a required minimum—or *ceiling pre-emption*—establishing a limit at which cities can't surpass. It is most often the ceiling pre-emption that limits public health action. Pre-emption language is not always explicit state law and is evident in other phrasing, for example, giving states the "sole authority" to regulate or preventing local governments from passing laws that are "more stringent" than state law.[24]

Policymaker Use of Research and Evidence

Policymaker uptake of research and evidence is perhaps the greatest challenge to making evidence-informed policy at the local level. As we will discuss further in Chapter 15, conducting sound research will not affect policy if it is not read, understood, and acted upon by those with decision making power.

In their 2015 *Lancet* commentary, Brownell and Lamberto (p. 2445)[25] ask why more science doesn't make its way into the hands of policymakers, stating:

> Evidence-based policy making is an important aspirational goal, but only a small proportion of research has the policy impact it might have. Most researchers are not trained to create policy impact from their work, engagement with policy makers is not encouraged or rewarded in most settings, and the communication of scientific findings occurs within the academic community but rarely outside it. There are exceptions, but little is done to systematically link scholarship to policy.

They propose a four-step model that develops strategic science with a policy impact.[25] Rather than researchers starting with questions of interest to them and then disseminating to those they believe should listen, the authors propose first identifying the key decision makers and then creating a mechanism for reciprocal information-sharing between researchers and these change agents. The second step is to develop strategic questions of mutual interest in a collaborative process between researchers and policymakers. Then researchers undertake strategic studies based on those questions. The final step is communicating these findings in a way that strengthens the bridge between policy and practice, which may follow a model similar to that described in Box 14.4.

Box 14.4 BRIDGING THE GAP BETWEEN URBAN PUBLIC HEALTH KNOWLEDGE AND POLICY

José G. Siri and Katherine Indvik

The gap between knowledge and policy is among the most persistent challenges to urban health. The widespread demand for policy-relevant evidence generally rests on the assumption that good evidence leads to good action, but reality is seldom so simple. The policy process is complex and influenced by multiple factors, even when current and relevant scientific evidence exists. As a result, urban policies are rarely optimal for health, and even the most pertinent evidence can take years to inform effective action.

Understanding barriers to the translation of knowledge to policy (KtP) can suggest pathways for improving this process. These barriers arise from the goals, assumptions, incentives, and constraints of both knowledge producers (e.g., researchers) and knowledge users (e.g., policymakers), and from the interfaces between these actors. Public health researchers and practitioners hoping to influence policy processes should consider each of these broad domains.

On the supply side, the knowledge produced by research communities is often not the knowledge needed by policymakers. Policymakers are rarely consulted during research design, and, as such, researchers often lack a clear perception of the needs and incentives that constrain policy processes, specific questions of relevance to policy making, and the types of information most likely to be applied in practice. Moreover, professional incentives within the academic community—such as those that determine what research is funded or published or which professionals advance within their fields—may favor basic and/or siloed research, which, in turn, tends to be less useful for policy than applied, interdisciplinary analysis.

Public health researchers can generate more relevant knowledge through genuine transdisciplinary engagement that incorporates policymakers throughout the research process. Moreover, by tracking the policy agenda (e.g., by monitoring political media or establishing direct communication with local political actors) and staying abreast of trends in knowledge and opinion among the general public and relevant stakeholder groups, researchers can position themselves to deliver knowledge where and when it will have greatest impact. More broadly, research ecosystems should be modified to incentivize production of the kind of knowledge that policymakers need, emphasizing applied, interdisciplinary research, valuation of the health, social and economic costs and (co-)benefits of particular policies and interventions, and provision of decision-support tools that specify the consequences of alternate policy scenarios, including opportunity costs and likely winners and losers. Tailoring research to local needs by including local knowledge and adopting place-based methods can also make outputs more relevant to policymakers.

On the demand side, many factors may limit how likely knowledge users are to make use of relevant information. Political actors usually have obligations, direct or implied, to a range of stakeholders, including donors, private sector lobbies, and the public and, as a result, must evaluate actions in terms of their distributed impacts. These actors generally operate within fixed budgets, over relatively short time horizons. They may lack the necessary skills or resources to access or interpret scientific literature or simply be unaware that relevant information exists. Moreover, they may see researchers as impractical and not consider them trusted sources of information.

Formal measures can be taken to improve the uptake of public health knowledge in urban policy, for example, by requiring consultation with experts throughout policy creation, mandating the adoption of health as a key performance indicator across government sectors, or requiring health impact assessments for urban development. Capacity-building efforts aimed at policymakers can improve their awareness of the potential benefits of effective knowledge translation and their ability to locate, access, interpret, and apply scientific information.

KtP translation often fails due to a lack of effective links between knowledge suppliers and knowledge users. Formal mechanisms or structures to ensure such connections are rare, especially at the local level where most actions take place, and are often highly vulnerable to political turnover. Even where potential linking mechanisms exist, effective communication can be hindered by adverse professional incentives or the jargon and perspectives specific to different sectors or disciplines. Furthermore, poor communication practices may limit the effective application even of highly-relevant knowledge. Such practices include formats that are relatively inaccessible to policymakers (e.g., scientific journal articles), that are wrongly targeted (i.e., to audiences with little power to influence policy making), or that are poorly timed and therefore fail to align with current policy agendas.

To address these issues, public health researchers should aim to build long-term relationships of mutual trust and respect with local policymakers and the civil servants and public sector practitioners who support them. Researchers should be aware of and anticipate changes in the policy agenda, positioning themselves to take advantage of policy windows. They should understand who, in a given system, has the power to act, and communicate messages simply and clearly to those who can use them. Key messages should be highlighted and easily identifiable. Researchers should seek to influence policy through the wider system, engaging with the public and building relationships with knowledge brokers likely to be effective at the relevant scale (e.g., UN agencies, city networks, advocacy organizations, or community groups). At the project level, knowledge-policy linkages can be created through meaningful transdisciplinary engagement. At the system level, knowledge can be embedded in policymaking structures (e.g., by creating positions for experts within governance) or mechanisms can be introduced to foster regular contact between knowledge suppliers and knowledge users.

Failures in KtP translation are undoubtedly a major barrier to achieving desired public health outcomes in cities worldwide. Nevertheless, KtP can be improved through actions readily available to researchers and policy actors. A more systematic approach to KtP planning has the potential to increase the effectiveness of public health research and practice and improve health and well-being for all.

Politics and Political Feasibility

In addition to the challenges presented by jurisdiction and governance constraints in urban health policymaking, it is equally critical to understand the importance of the political context and political feasibility in effecting policy change. While public health science itself may strive to be apolitical, the policymaking process is inherently a political process. It is critical to understand the political environment and context for policy change to understand the likelihood of a given policy being enacted and successfully implemented. This is not specific to urban areas, although cities have to operate both within their own political climates and contexts as well as in the hierarchy in which they reside.

As Friedan (p. 592)[26] discusses in his framework for health impact pyramid,

Interventions that address social determinants of health have the greatest potential public health benefit. Action on these issues needs the support of government and civil society if it is to be successful. The biggest obstacle to making fundamental societal changes is often not shortage of funds but lack of political will.

Understanding the political context and political feasibility is multifaceted. It begins by simply knowing who the actors and the processes for creating policy change are. Knowing the structure of the local government, elected officials and other decision makers, boards of health, and community advisory boards that influence policy is a necessary first start, followed by knowledge of the policymaking process itself—legislative and budget season, hearing schedules, and election cycles. Knowing—and appreciating—the political context in a city is critical to policy success; understanding upcoming elections and the electability of a policy champion may help inform the opportunities and constraints in moving a policy forward. Similarly, being aware of other major policy initiatives at the city level can inform the attention that will be paid to a particular urban health policy goal. It is not enough for urban health researchers to provide the science; we need to be aware of and engage in the policy process to see that work lead to action.

Policy Implementation

Creating policy is only the first step. Policy itself presents a theoretical solution to a problem. Policy implementation happens after a given policy or piece of legislation is adopted. Successful policy implementation is dependent upon a number of factors, including clear policy goals, committed and skillful leadership, and, most important, sufficient financial resources.[27] Policy implementation often requires coordination between government agencies and between government and those most impacted by the policy itself. Policies are only as strong as the commitment behind them—politically and financially—to ensure their success. For example, a city policy to limit tobacco sales to minors will only work if there are sufficient staff allocated to inspect establishments and regulate their sales. Policies that establish bike lanes on busy streets can only reduce fatalities if bike lanes are actually designated and enforced.

MEASURING AND EVALUATING POLICY: HOW DO WE KNOW IF IT WORKS?

Finally, creating and implementing policy is insufficient if we do not learn from policies once they are in place. Understanding policy processes and their implementation is critical to policy innovation and success in the long term.

Policy Surveillance

Policy surveillance defined formally as "the systematic tracking of policies of public importance"[1] is an important mechanism for understanding the scope of polices that can impact health. The description of when and where policies have been implemented can provide insight into the processes driving policy adoption and can suggest thematic or geographic areas for future policy development (via research dissemination or advocacy).[2]

There are several major US-based policy surveillance resources that can be used to understand the breadth of urban health policy. LawAtlas.org, associated with Temple University's Beaslely School of Law's Center for Public Health Law Research, houses over 100 policy surveillance maps in over 20 areas of public health. Funded primarily by the Robert Wood Johnson Foundation, it includes data sets supported through funding from multiple other government and nongovernment sources. LawAtlas also provides instruction on the use of policy surveillance data for particular surveillance questions. Additional policy surveillance resources include PDAPS.org; the National Institute on Drug Abuse–funded Prescription Drug Abuse Policy System; and CityHealth. org, maintained by the DeBeaumont Foundation to catalogue evidence-based policy change in select US cities.[28]

For surveillance of upstream influences on the urban environment, an advantage of legislative action is that the public record is accessible. Several organizations have undertaken steps to compile laws relevant to urban health, as was done by Milwaukee with a report titled "An Apple A Day: How Obesity Impacts Milwaukee and an Analysis of Prevention Strategies From Other Cities."[29] Some specific policy surveillance resources exist around topics such as energy efficiency,[30] child care,[31] tobacco control[32] (see also the Tobacco Control scale[33]), food environment policy,[34] occupational safety,[35] and environmental health.[36] For other topics, even if there is not an actively maintained database, there may nonetheless be a snapshot provided by published papers, as is the case for legislative approaches to the changing the food environment.[37,38]

Formal laws and published regulations are not the only sources of policies in cities. The Urban Health Collaborative's Policy Surveillance Project[39] has begun to characterize the presence of promising or effective policy, programmatic, and budgetary initiatives to promote health equity. The Big Cities Health Coalition, which represents the health leaders of the largest cities in the most urban areas of the United States, regularly monitors policy actions of their members and works to share best practices in public health policies across cities.

Policy Evaluation

Engagement in policy is not only informing and influencing policy, it is also about studying and understanding it. We study policy for a variety of reasons: to understand the origins and goals of policies and programs, to understand why particular policies are selected over alternative possibilities, to anticipate and diagnose problems in policy implementation and performance, and to determine the health or other impact of policies. Evaluation results can be used to determine how policy design and implementation can be improved. Put simply, we study policy to understand why things are the way they are and how we can make them better.

The CDC[40] defines policy evaluation as the application of "evaluation principles and methods to examine the content, implementation or impact of a policy. Evaluation is the activity through which we develop an understanding of the merit, worth, and utility of a policy." The CDC's policy evaluation framework describes three phases in evaluating the policy process:

- Evaluation of the policy content: does the policy itself articulate the goals and the logic for why and how the policy will produce intended change?
- Evaluation of Policy Implementation: was the policy implemented as intended
- Evaluation of Policy Impact: Did the policy produce the intended outcomes and impact.

As we discuss in Chapter 9, there are multiple methods of policy evaluation depending upon the evaluation question at hand. In his article "Asking the Right Questions: Research of Consequence to Solve Problems of Significance,"[41] Thomas Farley, Philadelphia's health commissioner, makes two critical recommendations for evaluation of health policies in cities. The first is to invest in observational studies of health policies across cities—learning about variations in policy, in environment, and in health outcome—to inform future activities. While methodologically strong studies of policy effects are most desirable, Farley points out the value of even single examples of policy successes, particularly in boosting public opinion or political feasibility. Second, measuring side effects of policies themselves and learning not only whether or not the policy had its desired effect, but what the effects are that may not have been anticipated or planned for in the original intent. Understanding the "side effects" of policies can help inform future policy action. For example, does adding trees in certain neighborhoods with the intent of reducing heat also lead to increases in asthma triggers? Does the introduction of a beverage tax cause people to cross city borders to make purchases, causing an unintended economic impact?

CONCLUSION

The marriage of urban health research with the power of problem-solving at the local level is what can enable evidence-based, politically powerful change to improve urban population health. Engagement of multiple stakeholders is critical to developing, implementing and evaluation policy in cities.

Policy is a critical tool for cities to take what we have learned in research and turn it into action that can improve health. Despite challenges in jurisdiction, governance, and politics, policy provides an opportunity to have direct impact on a full population.

REFERENCES

1. Policy. *Merriam-Webster Dictionary*. https://www.merriam-webster.com/. Accessed June 25, 2020.
2. Policy. In: *Cambridge Academic Content Dictionary*. New York: Cambridge University Press; 2019.
3. Centers for Disease Control, Prevention Office of the Associate Director for Policy and Strategy. Definition of policy. Last reviewed May 29, 2015; https://www.cdc.gov/policy/analysis/process/definition.html.
4. OECD Regional Development Ministerial. *Megatrends: Building Better Futures for Regions, Cities and Rural Areas*. Athens: OECD; 2019.
5. Rudolph L, Caplan J, Ben-Moshe K, Dillon L. *Health in All Policies: A Guide for State and Local Governments*. Washington, DC: American Public Health; 2013.
6. Frieden TR. A framework for public health action: The health impact pyramid. *American Journal of Public Health*. 2010;*100*(4):590–595.
7. Institute of Medicine, Committee on Public Health Strategies to Improve Health. *For the Public's Health: Revitalizing Law and Policy to Meet New Challenges*. Washington, DC: National Academies Press; 2011.
8. Frieden TR. The future of public health. *New England Journal of Medicine*. 2015;373(18):1748–1754.
9. Institute of Medicine. *For the Public's Health: Revitalizing Law and Policy to Meet New Challenges*. Washington, DC: The National Academies Press; 2011.
10. Katz B, Nowak J. *The New Localism: How Cities Can Thrive in the Age of Populism*. Washington, DC: Brookings Institution Press; 2017.
11. World Health Organization. WHO European Healthy Cities Network: Healthy Cities Vision. 2019; http://www.euro.who.int/en/health-topics/environment-and-health/urban-health/who-european-healthy-cities-network/healthy-cities-vision.
12. National Association of County City Health Officials. National profile of local health departments, United States, 2016, restricted-use level 2 data. Inter-University Consortium for Political and Social Research. 2018; https://doi.org/10.3886/ICPSR37145.v1.
13. City of Philadelphia. Philadelphia Lead Paint Disclosure and Certification Law. In: Philadelphia Co, ed. *Title 6, Chapter 6, Section 6-8002011*.

14. City of Philadelphia. The Philadelphia lead disclosure & certification law: What tenants need to know. June 2016; https://www.phila.gov/media/20181108140933/What-Tenants-Need-to-Know_6_16.pdf.

15. American Public Health Association. Policy statement 20167: Improving health by increasing the minimum wage. Policy no. 20167. November 1, 2016. https://www.apha.org/policies-and-advocacy/public-health-policy-statements/policy-database/2017/01/18/improving-health-by-increasing-minimum-wage

16. Leigh JP, Du J. Effects of minimum wage on population health. Health Affairs Policy Brief. October 4, 2018. https://doi.org/10.1377/hpb20180622.107025.

17. C40 Cities. https://www.c40.org/. Accessed June 25, 2020.

18. Corburn J, Curl S, Arredondo G, Malagon J. Making health equity planning work. *Journal of Planning Education and Research*. 2015;35(3):265–281.

19. City of Richmond California. Environment and Health Initiatives. *City of Richmond, California website* 2018; http://www.ci.richmond.ca.us/1610/Environment-and-Health-Initiatives. Accessed June 25, 2020.

20. City of Richmond, California. Health in All Policies strategy, 2013–14. 2015; http://www.ci.richmond.ca.us/2575/Health-in-All-Policies-HiAP. Accessed June 25, 2020.

21. Corburn J, Griffin JS. Richmond, California: Health Equity in All Urban Policies. In: Galea S, Ettman CK, Vlahov D, eds. *Urban Health* (pp. 323–329). New York: Oxford University Press; 2019.

22. Russell JD, Bostrom A. *Federalism, Dillon Rule, and Home Rule*. American City County Exchange. January 2016; https://www.alec.org/app/uploads/2016/01/2016-ACCE-White-Paper-Dillon-House-Rule-Final.pdf

23. National League of Cities. State preemption of local authority continues to rise, according to new data from the national league of cities. 2018; https://www.nlc.org/article/state-preemption-of-local-authority-continues-to-rise-according-to-new-data-from-the.

24. National League of Cities. *City Rights in an Era of Preemption: A State-by-State Analysis*. National League of Cities. April 2, 2018; https://www.nlc.org/resource/city-rights-in-an-era-of-preemption-a-state-by-state-analysis

25. Brownell KD, Roberto CA. Strategic science with policy impact. *The Lancet*. 2015;385(9986):2445–2446.

26. Frieden TR. A framework for public health action: the health impact pyramid. *Am J Public Health*. 2010;100(4):590–595. doi:10.2105/AJPH.2009.185652

27. Salvesen D, Evenson KR, Rodriguez DA, Brown A. Factors influencing implementation of local policies to promote physical activity: A case study of Montgomery County, Maryland. *Journal of Public Health Management and Practice*. 2008;14(3):280–288.

28. Temple University Center for Public Health Law Research. Policy Surveillance Program. http://publichealthlawresearch.org/content/policy-surveillance-program. Accessed June 25, 2020.

29. Spahr C, Henken R. An apple a day: How obesity impacts Milwaukee and an analysis of prevention strategies from other cities. Public Policy Forum. 2016; https://wispolicyforum.org/research/an-apple-a-day-how-obesity-impacts-milwaukee-and-an-analysis-of-prevention-strategies-from-other-cities/

30. American Council for an Energy-Efficient Economy. Policy database. http://database.aceee.org/. Accessed June 25, 2020.

31. Giannarelli L, Minton S, Durham C; US Department of Health and Human Services, Administration for Children and Families, Office of Planning, Research

and Evaluation. Child Care and Development Fund (CCDF) Policies Database, 2009. Inter-University Consortium for Political and Social Research. 2011; https://doi.org/10.3886/ICPSR32261.v1. Accessed June 25, 2020.

32. Campaign for Tobacco-Free Kids. Tobacco control laws. https://www.tobacco-controllaws.org/. Accessed June 25, 2020.

33. Joossens L, Raw M. The Tobacco Control Scale: A new scale to measure country activity. *Tobacco Control*. 2006;15(3):247–253.

34. Vandevijvere S, Dominick C, Devi A, Swinburn B. The healthy food environment policy index: Findings of an expert panel in New Zealand. *Bulletin of the World Health Organization*. 2015;93(5):294–302.

35. International Labour Organization. ILO Global Database on Occupational Safety and Health Legislation (LEGOSH). http://www.ilo.org/dyn/legosh/en/f?p=14100:1:::NO:::. Accessed June 25, 2020.

36. National Conference of State Legislatures. Environmental Health State Bill Tracking Database. March 25, 2020; http://www.ncsl.org/research/environment-and-natural-resources/environmental-health-legislation-database.aspx#resource.

37. Downs SM, Thow AM, Leeder SR. The effectiveness of policies for reducing dietary trans fat: A systematic review of the evidence. *Bulletin of the World Health Organization*. 2013;91(4):262–269H.

38. Story M, Kaphingst KM, Robinson-O'Brien R, Glanz K. Creating healthy food and eating environments: Policy and environmental approaches. *Annual Review of Public Health*. 2008;29:253–272.

39. Drexel University Urban Health Collaborative. Urban Policy and Program Surveillance Project. https://drexel.edu/uhc/projects/themes/urban-policy-program-surveillance-project/.

40. National Center for Injury Prevention and Control. Step by step—evaluating violence and injury prevention policies. Brief 1: Overview of policy evaluation. Centers for Disease Control and Prevention. 2013; https://www.cdc.gov/injury/pdfs/policy/Brief%201-a.pdf

41. Farley TA. Asking the right questions: Research of consequence to solve problems of significance. *American Journal of Public Health*. 2016;106(10):1778–1779.

CHAPTER 15

Dissemination of Urban Health Research to Maximize Impact

JENNIFER KOLKER, CLAIRE SLESINSKI,
AMY CARROLL-SCOTT, AND JONATHAN PURTLE

BACKGROUND

As those committed to improving urban public health, we have a responsibility to translate and disseminate what we know about urban health to those who make decisions about urban health, with the input of those who are most impacted by those decisions. Research needs to be communicated in a way that works for the decision maker and not the researcher. We need to communicate in a variety of ways—verbal, written, print, online—that appeal to multiple audiences.

Having introduced the diverse perspectives and potential partners relevant to the scope of urban health, we focus here on the range of tools, formats, and best practices suited to the goals of sharing emerging and established evidence with a range of different urban health audiences. In doing so, we ideally both provide and receive valued information that serves to maintain and grow partnerships over time. In Chapter 12 we reviewed the many stakeholders and actors in urban public health. Chapter 13 focused on the role of community members in both research creation and dissemination of findings, and Chapter 14, on the critical role that policy can play in improving health in cities. Building on prior chapters, we now focus on the importance of dissemination and translation of research and evidence to those who make—and live with—decisions about urban public health.

Jennifer Kolker, Claire Slesinski, Amy Carroll-Scott, and Jonathan Purtle, *Dissemination of Urban Health Research to Maximize Impact* In: *Urban Public Health*. Edited by: Gina S. Lovasi, Ana V. Diez Roux, and Jennifer Kolker, Oxford University Press (2021). © Oxford University Press 2021. DOI: 10.1093/oso/9780190885304.003.0015.

Urban health issues are relevant to more than half of the world's population, and urban health as a field incorporates knowledge and evidence from many disciplines. Because of this, urban health research generates insights and knowledge that, by nature, should be shared widely with many stakeholder groups globally.

Those living in cities have a vested interest in the findings of urban health research and the documented impact of urban health interventions and policies. Often, the public is providing the funding for research and interventions through their tax dollars. Just as frequently, data for such research and interventions are collected from community members who have a right to know the outcome of the research that was dependent on their participation. The field of urban health depends on the willingness of city residents to contribute to research and voice their support for the work of policymakers who implement urban health programs. More important, researchers have an ethical responsibility to disseminate their findings to the public and specifically to study participants.[1-4]

Urban health professionals find themselves embedded in networks through which information flows in multiple directions and in multiple forms. Traditional modes of publishing in peer-reviewed journals are only one of many strategies needed to disseminate urban public health research (see Boxes 15.1 and 15.2). Work that addresses pressing urban health questions can have broader impact by tailoring the communication formats to meet the needs of each of the relevant audiences, which requires listening as well as telling, joining conversations and serving as an ambassador for data and evidence.

Box 15.1 PRODUCING THE "RIGHT" KIND OF URBAN HEALTH EVIDENCE

Adriana C. Lein

To researchers, evidence that is "right" withstands the scrutiny of peer-review and conforms to scientific best practices. However, to policymakers facing numerous pressures—constituents, public opinion, election cycles, party platforms, and opponents, to name a few—the "right" evidence might provide a clear and actionable solution to a problem of high-relevance in their area or guide implementation or adaptation of an intervention.[5,6] Unfortunately, despite the potential for evaluations to be both rigorous and policy relevant, there is a dearth of research evaluating policies and interventions.[7]

Data infrastructure to better meet the needs of policymakers would include data that is at the local level and presentable in terms of socioeconomic indicators and urban health equity indicators that can capture the dynamic relationships between social, physical and economic measures, monitor community assets, and track policy decisions should be prioritized to integrate evidence into policy.[5,8] Such data could allow for comparisons of intracity differences and inform local level decisions and critically important. Yet, most large-scale efforts of drivers of disease burden have been undertaken at global and regional levels where country-level data may be more readily aggregated.[8]

Studies of policymakers preferences and information needs have shown that evaluative evidence that communicates the "effective ingredients" of interventions and the cascading effects of urban inequities and policy decisions are most valuable and sought after.[6,8,9]

Policymakers and other decision-makers are most likely to be interested in and consider evidence that is topical, aligned with the priorities of their policy agendas, and packaged in formats that can be readily applied.[5,10] One way to accomplish this is to involve policymakers and other relevant stakeholders throughout the research process (i.e., design, implementation, interpretation and evaluation). These efforts encompass collaborative research, translational T2 research, participatory research, co-production of knowledge, and practice-oriented research and may be discussed under the umbrella of "integrated knowledge translation."[10–12]

Transdisciplinary research, distinct from multidisciplinary or interdisciplinary research, in its abilities to work across barriers between siloed schools of thought and practice[11] is one approach gaining empirical support for its suitability to urban health and health equity agendas.[13,14] Urban health and public health challenges are by nature multidimensional. Solutions should be considered in the context of overarching trends, policy developments and actions that influence the actions of multilevel actors.[15,16] In this way, multisectoral research, which is predicated on harnessing collaborative teams of combined expertise from policy and research domains alongside community members,[17] holds promise for developing rigorous and sustainable solutions and succeeding in health promotion through multisectoral channels.[13]

For the purposes of this chapter, we define *dissemination* as the targeted distribution of research results or other information (e.g., surveillance or ecological data, intervention materials) to a specific audience using tailored strategies and communication channels. Effective dissemination of research

Box 15.2 HOW PEER-REVIEWED MANUSCRIPTS FIT WITHIN URBAN HEALTH RESEARCH DISSEMINATION

Gina S. Lovasi

The formality of developing manuscripts for peer-reviewed journals takes time, and even more so if adopting the unfamiliar conventions of another scientific discipline. Informal ways of sharing observations and data visualizations, such as blog posts, are much faster and less onerous than writing for peer-reviewed journals. The time between conceiving of a specific manuscript idea and having a citable publication is often two years or more, assuming that funding and data have already been secured. A substantial portion of this time can be after submission to the journal that ultimately accepts the article.

For time-sensitive topics, or those with current policy relevance, this slow pace is often misaligned with the broader goal of many urban health projects to provide timely evidence to local partners. Indeed, there are instances where a peer-reviewed publication is not the right choice or needs to be combined with an earlier dissemination product that is of use to multiple audiences.

However, peer-reviewed manuscripts remain an important way to formalize the sharing of knowledge from research projects. In some organizational contexts, the methods and results of research are considered proprietary, and full public disclosure and knowledge sharing might be avoided to protect the organization's comparative advantage. In contrast, many urban health investigators engaged in the peer-review system prioritize transparency of research methods, careful vetting of research, and sharing of insights toward the ends of building a strong and shared evidence base. The sharing of research methods and results is also used in disciplinary training and in our understanding of the research process itself. Ideally, the peer-review process steers the field toward cumulative knowledge with useful replication and elaboration over time. Where one paper may review the literature and articulate a gap, subsequent papers describe a strategy for answering one interesting question within that gap and provide a provisional answer. Additional work can then contradict, support, or add nuance to this initial answer. Eventually, the gap may be closed, or focal questions will shift, and thus the landscape gradually shifts, creating new understandings and opportunities.

Writing manuscripts for peer-reviewed journals is also linked to professional development goals and institutional incentive structures, used as a marker of one's visible contributions to recorded knowledge. Well-cited works are further viewed as demonstrating one's influence on the thinking or practice of other researchers. Publishing, and particularly publishing in well-regarded peer-reviewed journals, plays an important role in building a verifiable reputation in ways that matter for individual career opportunities, partnership opportunities, and future funding.

Ideally, policy-relevant peer-reviewed articles will have accompanying formats such as a fact sheet, infographic, or policy brief that can extend reach to nonresearch audiences. Adapting a paper to a more accessible format can be an efficient and direct way of communicating what is in an article while adjusting the language, length, and visuals to be more useful to policy and community audiences.

evidence has two primary goals—to inform and educate and to facilitate positive change. Dissemination, then

- Focuses on diffusing existing knowledge to urban health audiences with a stake in the content or issue (e.g., community members, policymakers, thought leaders).
- Focuses on effective strategies for getting this information and knowledge to the right urban health audiences in the right ways to ensure their most effective use of it.

Inherent in research translation and dissemination is that the responsibility rests with the communicator. As urban health researchers, we are often frustrated that the science is overlooked, not understood, or simply ignored. While this is often true, it is also the case that research is often disseminated in ways that are not useful for understanding or decision-making by the very audiences we are trying to reach. Research needs to be communicated in a way that works for the audience and not only for the researcher. While the principles and platforms we discuss in this chapter are not unique to urban health, the complexity of urban systems require particular attention to the methods and modes of effective dissemination.

PLANNING AND DESIGNING FOR DISSEMINATION

Dissemination of research to urban residents and decision makers should be deliberate, planned, and budgeted for at the outset of scientific work. Too often, researchers think about dissemination only after the work is completed. Instead, researchers should identify at the start how results may be used by various urban health audiences, which can then help direct products to be more effective and potentially guide aspects of research to meet urban health goals. Before research begins, investigators should

- Identify the audience(s) for the research to reach (i.e., identifying the different types of decision makers and their roles);
- Identify the types of dissemination products that will be most effective for these audiences;
- Identify the types of data that will be collected that targeted audiences are seeking and need to support their work; and
- Build relationships and establish partnerships in the cities being studied to shape the content and framework for the research.

In their chapter "Designing for Dissemination in Chronic Disease Prevention and Management," Owen et al.[18] propose a framework of principles for designing research for dissemination. This framework includes three specific process steps for effective dissemination:

- Engage key stakeholders for research through audience research.
- Identify models for dissemination efforts.
- Identify the appropriate means of delivering the message.

Identifying and Defining Audiences

The first step in determining dissemination plans and products is to identify the audience(s). The audience for dissemination varies depending on the type of evidence produced and the desired impact of the scientific knowledge generated. As strategic audiences are identified, these fundamental questions should be addressed:

1. Who will be interested in research findings? What group can most benefit from receiving and understanding the evidence that has been produced? Urban residents, policymakers, thought leaders, government managers, etc.?
2. Who will be able to take action with research findings and make a difference in urban health? Who can most efficiently and effectively create change based on this research? Who can maximize the impact of the evidence?

Potential audiences for dissemination are broad and diverse. For the purposes of this chapter, we divide our audiences into two primary areas: policymakers/decision makers and community residents/leaders. We will go into detail on each later in this chapter, recognizing that there is obvious overlap and connection between the two.

Once audiences have been defined, a next step is to identify the *relevant knowledge and attitudes* among the target audience about the specific topic of research, understanding if they have prior beliefs or biases that will influence how they receive research findings. Next, it is critical to understand *informational preferences and needs* of the audience related to this specific topic. Target audiences may prefer to receive relatable narrative stories, cost-effectiveness data, or concrete recommendations for action. Surveys, key informant interviews, and focus groups can all be used to gather this type of information; ideally data collection strategies to meet audience needs and preferences will have been considered during dissemination and research planning. Finally, it is important to also understand which material, platform, or medium is optimal for the intended audience. There are many options from which to choose to disseminate to both of these audiences as well as to other researchers, some examples of which are discussed later in this chapter.

When selecting the methods and platforms for dissemination of research results, it is important to consider the following questions:

- Where does my audience usually look for this type of information?
- Through what platforms does my audience usually engage with their trusted sources of information?
- What's the best method for communicating the specific information I plan to disseminate?

DISSEMINATION TO POLICY AUDIENCES AND DECISION MAKERS

Decision makers comprise multiple audiences and are influenced by multiple audiences. Referring to Chapter 12 will help to define audiences, and Chapter 14, knowing what change you are hoping to make and how that change will be made will influence the decision makers you choose and the products needed to reach them.

Many stakeholders, decision makers, and thought leaders do not read academic journals or use them to inform their work. This is due to a variety of reasons; many do not have access to these sources, although there has definitely been a movement in recent years toward more and more open access. Peer-reviewed articles are often too dense and jargon-filled for many working in public health practice or in other decision-making roles. Finally, urban health decision makers want information that is tailored to their local contexts and that recommend specific actions that they can take—translating sound research into options for action. Most decision makers know what the problems are; they need evidence-based solutions.

As Brownell and Lamberto (p. 2445)[19] said in their 2015 *Lancet* commentary,

evidence-based policy making is an important aspirational goal, but only a small proportion of research has the policy impact it might have. Most researchers are not trained to create policy impact from their work, engagement with policy makers is not encouraged or rewarded in most settings, and the communication of scientific findings occurs within the academic community but rarely outside it. There are exceptions, but little is done to systematically link scholarship to policy.

As discussed in Chapter 14, decision maker uptake of science to inform policy is lacking. Much has been written about the gap between public health knowledge and the use of that knowledge in policy and decision-making and challenges in effective dissemination of knowledge (see Table 15.1), often referred to as "translation gap."[20] There is a growing body of evidence on effective translation and dissemination and the tools that work best in communicating to decision makers on public health. As Brownson and colleagues (p. 103)[20]

Table 15.1 BARRIERS TO POLICYMAKER AND COMMUNITY USE OF RESEARCH EVIDENCE

Barriers to Policymaker Use of Research Evidence	Barriers to Community Use of Research Evidence
Lack of trust in the sources of research evidence	Lack of trust in the sources of research evidence
Research evidence fails to reach policymakers	Research evidence fails to reach community leaders and members
Presentation of research evidence is unclear and not compelling	Presentation of research evidence is unclear and not compelling
Publications require understanding of research terminology & methods	Publications require understanding of research terminology & methods
Need information in real time and a research/academic timeline doesn't fit	Need information in real time and a research/academic timeline doesn't fit
Research evidence is not policy relevant	Research evidence is not relevant to their own community context
Policymaking is political	Community had no role in shaping research questions and so distrust its results and messages
Politics are driven by values more than evidence	

Source: Purtle et al.[21]

discuss in *Getting the Word Out: New Approaches for Disseminating Public Health Science*, there are several accepted findings in the dissemination of public health research to decision-making audiences:

1. Passive approaches to dissemination are largely ineffective because uptake does not happen spontaneously.
2. Stakeholder engagement in research and evaluation processes is likely to enhance dissemination.
3. Dissemination of research to nonscientists is enhanced when messages are framed in ways that evoke emotion and interest and demonstrate usefulness.
4. At an agency level (e.g., health departments, community-based organizations), dissemination approaches should be time-efficient, consistent with organizational climate, culture, and resources, and aligned with the skills of staff members.
5. Dissemination to policy audiences needs to take into account unique characteristics of policy makers as dissemination targets (e.g., time horizons, need for local data).
6. The objective of research dissemination is to inform action or decisions; measures of academic impact often differ significantly from the markers of importance to practice and policy audiences.

A survey of mayors and health commissioners of all US cities with a population ≥50,000 was conducted in 2016 to inform the design of strategies to disseminate evidence about health disparities to city policymakers.[22] The survey was completed by 230 mayoral officials and 305 health commissioners. The survey found that 41.6% of mayoral officials and 61.1% of health commissioners officials strongly agreed that health disparities existed in their city, while 30.2% of mayoral officials and 8.0% of health commissioner officials believed that city policies could have little or no impact on disparities. These results highlight a need to better dissemination of evidence about the existence of heath disparities and potential of city policies to address them to these policymaker audiences. The survey also found that opinions about urban health disparities varied significantly by the ideology of city policymakers. For example, liberals were more much likely than conservatives to strongly agree that disparities exist. This finding suggests that there might be value in developing and tailoring separate dissemination materials for liberal and conservative city policymakers.

The survey also assessed mayoral officials' perceptions of the importance of different features of research evidence that is disseminated to them and the trustworthiness of evidence from different sources.[23] The features of disseminated evidence most frequently identified by mayoral officials as "very important" were evidence telling a story, being concise, and being relevant to their constituents. The sources of evidence that were perceived as "very trustworthy" most frequently were universities, followed by philanthropies, industry, constituents, and advocacy groups.

TYPES OF DISSEMINATION PRODUCTS FOR POLICY AUDIENCES

There are multiple platforms for disseminating urban health research in a way that is useful to decision makers and nonacademic audiences. Numerous resources are available to provide guidance and examples. The Purdue Online Writing Lab (OWL) at Purdue University (https://owl.purdue.edu) is a resource for a variety of written products that support dissemination of research into practice.

White papers are an often-used format for distilling research into a more summative piece which may be directed at decision makers among other audiences. White papers can vary in length, focus depth, and technicality: they can be simple and convey critical information or be as dense as a peer-reviewed paper. Examples of white papers abound on the Internet and familiarizing oneself with the range of types and formats is a great first step in learning how to write one. What white papers typically share is a desire to convince their audience of a particular path to choose. At the same time, white papers should be objective in presenting facts and present all information, even if you are trying to convince the audience of a particular point. They will ideally use graphics/visuals.

Issue, evidence, and policy briefs are generally shorter pieces than white papers, and the goal is brevity and a clear message. Wong and colleagues[24] propose a four-step process, which we adapt for the context of urban health: (i) define the problem with attention to the audience's perspective, (ii) state one to three policy actions that could address the problem, (iii) use data (one to two tables/figures) to make your case, and (iv) identify health implications of both action and inaction. They define policy briefs as providing "focused discussion of an action to achieve intentional and purposeful movement (p. 21)."[24] The central role of a potential policy action differentiates this type of writing from an issue brief. Reaching the audience with a clear message in such a short document is challenging. The main conclusion should be stated upfront, and the tone should be measured and balanced. Briefs are used by many sectors to convey a summary of research and data. For example, the Philadelphia Department of Public Health's CHART series, which "highlights under-reported or under-appreciated public health issues in an effort to kick-start a conversation."[25] Funders, such as the Robert Wood Johnson Foundation, Pew Charitable Trusts and Commonwealth, all publish issue and policy briefs that summarize research and program evaluation for a broader audience, many of which are focused on issues of urban health. And, of course, these are joined by publications by large organizations such as the Urban Institute and World Health Organization.

Public testimony—usually delivered orally with a written submission for the record—is a powerful policymaker communication tool. Often used in government hearings for decision makers with a public audience, testimony needs to convey critical information to a lay audience, and the testifier needs to be prepared to answer questions, which can be both scientific and political in nature. Everything communicated in a testimony (and the question-and-answer period) is part of the public record and, depending on the topic and setting, can receive press coverage. Reports to funders can contain not only expenditure and programmatic details but also be a mechanism for educating the funder and disseminating findings and results (which can help to secure future funding) and provide an avenue to begin to write about the work being conducted—often referencing or laying the groundwork for presentations or publications directed at other audiences (see Box 15.3).

Box 15.3 PUBLIC TESTIMONY BEFORE PHILADELPHIA CITY COUNCIL

Marla Gold

Good morning, Chairwoman Blackwell and the members of the Finance Committee. I am Dr. Marla Gold, Dean Emerita and Professor of Health Management and Policy at the Drexel Dornsife School of Public Health. Thank you for the opportunity to give testimony on Bill No. 180522, which if enacted, would effectively overturn significant portions of the tobacco retail permit regulation passed by the Board of Health in 2016.

As a member of the Board of Health and a public health leader in Philadelphia, I, along with my fellow Board members, carefully reviewed the evidence before we approved the tobacco retail permit regulations. You know that tobacco use is responsible for more deaths in Philadelphia than any other cause. We found that a higher density of tobacco retail is associated with teen smoking initiation and with lower rates of quitting among chronic smokers. More tobacco retailers in an area translates to more young people initiating smoking. More tobacco retailers in an area translates to less Philadelphians who smoke being able to quit.

We also reviewed solid evidence of marked inequities between neighborhoods in Philadelphia. Our low-income neighborhoods and particularly schools in those neighborhoods have up to 3 times as many tobacco outlets per capita as higher income neighborhoods.

The City's tobacco permit law, which requires a permit for each owner at each location, specifically gives the Board of Health the authority to regulate permits based on public health needs. The public health need in the case of *these* permit regulations is the need to save lives; the need to decrease smoking rates and associated disease and death rates connected to smoking in Philadelphia. On behalf of the Board of Health, I strongly support these regulations as passed. In the 2 years since they were passed, they have already started to improve the equity of our neighborhoods and protect teens from a major cause of illness and death.

Overturning these regulations has two very negative consequences. First, it will add hundreds of tobacco sales outlets in low-income neighborhoods, which will increase smoking rates and harm the health of Philadelphia residents. Second, it would set a dangerous precedent that whenever the Board of Health adopts regulations to protect residents from a health threat, such regulations can be overturned by political action. This precedent may hurt our ability to respond to the next epidemic that hits Philadelphia.

In closing, like you, I and my colleagues on the Board of Health are dedicated to making our City the best in the nation. Being the best involves health, education, the business community and much more. In this case, we thoroughly reviewed the science and health evidence, took all steps involved in writing regulations including taking into account community feedback garnered at hearings. In the end, we developed tobacco permit regulation based on keeping Philadelphians, particularly young people here, safe, healthy and alive. Thank you.

Conference presentations and posters can reach an audience who would not have read a peer-reviewed article, thereby giving it more reach. They also convey information that is not (or not yet) in peer-reviewed literature and can enhance discussion about an issue in a broader setting with an engaged audience. Conference presentations often take less time to prepare than an article and are less rigorously reviewed. They can also provide opportunity for collaboration and the marrying of research and practice—such as a panel with a researcher and practitioners together.

The Challenge of Timing

The timing of dissemination to policymakers and decision makers is often difficult to optimize. As researchers, we often feel we can't translate or disseminate until our research is completed, which may be long past the timing needed to make critical policy decisions. Indeed, it has been long-established that there is an evidence–practice gap, where it sometimes takes more than a decade for research results to be integrated into practice.[26,27] Decision makers want answers to questions immediately, as policy, budgets, and the political winds shift quickly. There needs to be a balance, then, between upholding scientific integrity while providing research findings in real enough time that they are useful. The most perfect results are of no use if they appear long after decisions have been made.

DISSEMINATION TO COMMUNITY ACTORS

One of the biggest challenges to engaging community actors in urban public health research is that research evidence fails to reach them. There are two different kinds of failures that are often experienced:

- research results are often never communicated back to community stakeholders, and
- research results are often only communicated in scientific journals or using language and framing results in ways that meet the expectations and preferences only of other scientists.

The data or results that community actors usually want from research that occurs within their community are often very different than that for policymakers and decision makers. Community actors seek descriptive data that documents the extent of community health or underlying social inequities or explicit community health needs for advocacy purposes or provides formative information such as assets or resident preferences upon which programs or policies can be built. Community actors often want a blend of quantitative and qualitative data as well—quantitative to document the inequities or needs and qualitative to include lived experience with those needs (see the discussion of qualitative and mixed methods research in Chapter 6).

Community actors are usually only interested in causality insofar as it clarifies formerly unknown causes of local health issues for prevention purposes; however, this is rare as prevalent community health issues usually have known or suspected causes. In fact, the audiences outside of academia (e.g., funders, policymakers, community members) are not typically convinced by novel methods and want instead to be shown that this community has inequities or needs or requires new programming, based on proven measures or using long-established benchmarks. Therefore, the descriptive evidence that community actors want to be produced from research are fundamentally very different than what their researcher partners' may initially envision. Data about a particular community's health needs and potential solutions are often not novel enough to be of interest to scientific journals.

Urban researchers and practitioners who want their results to be translated into community action or policy change need to consider dissemination strategies specific to these urban health actors. Data literacy is a very real barrier to the uptake of scientific evidence among community actors in urban health,[14] and so dissemination products tailored to community actors and audiences should emphasize user-friendly data visualizations and graphics and avoid or define scientific jargon in plain language (see Table 15.2 for tips to make dissemination products clear and compelling).

When community organizations and community leaders are engaged in research, one of the first things they request in terms of results dissemination is that results be shared with participants.[29,30] They will want to see these same results but will want the results reported back to them in a live presentation where they can ask clarifying questions and request to see information in new ways (e.g., What were differences by neighborhood or police/legislative district? How did results differ among resident population groups?). These same community leaders may request further dissemination products to assist with translating the information for current program planning processes, grant-seeking strategies, or policy debates or other advocacy opportunities. This is exactly what translation looks like in a local urban community, and these dissemination opportunities are exactly what researchers should plan for and be responsive to.

Some possible products that could result from such a continued collaboration could include reports (whether brief reports or longer white papers), press releases, websites, or social media strategies building upon any of these products.

Table 15.2 TIPS FOR EFFECTIVE DISSEMINATION

To Make Dissemination Products More	Tips
Clear	Use clear, concise, and simple "lay" language (i.e., make sure your nonresearcher friends could understand)
	Define jargon/high literacy terms; focus in on your culprits and address them
	Include easy-to-navigate table of contents and page numbers and headers for longer reports
Compelling	Use narrative language (e.g., quotes, testimonials, case studies) to increase attention and retention
	Use whole numbers rather than percentages and decimal places
	Use less data imbedded within text

Another important community dissemination product is the community forum. Community forums, also known as community town hall meetings or community conversations, arise from a commonly used data collection method in community-based research.[31] Community forums, like focus group discussions, are a series of discussions focused on a defined topic. However, instead of including 8 to 12 participants as is typical of focus groups, community forums are set up as a public meeting with the explicit purpose of engaging multiple types of stakeholders on the given health issue to allow for broad community participation and the gathering of multiple perspectives at once. As with focus group discussions and community partner meetings (see Chapter 13), skilled moderation is important. In contrast to focus group discussions, the purpose of a community forum is often to share results and build data literacy through educational content. In community-partnered research, this can include research results for the purpose of eliciting discussion, interpretation, and strategic planning next steps. Therefore, the end result of community forums is to draw meaning from the data and produce action items that will turn results into solutions.

The Challenge of Timing

As with policymakers and decision makers, timeliness is a challenge for researchers in dissemination to community audiences. Community actors do not think in terms of long-term benefits to something that is causing research burden or exhaustion today. If they were convinced that a research partnership would provide benefit to their community, they want to see the immediate benefits of the data collected. They know how quickly community demographics, health priorities, and potential solutions can change. Therefore, the academic process, with known lag times between research completion and publication,[32] is challenging to fit with this reality.

Timeliness is of utmost importance in this phase of dissemination, so that organizations, community leaders, and residents can immediately realize the practical benefits of the data and research results. Since dissemination is largely descriptive and occurring in presentation and nonpublished formats, this type of dissemination can occur earlier in the researchers' analytic plan and can occur without violating any copyright laws or embargoes that will govern its eventual publication in peer-reviewed journals.

Another one of these community dissemination requests may entail actual data-sharing if community-based organizations (CBOs) have the capacity for analyzing their own data to pursue their own research questions. Depending on the institutional review board, data use agreement, or other rules governing the data produced by the research, this may look like an aggregate data request or a de-identified individual record-level data request. Some more sophisticated CBOs may request data-sharing as a part of a memorandum of understanding governing the entire research partnership. The benefits of data-sharing are that it acknowledges the co-creation of knowledge and that it allows community actors to extract information out of the research that can create immediate action and benefit to community health.

Lastly, it should be mentioned that even in the age of open access to many journals and Google Scholar, there are still scientific journals that CBOs cannot access. Evidence shows that CBOs do conduct literature reviews to inform their program planning.[33] Thus, academic research partners should consider open-access publications and sharing strategies for accessing prior literature (see Chapter 10) with key CBO partners to help increase community access to scientific evidence.

DIGITAL DISSEMINATION AND SOCIAL MEDIA

Social media may be one of the cheapest and easiest ways to reach a large and diverse audience. According to Pew Research, 73% of US adults have used YouTube, 69% use Facebook, and 37% use Instagram (see Figure 15.1).[34] About 75% of Facebook users visit the site every day.

There are several ways to use social media to disseminate research, and the content shared will vary from platform to platform. Social networks, like

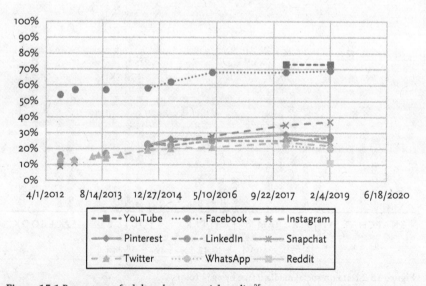

Figure 15.1 Percentage of adults who use social media.[35]
Source: Pew Research Center. Social media fact sheet. June 12, 2019; https://www.pewresearch.org/internet/fact-sheet/social-media/.

Facebook, Twitter, and LinkedIn work well for sharing a range of content on a public platform. Media-sharing networks include platforms for sharing images (Instagram) and video (Instagram and YouTube). Each has users of different demographics, which may also influence selection, and the time before content is considered out of date is of particular importance in the social media world.

City health departments, especially those in large cities, are becoming more active on social media, using the platform as a way to disseminate public and urban health information and messages.[36] New York City's Department of Health and Mental Hygiene's Twitter account, @nycHealthy, has tweeted 21,900 times and is followed by 45,800 other Twitter users (as of June 3, 2019). Mexico City's secretariat of health is also on Twitter and has tweeted 22,700 times to its 60,000 followers. National governments are also taking advantage of these audiences. The US Centers for Disease Control and Prevention has a Twitter account specifically focused on environmental health, @CDCEnvironment, which boasts 21,700 followers. Public Health England, the United Kingdom's public health agency, has 187,000 Twitter followers.

When deciding how to use social media for dissemination, an important first step is to find out which social media platform your audience uses before investing time in a social media strategy. As shown in Figure 15.2, nearly 50% of US adults over the age of 65 use Facebook, only 3% use SnapChat.

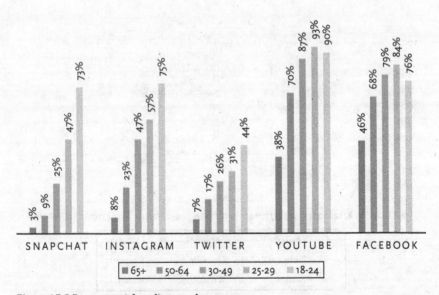

Figure 15.2 Data on social media usage by age group.
Source: Perrin A, Anderson M. Share of U.S. adults using social media, including Facebook, is mostly unchanged since 2018. Pew Research Center. April 10, 2019; https://www.pewresearch.org/fact-tank/2019/04/10/share-of-u-s-adults-using-social-media-including-facebook-is-mostly-unchanged-since-2018/.

Meanwhile, 75% of adults aged 18 to 24 use Instagram. These patterns are likely to vary drastically across countries, regions, and cultures and will likely change over time.

Blogging has been around since the mid-1990s, and more and more professionals have turned to blogging as a way to share perspectives on news, science, and research. Blogging can be helpful for disseminating urban health evidence to specific audiences interested in a niche topic. Blog posts can also serve as a useful platform for sharing research in a format that can be easily shared and understood by nonscientists through social media and websites. There are now many topic-specific blogs and sites that post content daily from scientists and researchers, including those featuring urban health and public health researchers and practitioners. This includes many well-established sites that frequently allow guest authors to contribute. ScienceBlogs.com and the Scientific American blog share writing about all types of scientific research. There are several established blogs that focus on urban issues, such as City Fix, CityLab, and New Geography. Some sites have adopted a news/blogging hybrid format and post content about a wide variety of topics, such as The Conversation (which only accepts writing from researchers and academics). City-specific sites like Gothamist (focused on New York City), DCist (focused on Washington, DC), or CityWatch (focused on Los Angeles). Other blogs focus on specific cities or regions, such as SustainableRome.net, TheTehranTimes.net, and AfricanUrbanism.net (which focuses on West African cities).

Podcasts are a similarly effective way to engage nonresearchers in public health research and practice. Since the 2000s, podcasts have gradually become more and more popular with all kinds of audiences. Podcasts, some of which began as shows broadcast solely on FM radio, such as This American Life, Serial, Radiolab, and Dan Carlin's Hardcore History have long-standing followings, while new podcasts emerge on what seems like a daily basis. There are several podcasts that routinely focus on urban issues, including The Uncertain Hour, from Marketplace; Placemakers, from Slate; 99 Percent Invisible, from Radiotopia; The Urbanist and Tall Stories, from Monocle 24; Third Wave Urbanism; and Candidate Confessional.[37] The International Society for Urban Health has its own podcast, ISUH Conversations.[38] The American Public Health Association has four different podcasts: The Get Ready Report, The Nation's Health, Healthy You, and Healthy Communities.[39]

All forms of dissemination can lend themselves to some sort of data visualization—either as a component of a written product or as the main piece of a website. The use of visualizations and infographics can help to convey complex information quickly and clearly and can appeal to those who are more visually inclined. Data stories—a series of data visualizations focused on answering a specific question—can break down institutional silos, build participant expertise, and expand dissemination of the findings, especially when developed through a collaborative process.

MONITORING AND TRACKING THE REACH OF DISSEMINATION

Once dissemination activities are underway, there are several reasons why monitoring and tracking the "reach" (the number of people who have interacted with your dissemination materials) of dissemination could be beneficial. Monitoring and tracking can refine the approach to better meet dissemination goals; provide important performance metrics for the funders of research; help gather evidence of research impact, which can be used in future fundraising efforts; and help clarify and inform ways to improve future dissemination efforts.

There are many ways to track the reach of dissemination efforts that do not require any significant financial investment. These include

- Mentions of evidence in legislative meetings which are recorded for public record.
- Visits to websites and downloads of materials.
- Email opens of dissemination newsletters, and the rate at which newsletter recipients open links within the newsletter.
- Social media engagement metrics.
- News media coverage related to your research.

Additional mechanisms for evaluating the impact of dissemination efforts (which require an investment of resources) include key informant interviews, focus groups, or a survey among your intended audience to understand whether they have been reached by your research can provide robust and comprehensive information on how well your dissemination strategy has worked.

CONCLUSION

For research in urban health to truly lead to change, that research and knowledge needs to be translated and disseminated to the very people who live in the cities being studied and who make public health decisions. As we have discussed in this chapter, dissemination needs to be inclusive and deliberate with a clear framework and goal. Dissemination needs to be tailored to multiple audiences, with products developed specifically to meet the needs of those audiences. Those products should be tested, and outcomes of dissemination should be monitored, and dissemination adjusted in response. Urban communities who are engaged in research efforts, understand research results and are able to use research evidence to guide decisions and actions will be poised to make sustainable changes to improve health.

REFERENCES

1. World Medical Association. Ethical principles for medical research involving human subjects. *European Journal of Emergency Medicine.* 2001;8(3):221–223.
2. Berwick DM. Disseminating innovations in health care. *JAMA.* 2003;289(15): 1969–1975.
3. Emanuel EJ, Wendler D, Grady C. What makes clinical research ethical? *JAMA.* 2000;283(20):2701–2711.
4. Chan A-W, Tetzlaff JM, Altman DG, Laupacis A, Gøtzsche PC, Krleža-Jerić K, Hróbjartsson A, Mann H, Dickersin K, Berlin J, Doré C, Parulekar W, Summerskill W, Groves T, Schulz K, Sox H, Rockhold FW, Rennie D, Moher D. SPIRIT 2013 Statement: Defining standard protocol items for clinical trials. *Ann Intern Med.* 2013;158(3):200-207.
5. Martens PJ. The right kind of evidence—integrating, measuring, and making it count in health equity research. *Journal of Urban Health.* 2012;89(6):925–936.
6. O'Campo P. Are we producing the right kind of actionable evidence for the social determinants of health? *Journal of Urban Health.* 2012;89(6):881–893.
7. Bonneux L. From evidence based bioethics to evidence based social policies. *European Journal of Epidemiology.* 2007;22(8):483–485.
8. Corburn J, Cohen AK. Why we need urban health equity indicators: Integrating science, policy, and community. *PLoS Medicine.* 2012;9(8):e1001285.
9. Armstrong R, Doyle J, Lamb C, Waters E. Multi-sectoral health promotion and public health: The role of evidence. *Journal of Public Health (Oxford, England).* 2006;28(2):168–172.
10. Gagnon ML. Moving knowledge to action through dissemination and exchange. *Journal of Clinical Epidemiology.* 2011;64(1):25–31.
11. Lapaige V. "Integrated knowledge translation" for globally oriented public health practitioners and scientists: Framing together a sustainable trans-frontier knowledge translation vision. *Journal of Multidisciplinary Healthcare.* 2010;3:33-47.
12. Graham ID, Tetroe J. How to translate health research knowledge into effective healthcare action. *Healthcare Quarterly (Toronto, Ont).* 2007;10(3):20–22.
13. Kirst M, Schaefer-McDaniel N, Hwang S, O'Campo P. *Converging Disciplines: A Transdisciplinary Research Approach to Urban Health Problems.* New York: Springer-Verlag; 2011.
14. Rashid JR, Spengler RF, Wagner RM, et al. Eliminating health disparities through transdisciplinary research, cross-agency collaboration, and public participation. *American Journal of Public Health.* 2009;99(11):1955–1961.
15. Diez Roux AV, Slesinski SC, Alazraqui M, et al. A novel international partnership for actionable evidence on urban health in Latin America: LAC-Urban Health and SALURBAL. *Global Challenges.* 2019;3(4):1800013.
16. United Nations Human Settlements Programme; World Health Organization, Kobe Centre. *Global report on urban health: Equitable healthier cities for sustainable development.* Kobe, Japan: WHO Kobe Centre; 2016.

17. Rosenfield PL. The potential of transdisciplinary research for sustaining and extending linkages between the health and social sciences. *Social Science & Medicine*. 1992;35(11):1343–1357.

18. Owen N, Goode A, Sugiyama T, et al. *Designing for Dissemination in Chronic Disease Prevention and Management*. New York: Oxford University Press; 2017.

19. Brownell KD, Roberto CA. Strategic science with policy impact. *The Lancet*. 2015;385(9986):2445–2446.

20. Brownson RC, Eyler AA, Harris JK, Moore JB, Tabak RG. Getting the word out: New approaches for disseminating public health science. *Journal of Public Health Management and Practice*. 2018;24(2):102–111.

21. Purtle J, Peters R, Brownson RC. A review of policy dissemination and implementation research funded by the National Institutes of Health, 2007–2014. *Implementation Science*. 2016;11:1.

22. Purtle J, Henson RM, Carroll-Scott A, Kolker J, Joshi R, Diez Roux AV. US mayors' and health commissioners' opinions about health disparities in their cities. *American Journal of Public Health*. 2018;108(5):634–641.

23. Purtle J, Henson RM, Carroll-Scott A, Kolker J, Roux AD. US mayors' evidence dissemination preferences: towards evidence-based city policies. Paper presented at: 10th Annual Conference on the Science of Dissemination and Implementation 2017; Arlington, VA.

24. Wong SL, Green LA, Bazemore AW, Miller BF. How to write a health policy brief. *Families, Systems, & Health*. 2017;35(1):21–24.

25. Philadelphia Department of Public Health. CHART. 2020; https://www.phila.gov/departments/department-of-public-health/data/chart/. Accessed June 23, 2020.

26. Dilling JA, Swensen SJ, Hoover MR, et al. Accelerating the use of best practices: The Mayo Clinic model of diffusion. *Joint Commission Journal on Quality and Patient Safety*. 2013;39(4):167–176.

27. Kristensen N, Nymann C, Konradsen H. Implementing research results in clinical practice: The experiences of healthcare professionals. *BMC Health Services Research*. 2016;16:48.

28. Carroll-Scott A, Toy P, Wyn R, Zane JI, Wallace SP. Results from the Data & Democracy initiative to enhance community-based organization data and research capacity. *American Journal of Public Health*. 2012;102(7):1384–1391.

29. Johnson JC, Hayden UT, Thomas N, et al. Building community participatory research coalitions from the ground up: The Philadelphia Area Research Community Coalition. *Progress in Community Health Partnerships: Research, Education, and Action*. 2009;3(1):61–72.

30. Martin del Campo F, Casado J, Spencer P, Strelnick H. The development of the Bronx Community Research Review Board: A pilot feasibility project for a model of community consultation. *Progress in Community Health Partnerships: Research, Education, and Action*. 2013;7(3):341–352.

31. Noonan EJ, Sawning S, Combs R, et al. Engaging the transgender community to improve medical education and prioritize healthcare initiatives. *Teaching and Learning in Medicine*. 2018;30(2):119–132.

32. Powell K. Does it take too long to publish research? *Nature News*. 2016; 530(7589):148.

33. Humphries DL, Carroll-Scott A, Mitchell L, Tian T, Choudhury S, Fiellin DA. Assessing research activity and capacity of community-based organizations: Development and pilot testing of an instrument. *Progress in Community Health Partnerships: Research, Education, and Action*. 2014;8(4):421–432.

34. Perrin A, Anderson M. Share of U.S. adults using social media, including Facebook, is mostly unchanged since 2018. Pew Research Center. April 10, 2019; https://www.pewresearch.org/fact-tank/2019/04/10/share-of-u-s-adults-using-social-media-including-facebook-is-mostly-unchanged-since-2018/.

35. Pew Research Center. Social media fact sheet. June 12, 2019; https://www.pewresearch.org/internet/fact-sheet/social-media/.

36. Harris JK, Mueller NL, Snider D. Social media adoption in local health departments nationwide. *American Journal of Public Health*. 2013;103(9):1700–1707.

37. Kinney J. 7 podcasts urbanists should be listening to now. Next City. January 26, 2017. https://nextcity.org/daily/entry/7-podcasts-urbanists-should-be-listening-to-now. Accessed June 24, 2020.

38. International Society for Urban Health. Welcome to the ISUH Conversations Podcast. https://isuh.org/isuh-conversations-podcast/. Accessed June 24, 2020.

39. American Public Health Association. Podcasts. https://www.apha.org/news-and-media/multimedia/podcasts. Accessed June 24, 2020.

Concluding Remarks

We set out in this text to articulate a range of foundational concepts, research tools and engagement strategies relevant to urban health, all with the intent to provide both knowledge and skills to have an impact on population health in cities across the globe. We hope the four inter-related parts of the book have helped to introduce such a toolkit and enticed you to ponder other questions along the way. To summarize our thinking on this, one might now say that for urban health training, we would expect emerging professionals be ready to:

- Work across disciplinary and sectoral lines and within diverse partnerships to articulate the scope and purpose of research projects, and to help to secure the financial, personnel, and network-based resources needed for success.
- Launch and follow-through with efforts to identify, collect, analyze, and synthesize data on how urban contexts affect population health outcomes, with awareness of common challenges and limitations faced when unpacking the study question and generating compelling answers.
- Identify and develop the partnerships necessary to create actionable interventions and policy, and work across sectors—both within and outside of traditional public health—to improve health outcomes.
- Communicate clearly, creatively, and to multiple audiences about urban health knowledge in a format that meets each audience's needs and creates opportunities for input.

Urban health can be improved. We have seen examples that highlight how creative solutions can reduce health hazards and barriers to healthy lifestyles. More stories of success and resilience continue to emerge, giving us a basis for continued optimism. We hope the readers of this text will be successful

Concluding Remarks In: *Urban Public Health*. Edited by: Gina S. Lovasi, Ana V. Diez Roux, and Jennifer Kolker,
Oxford University Press (2021). © Oxford University Press 2021. DOI: 10.1093/oso/9780190885304.003.0016.

in convening partners and articulating the value of urban health; generating timely and convincing knowledge for use by stakeholders at local, national, regional, and global levels; and enacting changes to urban contexts that benefit health and improve health equity.

Yet urban health improvements are not inevitable. The fragility of our urban systems has been underscored by disasters ranging from localized storm events to the special vulnerability of cities to the recent COVID-19 pandemic. These urban health threats have also made even more visible the fundamental drivers of health inequities in cities linked to living and working conditions and the need to address these determinants to improve urban health. The successful translation of our growing knowledge base into effective action requires thoughtful and sensitive communication, and attention to multiple perspectives. It will also require intersectoral partnership and addressing the structural determinants of health and health inequities in cities including economic processes and racism.

Particular attention is needed to integrate what we know about health inequities as we build evidence and take action to benefit population health. For urban health, this means that our expanding evidence base and actions to protect the health of local populations will not automatically reduce the stark urban health inequities. Direct and sustained attention to the environments, perspectives, and health needs of socially or economically disadvantaged populations improves our chances of ensuring that the work of urban health benefits all.

While this text cannot possibly cover all of the topics that come into play while working in an area as complex and dynamic as urban health, we are eager to remain active in a conversation about how to further optimize practice and impact. We hope you can use the preceding chapters to guide a process of thoughtfully engaging in impactful urban health research, and using both existing and emerging evidence for action. We have reiterated throughout the importance of matching solutions to the needs and constraints of the current situation, and of attending to the process for changing city environments—not only the *what*, but also the *how* of changing places to benefit health.

We resist expert status, as that would mean we are done. Instead, as individuals and as a field we continue to develop knowledge, skill, and insight. We need to maintain our flexibility, our humility, and our openness to new knowledge and challenges to our own thinking as we strive to move forward in the field.

The centrality of both data and action to our task are clear, but both are nurtured and used to maximal effect by locally embedded teams, within multicity networks that allow sharing of lessons and strategies. Together, our task is to build a rigorous evidence base with both local and global relevance to guide decision-making at multiple levels toward a healthy future for all in our cities.

ACKNOWLEDGMENTS

Just as numerous interrelated individuals and organizations shape the systems that matter for the health of urban residents, numerous organizations and individuals have had a hand in shaping this book. We are grateful to all who informed our thinking or played a role in the development of *Urban Public Health: A Research Toolkit for Practice and Impact*.

We would like to first thank those who have financially supported the collaborative research projects that informed this work. Particular appreciation goes to Dana and David Dornsife for their generous gift to the Dornsife School of Public Health at Drexel University. In particular, we recognize the US federal funding and foundation funding we have received through the National Institutes of Health (NIHHD, NIA, NICHD, NHLBI, and NIEHS), the US Department of Education, the Environmental Protection Agency, the Commonwealth Universal Research Enhancement (C.U.R.E) program funded by the Pennsylvania Department of Health, Wellcome Trust's Our Planet Our Health Programme, the Robert Wood Johnson Foundation, the de Beaumont Foundation, and the Philadelphia Department of Public Health.

Appreciation is also due to the many colleagues and trainees who have helped us to learn about and advance the field of urban health. The students, staff, faculty, and visiting scholars affiliated with the Drexel University Urban Health Collaborative at the Dornsife School of Public Health have inspired and supported us in this effort. Particular thanks go to the teams from the following projects: SALURBAL, the Pediatric Big Data Project with Children's Hospital of Philadelphia, Retail Environment and Cardiovascular Disease, West Philadelphia Promise Neighborhood, and the Big Cities Health Coalition for their valuable contributions. Colleagues, staff, and students engaged in the Pennsylvania Public Health Training Center and the Columbia University Mailman School of Public Health's Urban+Health Initiative also contributed importantly to our thinking about the topics reflected in this book. The faculty and students at the Dornsife School of Public Health—with whom we collaborate, teach, and mentor—contributed to our thinking about how we frame urban health within the greater context of public health. Thanks also to the editorial team at Oxford University Press and to anonymous peer reviewers who shaped the scope and tone of this book for the better.

Particular thanks go to Vaishnavi Vaidya for coordinating our efforts and to Kathleen Escoto for helping us stay organized in our use of references and figures. We also recognize the valuable contributions of many others who have supported our efforts, including not only those named as chapter coauthors or other contributors, but also the many people in our personal and professional lives who support our endeavors and make the journey worthwhile. In the interest of brevity, we highlight only those most crucial to our ability to write this book: Amy Auchincloss, Tanisha Barnes, Jody Bayer, Autumn Ciarrocchi, Alex Ezeh, Christopher B. Forrest, Dennis Gallagher, Sarah Greer, Allison Groves, Phil Hurvitz, Felice Le Scherban, Kathleen Livengood, Laszlo Lovasi, Leah Schinasi, Kari Moore, Alex Quistberg, Puja Upadhyay, and Mike Yudell.

ABOUT THE AUTHORS

Gina S. Lovasi, Jennifer Kolker, and Ana V. Diez Roux each have leadership roles with the Urban Health Collaborative at Drexel University in Philadelphia, Pennsylvania, where they share an aspiration to invest in collaborations that productively bring together diverse community and professional perspectives, to conduct rigorous and relevant place-based research and to thoughtfully engage with partners whose actions can benefit urban residents locally and globally.

Contributors from within and beyond the Drexel University Urban Health Collaborative have generously shared their work and insights within these pages, greatly enhancing the range of ideas and experience available to readers.

INDEX

Tables, figures and boxes are indicated by *t*, *f*, and *b* following the page number.

Movement of Healthy Cities,
Municipalities and Communities of
the Americas (PAHO), 48
Moving to Opportunity Experiment, 96
multicollinearity, 202–205
multilevel models (MLM), 200
multiple study designs, 222t
multisectoral approaches, 63–67, 260–261
multivariable descriptive analysis,
197–198

naming conventions
file naming, 186–187
for variables, 182
National Association of City and County
Health Officials (NACCHO), 254
National Center for Health Statistics
(US), 7b–8b
National Establishment Time Series, 120
National Health and Nutrition
Examination Survey, 169
National Institute for Health and Care
Excellence (NICE)
Checklist, 221b, 222t
evidence guidelines, 224
National Institute on Drug Abuse, 309
National Institutes of Health (NIH)
Clinical and Translational Science
Awards Consortium, 277–278
LandCare program (Philadelphia),
208b–209b
National League of Cities, 163b
National Neighborhood Indicators
Partnership, 115
National Profile of Local Health
Departments, 254
National Resource Network, 163b
The Nation's Health podcast, 331
NCDs. see noncommunicable diseases
needs assessments, community health,
159, 257
neglect, 109, 110t
neighborhood interventions, 299
Neighborhood Recovery Program
(Recuperación de Barrios), 94
neighborhoods
assessment domains and indicators,
114–118
definition of, 13–17, 15t, 17t,
113, 113f

gentrification, 96–100, 97b–98b
health inequities across, 58–59, 58f,
80–81, 82f
key considerations, 17t
personalized definitions, 113, 113f
physical disorder in, 109, 110t
Neighborhoods United Against Violence
website, 271b
nested conceptualizations, 56, 57f
network analysis, 237
networks
academic and scientific, 49
of cities, 48
New Geography, 331
New Urban Agenda (UN Habitat),
21b–22b, 46–47, 296b–297b
New York Academy of Medicine, 220, 224
New York City, New York
Department of Health and Mental
Hygiene, 330
mortality rates, 202, 203f
New York City Community Air Survey
(NYCCAS), 109, 120, 122, 123b–124b
New York Restoration Project, 147–148
New York University (NYU), 163b
New Zealand, 35b
Newcastle-Ottawa Scale (NOS), 222t
NGOs (nongovernmental organizations),
252, 253t, 258
NICE (National Institute for Health and
Care Excellence), 221b
Nigeria, 9t
99 Percent Invisible podcast, 331
noncommunicable diseases, 41–42
example outcomes and measurements,
156, 157t–158t
nongovernmental organizations (NGOs),
252, 253t, 258
nonlinearity, 200–205
associations, 201, 201f
effects, 231b
Normalized Difference Vegetation Index,
122, 193b
North Africa, 35b, 76–77, 78f
North America, 27–28, 29f, 33, 34f
notifiable illness, 169
Nutrition Environment Measures
Survey, 125
nutrition services, 256t
NVivo software, 150b